T0348729

Management of Benign Pancreatic Disease

Editor

JOHN M. PONEROS

GASTROINTESTINAL ENDOSCOPY CLINICS OF NORTH AMERICA

www.giendo.theclinics.com

Consulting Editor
CHARLES J. LIGHTDALE

October 2018 • Volume 28 • Number 4

ELSEVIER

1600 John F. Kennedy Boulevard • Suite 1800 • Philadelphia, Pennsylvania, 19103-2899

http://www.theclinics.com

**GASTROINTESTINAL ENDOSCOPY CLINICS OF NORTH AMERICA Volume 28, Number 4
October 2018 ISSN 1052-5157, ISBN-13: 978-0-323-64225-5**

Editor: Kerry Holland
Developmental Editor: Donald Mumford

Gastrointestinal Endoscopy Clinics of North America (ISSN 1052-5157) is published quarterly by Elsevier Inc., 360 Park Avenue South, New York, NY 10010-1710. Months of issue are January, April, July, and October. Business and Editorial Offices: 1600 John F. Kennedy Blvd., Suite 1800, Philadelphia, PA, 19103-2899. Periodicals postage paid at New York, NY and additional mailing offices. Subscription prices are $349.00 per year for US individuals, $593.00 per year for US institutions, $100.00 per year for US students and residents, $385.00 per year for Canadian individuals, $702.00 per year for Canadian institutions, $474.00 per year for international individuals, $702.00 per year for international institutions, and $245.00 per year for Canadian and foreign students/residents. To receive student/resident rate, orders must be accompanied by name of affiliated institution, date of term, and the *signature* of program/residency coordinator on institution letterhead. Orders will be billed at individual rate until proof of status is received. Foreign air speed delivery is included in all *Clinics* subscription prices. All prices are subject to change without notice. **POSTMASTER:** Send address change to *Gastrointestinal Endoscopy Clinics of North America*, Elsevier Health Sciences Division, Subscription Customer Service, 3251 Riverport Lane, Maryland Heights, MO 63043. **Customer Service: 1-800-654-2452 (US). From outside the United States, call 1-314-447-8871. Fax: 1-314-447-8029. E-mail: JournalsCustomerService-usa@elsevier.com (for print support) or JournalsOnlineSupport-usa@elsevier.com (for online support).**

Reprints. For copies of 100 or more, of articles in this publication, please contact the Commercial Reprints Department, Elsevier Inc., 360 Park Avenue South, New York, NY 10010-1710. Tel. 212-633-3874; Fax: 212-633-3820; E-mail: reprints@elsevier.com.

Gastrointestinal Endoscopy Clinics of North America is covered in *Excerpta Medica, MEDLINE/PubMed (Index Medicus), and MEDLINE/MEDLARS.*

Contributors

CONSULTING EDITOR

CHARLES J. LIGHTDALE, MD
Professor of Medicine, Division of Digestive and Liver Diseases, Columbia University Medical Center, New York, New York, USA

EDITOR

JOHN M. PONEROS, MD, FASGE, NYSGEF
Associate Professor, Columbia University Vagelos College of Physicians and Surgeons, Acting, Clinical Chief, Division of Digestive and Liver Diseases, Acting, Director of Endoscopy, NewYork-Presbyterian Hospital, Columbia University Irving Medical Center, New York, New York, USA

AUTHORS

MAISAM ABU-EL-HAIJA, MD
Department of Pediatrics, University of Cincinnati College of Medicine, Division of Gastroenterology, Hepatology and Nutrition, Cincinnati Children's Hospital Medical Center, Cincinnati, Ohio, USA

JEFFREY MICHAEL ADLER, MD, MSc
Division of Digestive and Liver Disease, Instructor, Department of Medicine, Columbia University Irving Medical Center, Assistant Attending Physician, NewYork-Presbyterian Hospital, New York, New York, USA

VENKATA S. AKSHINTALA, MD
Division of Gastroenterology, Johns Hopkins Medical Institutions, Baltimore, Maryland, USA

DARWIN L. CONWELL, MD, MS
Department of Internal Medicine, Division of Gastroenterology, Hepatology and Nutrition, The Ohio State University Wexner Medical Center, Columbus, Ohio, USA

CHRISTOPHER J. DiMAIO, MD
Division of Gastroenterology, Icahn School of Medicine at Mount Sinai, New York, New York, USA

B. JOSEPH ELMUNZER, MD
Division of Gastroenterology and Hepatology, Medical University of South Carolina, Charleston, South Carolina, USA

JAMES J. FARRELL, MD
Professor of Medicine, Section of Digestive Disease, Yale School of Medicine, Director, Yale Center for Pancreatic Diseases, Yale University, New Haven, Connecticut, USA

TAMAS A. GONDA, MD
Division of Digestive and Liver Diseases, Assistant Professor, Department of Medicine, Columbia University Irving Medical Center, New York, New York, USA

FRANK G. GRESS, MD
Clinical Chief, Digestive and Liver Diseases, Columbia University Vagelos College of Physicians and Surgeons, New York, New York, USA

AVERILL GUO, MD
Department of Medicine, Columbia University Irving Medical Center, New York, New York, USA

AWS HASAN, MD
Department of Internal Medicine, Columbia University Irving Medical Center, New York, New York, USA

AYESHA KAMAL, MD
Division of Gastroenterology, Johns Hopkins Medical Institutions, Baltimore, Maryland, USA

JEREMY H. KAPLAN, MD
Division of Digestive and Liver Diseases, Department of Medicine, Columbia University Irving Medical Center, New York, New York, USA

FAY KASTRINOS, MD, MPH
Associate Professor of Medicine, Division of Digestive and Liver Diseases, Columbia University Irving Medical Center, Herbert Irving Comprehensive Cancer Center, New York, New York, USA

BONNA LEERHØY, MSc
Digestive Disease Center, Bispebjerg Hospital, University of Copenhagen, Copenhagen, Denmark

KAMRAAN MADHANI, MD
Clinical Instructor, Department of Medicine, Yale School of Medicine, New Haven, Connecticut, USA; Department of Medicine, Waterbury Internal Medicine Residency Program, Waterbury Hospital, Yale New Haven Hospital, Waterbury, Connecticut, USA

DAGMARA I. MOSCOSO, MS
Division of Digestive and Liver Diseases, Columbia University Irving Medical Center, New York, New York, USA

PATRICK I. OKOLO III, MD, MPH, FASGE
Professor of Medicine, Donald and Barbara Zucker School of Medicine at Hofstra/Northwell, Chief, Division of Gastroenterology, Lenox Hill Hospital, New York, New York, USA

JOHN M. PONEROS, MD, FASGE, NYSGEF
Associate Professor, Columbia University Vagelos College of Physicians and Surgeons, Acting, Clinical Chief, Division of Digestive and Liver Diseases, Acting, Director of Endoscopy, NewYork-Presbyterian Hospital, Columbia University Irving Medical Center, New York, New York, USA

AMIT H. SACHDEV, MD
Clinical Instructor of Medicine, Digestive and Liver Diseases, Columbia University Vagelos College of Physicians and Surgeons, New York, New York, USA

BETH SCHROPE, MD, PhD
Associate Professor, Department of Surgery, Columbia University Vagelos College of Physicians and Surgeons, New York, New York, USA

AMRITA SETHI, MD, MSc, FASGE
Division of Digestive and Liver Disease, Associate Professor, Department of Medicine, Columbia University Irving Medical Center, New York, New York, USA

STEVEN SHAMAH, MD
Advanced Endoscopy Fellow, University of Chicago Medical Center, CERT Division, Chicago, Illinois, USA

VIKESH K. SINGH, MD, MSc
Division of Gastroenterology, Johns Hopkins Medical Institutions, Baltimore, Maryland, USA

Contents

Acute pancreatitis is among the most common gastrointestinal disorders requiring hospitalization worldwide. Establishing the cause of acute pancreatitis ensures appropriate management and proper health care resource utilization. Causes of acute pancreatitis include biliary, alcohol use, hypertriglyceridemia, hypercalcemia, drug-induced, autoimmune, hereditary/genetic, and anatomic abnormalities. Fluid therapy remains the cornerstone of managing acute pancreatitis. This article provides a brief summary of current evidence-based practices in the diagnosis and management of uncomplicated acute pancreatitis.

Pancreatitis remains the most common and potentially devastating complication of endoscopic retrograde cholangiopancreatography (ERCP) pancreatitis. Recent advances in prophylaxis have improved but not eliminated this problem, underscoring the importance of ongoing research toward this goal. This article provides an evidence-based approach to post-ERCP pancreatitis prevention through patient selection, risk stratification, procedural technique, and multimodality prophylaxis, and discusses ongoing and future research initiatives in this important area.

Patients with recurrent acute pancreatitis (RAP) have few treatment options available to them to manage their symptoms or prevent progression to chronic pancreatitis. At present, endotherapy is typically pursued as a means to achieve symptom remission and reduce rates of recurrence, hospitalization, abdominal pain, narcotic use, and surgical intervention. However, evidence that endotherapy effectively alters the natural history of disease remains limited. This article reviews the recent literature on the efficacy of endoscopic intervention in the treatment of RAP with a focus on high-quality prospective randomized controlled studies. Additional studies are needed to corroborate these findings.

Since the original description of pancreatic fluid collections (PFCs) in 1761 by Morgagni, their diagnosis, description, and management have continued to evolve. The mainstay of therapy for symptomatic PFCs has been the creation of a communication between a PFC and the stomach, to enable drainage. Surgical creation of these drainage conduits had been the gold standard of therapy; however, there has been a paradigm shift in recent years with an increasing role of endoscopic drainage. The techniques of endoscopic drainage have evolved from blind fluid aspiration to include endoscopic necrosectomy and the placement of lumen-apposing metal stents.

Type 1 autoimmune pancreatitis (AIP) is an IgG-4–related systemic disease that can manifest as a pancreatic disorder or another disorder of presumed autoimmune origin. Type 2 disease is typically characterized by absent IgG-4–positive cells. As patients often present with acute pancreatitis, obstructive jaundice, or pancreatic mass, it is imperative to exclude malignancy, a more common diagnosis. AIP may respond to corticosteroids and has a strong association with other immune-mediated diseases. The recent literature suggests the benefit of immune-modulating therapy, including rituximab, although no consensus exists. This article covers the essentials of diagnosis but focuses primarily on the management of AIP.

Endoscopic pancreatic function testing assesses exocrine insufficiency and chronic pancreatitis. Indirect pancreatic function tests have limited sensitivity and specificity in early disease stages. Magnetic resonance cholangiopancreatography shows promise in detecting early changes as a direct measure of pancreatic function. This article summarizes the evolution of pancreatic function testing and highlights areas for future research, such as development of diagnostic biomarkers to stratify disease severity and targeted therapies to retard disease progression.

Pancreatic cystic lesions are a common clinical entity. The majority are neoplastic and have the potential for malignant transformation. To assist with patient management, a number of clinical guidelines have been developed over the past decade. However, controversies exist in regards to the various guidelines and treatment strategies they offer. This article reviews the various clinical guidelines for the management of pancreatic cysts, describes the limitations of these guidelines, and presents future directions for improvement in clinical decision-making for patients diagnosed with a pancreatic cystic neoplasm.

First described in the early 1980s, total pancreatectomy with autologous islet cell transplantation for the treatment of chronic pancreatitis is still only offered in select centers worldwide. Indications, process details including surgery as well as islet isolation, and results are reviewed. In addition, areas for further research to optimize results are identified.

GASTROINTESTINAL ENDOSCOPY CLINICS OF NORTH AMERICA

FORTHCOMING ISSUES

January 2019
Gastroparesis: Current Opinions and New Endoscopic Therapies
Qiang Cai, *Editor*

April 2019
The Endoscopic Hepatologist
Christopher J. DiMaio, *Editor*

July 2019
Inflammatory Bowel Disease
Simon Lichtiger, *Editor*

RECENT ISSUES

July 2018
Endoscopic Management of Gastrointestinal Bleeding
Ian M. Granlek, *Editor*

April 2018
Lumen-Apposing Stents
Jacques Van Dam, *Editor*

January 2018
Eosinophilic Esophagitis
David A. Katzka, *Editor*

RELATED CLINICS SERIES

Gastroenterology Clinics
Clinics in Liver Disease

Foreword

Management of Benign Pancreatic Diseases

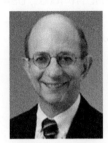

Charles J. Lightdale, MD
Consulting Editor

For generations, freshly minted surgical residents heard the advice: "eat when you can, sleep when you can...and don't mess with the pancreas." Times have changed. Gastroenterologists, interventional endoscopists, and surgeons have learned how to diagnose and treat benign pancreatic diseases with remarkable success. This issue of *Gastrointestinal Endoscopy Clinics of North America* highlights interventions using endoscopic ultrasonography (EUS) and endoscopic retrograde cholangiopancreatography (ERCP) for diagnosis and treatment of recurrent acute pancreatitis, autoimmune pancreatitis, and pancreatic cyst drainage. Another key article focuses on how to avoid post-ERCP pancreatitis. The management of acute pancreatitis using evidence-based decisions is the lead article, and other major areas covered include the role of genetics in pancreatitis, and the treatment of exocrine pancreatic insufficiency.

Pancreatic imaging using computed tomography and MRI has greatly enhanced management approaches to benign pancreatic diseases, but has also led to the detection of incidental asymptomatic pancreatic cystic neoplasms. A review of current guideline controversies in management of these cystic lesions, and the use of biomarkers obtained by EUS-guided fine-needle aspiration for risk stratification of cystic neoplasms, should be extremely helpful in deciding when to observe and when to surgically intervene. The role of interventional EUS in the pancreas is thoroughly covered, and a separate article presents the major new area of endoscopic cyst gastrostomy. Pancreatic pain can be unrelenting and debilitating, and EUS-guided celiac plexus block and neurolysis for pain relief are reviewed in depth. A final article covers the amazing surgical approach to severe pancreatic disease: total pancreatectomy with autologous islet cell transplantation.

The Editor for this issue of *Gastrointestinal Endoscopy Clinics of North America* is Dr John Poneros, a skillful and thoughtful leader in interventional endoscopy, who has gathered a remarkable group of experts to present a comprehensive review of current

Gastrointest Endoscopy Clin N Am 28 (2018) xiii–xiv
https://doi.org/10.1016/j.giec.2018.08.001
1052-5157/18/© 2018 Published by Elsevier Inc.

giendo.theclinics.com

approaches to the understanding and management of benign pancreatic diseases. Eat when you can and sleep when you can, and don't miss this terrific issue.

Charles J. Lightdale, MD
Department of Medicine
Columbia University Medical Center
161 Fort Washington Avenue
New York, NY 10032, USA

E-mail address:
CJL18@columbia.edu

Preface

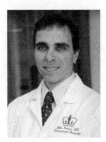

John M. Poneros, MD, FASGE, NYSGEF
Editor

The management of benign pancreatic diseases is one of the more difficult clinical problems that the practicing gastroenterologist faces. The management of acute and chronic pancreatitis and autoimmune pancreatitis and the evaluation and surveillance of incidentally found pancreatic cysts can be particularly vexing. Due to the relative scarcity of these conditions relative to the more common gastrointestinal problems, management of these clinical scenarios can be overwhelming for those who are not accustomed to these diseases. In addition, the management guidelines suggested by the various gastrointestinal societies change rapidly, confounding a practicing gastroenterologist's management even further. Finally, these can be a challenging set of patients to manage given that there are frequently issues of chronic pain and the specter of pancreatic cancer looms over their course.

In this issue of *Gastrointestinal Endoscopy Clinics of North America*, we have attempted to bring together various expert specialists to provide state-of-the-art reviews of the management of benign pancreatic disease. This issue grew out of the program of the first Pancreas Symposium held at New York Presbyterian Hospital/Columbia in 2017. Gastrointestinal endoscopists play a key role in the management of these disorders as they are frequently consulted to provide therapeutic and diagnostic interventions. Gastrointestinal endoscopic management of these disorders is highlighted in this issue. These articles are meant to be a practical resource to aid clinical decision making.

I would like to acknowledge the generosity of the Diller-von Furstenberg Family Foundation in helping establish the Pancreatitis Program at New York Presbyterian Hospital/Columbia.

Gastrointest Endoscopy Clin N Am 28 (2018) xv–xvi
https://doi.org/10.1016/j.giec.2018.07.001
1052-5157/18/© 2018 Published by Elsevier Inc.

giendo.theclinics.com

I would like to thank all the authors for their excellent contributions to this issue and Dr Lightdale for allowing me to serve as its Editor.

John M. Poneros, MD, FASGE, NYSGEF
Columbia University College of
Physicians and Surgeons
Division of Digestive and Liver Diseases
New York Presbyterian Hospital/Columbia
161 Fort Washington Avenue
Herbert Irving Pavilion
Room 1344
New York, NY 10032, USA

E-mail address:
jmp14@columbia.edu

Uncomplicated Acute Pancreatitis
Evidenced-Based Management Decisions

Venkata S. Akshintala, MD[a],*, Ayesha Kamal, MD[b],
Vikesh K. Singh, MD, MSc[c]

KEYWORDS

- Pancreatitis • Acute • Severity • Management

KEY POINTS

- Acute pancreatitis is among the most common gastrointestinal disorders requiring hospitalization.
- Early goal-directed fluid resuscitation with lactated Ringer solution remains the cornerstone of therapy the management of mild acute pancreatitis.
- Non-opioid analgesics should be considered in the management of pain in acute pancreatitis.
- A low-fat, low-residue diet can be used for initial re-feeding after resolution of nausea, emesis and abdominal pain.
- There is no role of prophylactic antibiotics in the setting of necrotizing pancreatitis.

INTRODUCTION AND EPIDEMIOLOGY

Acute pancreatitis (AP) is among the most common gastrointestinal disorders requiring hospitalization worldwide with an annual incidence of 13 to 45 cases per 100,000 persons.[1] In the United States, AP resulted in 275,000 hospitalizations in 2012 with aggregate costs of $2.6 billion.[2] Recent National Hospital Discharge Surveys suggests that although there has been an increase in AP admissions, the overall mortality rate has remained around 2%.[3]

Disclosure Statement: V.K. Singh: Consultant for Abbvie, Ariel Precision Medicine, and Akcea Therapeutics. All the other authors have no disclosures.
[a] Division of Gastroenterology, Johns Hopkins Medical Institutions, 1830 East Monument Street, Room 436, Baltimore, MD 21205, USA; [b] Division of Gastroenterology, Johns Hopkins Medical Institutions, 600 North Wolfe Street, Baltimore, MD 21205, USA; [c] Division of Gastroenterology, Johns Hopkins Medical Institutions, 1830 East Monument Street, Room 428, Baltimore, MD 21205, USA
* Corresponding author.
E-mail address: vakshin1@jhmi.edu

DIAGNOSIS OF ACUTE PANCREATITIS

According to the revised Atlanta classification, AP is diagnosed if two or more of the three clinical features listed at the top of **Table 1** are present.[4] There are additional considerations listed under each of these clinical features that are importance to the practitioner (see **Table 1**).

ELEVATION OF PANCREATIC ENZYMES WITHOUT ACUTE PANCREATITIS

Lipase is elevated to three times the upper limit of normal in many nonpancreatic conditions as summarized in **Table 2**.[5–7] In a large study of cardiovascular safety in patients with type 2 diabetes, 22.7% were noted to have asymptomatic amylase and lipase elevation.[8] Abdominal imaging should be considered when a patient without clear risk factors for AP presents with upper abdominal pain and elevated pancreatic enzymes because neither are specific for AP.

EVALUATION OF THE CAUSE OF ACUTE PANCREATITIS

Establishing the cause of AP ensures appropriate management and proper health care resource use. The two most common causes of AP are biliary (40%–70%) and alcohol use (25%–35%).[1,9] Other causes include metabolic factors, such as hypertriglyceridemia (HTG), hypercalcemia, drug induced, autoimmune, hereditary/genetic, and anatomic abnormalities.

Biliary Tract Stones and/or Sludge

Biliary tract stones and/or sludge are the most common cause of AP. Approximately 7% of the US adult population has gallstones but only 0.1% to 0.3% develop associated complications including acute cholecystitis, choledocholithiasis, or acute biliary pancreatitis.[10,11] All patients presenting with their first episode of AP should undergo abdominal ultrasonography.[12] If abdominal ultrasonography does not identify stones or sludge, an alanine aminotransferase greater than three times the upper limit of normal has greater than 95% positive predictive value for acute biliary pancreatitis.[13] Patients with elevated liver enzymes on Day 1 were found to have low risk of AP recurrence after cholecystectomy (9%), but the risk of AP recurrence is higher among those without elevated liver enzymes (34%) or in those without gallbladder stone/sludge (61%).[14]

The risk of pancreatitis among heavy users of alcohol ranges from 2% to 5%.[15,16] It should be highlighted that most heavy drinkers do not develop pancreatitis, which suggests that there are other factors that drive risk. Alcohol can modify the risk of AP from other etiologies including genetic mutations, hyperlipidemia, and drug-induced pancreatitis.[1] There is a dose-dependent relationship between alcohol and the risk of AP with various reports describing an increased risk of pancreatitis in individuals consuming greater than 14 beers per week.[16,17]

Smoking Tobacco

Smoking tobacco has been identified to be independent risk factor for pancreatitis. The risk is dose dependent, particularly with a 15 pack-year history.[18] However, with two decades of smoking cessation, the risk is noted to be reduced to the levels of never smokers.[19] Smoking is also known to modify risk of AP from other etiologies and combined use of smoking and alcohol can synergistically increase the risk of AP.[1]

Table 1
Diagnosis of acute pancreatitis

Clinical Features	Upper Abdominal Pain	Elevation of Amylase or Lipase ≥3 Times the Upper Limit of Normal	Abdominal Imaging
Considerations	• Most commonly localized to the epigastrium with or without radiation to the back. • Location of pain is nonspecific because of viscerosomatic sensory convergence in the spinal cord and can therefore be confused with other conditions that cause upper abdominal pain.	• Amylase has short half-life and is normal by 24 h but lipase can remain elevated for 8–14 d, longer in the setting of renal dysfunction. Lipase has higher sensitivity and because of wider window of detection is more suitable for delayed presentations. • Lipase alone is recommended for the diagnosis of AP.[80,81] • The reference range of lipase varies based on laboratory assay used. • Lipase levels should only be used to diagnose AP and should not be checked each day of hospitalization because it does not correlate with prognosis, clinical improvement, or disease severity.[82] • Higher triglyceride levels (>1000 mg/dL) are associated with higher lipase and lower amylase level because of interference with the lipase assay, and serial dilutions are needed for accurate measurements in this setting.[23]	• CECT is the most commonly used imaging modality in the setting of AP and has a sensitivity and specificity of more than 90% for the diagnosis of AP.[83] • Consider imaging to assess for other causes when there is diagnostic uncertainty or assess for complications especially when there is inadequate response to initial treatment. • Caution must be used when mild AP changes are reported on imaging studies because radiologists are not typically blinded to laboratory studies and this results in interpretation bias. • IAP/APA guidelines recommend the optimal timing and type of CECT.[68] • Among patients with renal insufficiency or with contrast allergy T2-weighted MRI is used to accurately diagnose pancreatic necrosis.[84]

Abbreviations: APA, American Pancreatic Association; CECT, contrast-enhanced computerized tomography; IAP, International Association of Pancreatology.

Table 2
Elevation of amylase and lipase in the absence of acute pancreatitis

Gastrointestinal	Nongastrointestinal
Elevated amylase or lipase	Elevated amylase or lipase
Gastroenteritis	Ectopic pregnancy
Peptic ulcer disease	Diabetes type 1 and type 2
Bowel perforation	Sarcoidosis
Bowel ischemia	Intracranial hemorrhage or traumatic brain
Bowel obstruction	injury
Pancreatic pseudocyst	Renal impairment
Cholangitis	Ruptured abdominal aortic aneurysm
Cholecystitis	Opioid analgesics
Post endoscopic retrograde	Elevated amylase
cholangiopancreatography	Parotitis
(without pancreatitis)	Macroamylasemia
Peritonitis	Ovarian cyst or cystic neoplasm
Celiac disease	Carcinoma of the lung

Hypertriglyceridemia

HTG is the third leading cause of AP in the United States and is identified as the cause of AP in up to 14% of AP cases, and up to 56% cases of AP during pregnancy.[20,21] HTG can result from primary (genetic) and secondary disorders of lipoprotein lipase metabolism. Frederickson type I (high chylomicrons), now known as familial chylomicronemia syndrome, type IV (high very-low-density lipoprotein), and type V (high chylomicrons and very-low-density lipoprotein) can cause severe HTG and increase the risk of AP. Secondary disorders including poorly controlled diabetes, medications, alcohol use, hypothyroidism, and pregnancy can result in HTG and AP. Triglyceride level of greater than 885 mg/dL was suspected to increase the risk of AP but a recent large epidemiologic study found that levels as low as 177 mg/dL are associated with an increased risk of AP but the absolute risk is still low.[22–24] The risk of AP at triglyceride levels greater than 1000 mg/dL is 5% and greater than 2000 mg/dL is 15%.[22] Approximately one-fourth of the adult population in the United States has triglycerides levels greater than 176 mg/dL.[25] Increasing triglyceride levels have been shown to positively correlate with the risk of persistent organ failure, regardless of the cause of AP, likely because of triglyceride-related lipotoxicity.[24] Although the initial treatment of severe HTG involves supportive measures commonly instituted in patients with AP, specific treatments, such as apheresis, heparin, and insulin, have also been used. It should be noted that HTG-mediated injury leading to AP has already occurred by the time a patient is admitted to the hospital; therefore, interventions to acutely reduce the triglyceride level, although commonplace, are not evidence based. Data from two large US health databases have shown that among the patients with severe HTG, reducing the triglyceride level to less than 200 mg/dL resulted in the lowest rates of recurrent AP on follow-up.[26] Long-term levels of triglycerides should be maintained less than 200 mg/dL through a combination of diet, exercise, fibrates, and omega-3 fatty acids.[27]

Pancreas Divisum

Pancreas divisum is the most common congenital anomaly in humans and is present in around 7% to 8% of the white population with more than 95% being asymptomatic.[28] Pancreas divisum does not modify the natural history of idiopathic recurrent

AP and is more likely to be an incidental finding.[29] No clear association between AP and pancreas divisum has been identified, in the absence of CFTR or SPINK1, or PRSS1 mutations.[30] Pancreatic endotherapy including repeated pancreatic duct stent placements and pancreatic sphincterotomies are therefore not recommended for patients with idiopathic AP and pancreas divisum.

Idiopathic Pancreatitis

Idiopathic pancreatitis is defined as AP where the cause is not apparent after history, laboratory, and imaging studies are obtained. Endoscopic ultrasound because of its higher sensitivity must be considered to evaluate for microlithiasis and ampullary or pancreatic cancer, particularly in patients who are older, smoke, and have new-onset diabetes and/or unexplained weight loss.[31] Hereditary/genetic pancreatitis is considered among patients in whom the cause continues to be unidentified, particularly in patients less than 35 years of age.[32]

CLASSIFICATION OF DISEASE SEVERITY AND RISK STRATIFICATION

After a diagnosis of AP is made, it is important to identify which patients either have or are at risk of severe AP. Severe AP occurs in 15% to 20% of patients with AP, which is the incidence reported from academic centers; however, the transfer of patients to these centers likely results in an overestimation of severe AP.[33] **Table 3** summarizes the definitions of disease severity in AP based on the most recent classification systems.[4,34,35] The revised Atlanta classification defines organ failure as a score of two or more in any one of the organ systems (renal, respiratory, and cardiovascular) using the modified Marshall scoring system. Clinicians should recognize that most patients with severe AP do not present with organ failure or local complications at the time of admission and these could develop as a result of inadequate resuscitation or lack of identification of early signs.[36] The ability to predict the severity of disease early in the course of hospitalization allows for triage to advanced level of care in the intensive care unit setting, aggressive fluid therapy, and enteral nutrition. Although there have been numerous clinical and radiologic scoring systems developed to predict the severity of AP, they are associated with high negative but low positive predictive value for severe AP.[37]

The bedside index for severity in AP scoring system consists of five parameters: (1) blood urea nitrogen greater than 25 mg/dL, (2) impaired mental status, (3) presence of the systematic inflammatory response syndrome (SIRS), (4) age greater than 60 years, and (5) pleural effusions.[38] A score of three or more in the first 24 hours has been

Table 3
Acute pancreatitis severity classification systems

Classification System	Disease Severity	Criteria
Atlanta Classification 1992	Mild	No organ failure and no local complications
	Severe	Organ failure and/or local complications
Revised Atlanta Classification 2007 (published 2013)	Mild	No organ failure and no local or systemic complications
	Moderate	Transient organ failure and/or local complications
	Severe	Persistent organ failure
Determinant-Based Classification 2012	Mild	No (peri)pancreatic necrosis and no organ failure
	Moderate	Sterile necrosis and/or transient organ failure
	Severe	Infected necrosis or persistent organ failure
	Critical	Infected necrosis and persistent organ failure

shown to be associated with a 5% to 20% risk of mortality.[38] Papachristou and colleagues[39] compared several scoring systems and found the prognostic accuracy of bedside index for severity in AP to be similar to other scoring systems but simpler to use. The simplicity of SIRS has also made it attractive as a single biomarker for assessing disease activity.[40] SIRS on Day 1 of admission has also been shown to predict severe AP with high sensitivity (85%–100%) and the absence of SIRS on Day 1 was associated with a high negative predictive value (98%–100%).[41] The recently developed and prospectively validated Pancreatitis Activity Scoring System uses organ failure, SIRS, abdominal pain, requirement for opioids, and ability to tolerate oral intake as a dynamic measure of disease activity in AP.[42]

INITIAL MANAGEMENT OF ACUTE PANCREATITIS
Indications for Early Discharge Versus Monitored or Intensive Level of Care

The incidence of early readmission in AP is high, occurring in 19% of patients.[43] On a multivariable analysis, moderate to heavy alcohol use (odds ratio, 10.1), discharge on less than a solid diet (odds ratio, 23.8), and persistent gastrointestinal symptoms, such as nausea/emesis (odds ratio, 44.2), were determined to be the strongest risk factors for early readmission. Among patients who require prolonged hospitalization, most are managed at specialty centers experienced in the management of AP. However, patients with severe AP should be appropriately triaged and considered for transfer to tertiary centers.

Fluid Therapy in Acute Pancreatitis Management

Fluid therapy remains the cornerstone of managing AP. The fluid losses are significant in AP and result from multiple factors inherent to the pathophysiology of AP, including third spacing, vomiting, reduced oral intake, respiratory losses, and diaphoresis. This is further compounded by the microangiopathic effects of cytokines and inflammatory mediators of AP leading to reduced vascular resistance similar to sepsis, resulting in reduced pancreatic blood flow, cellular death, and necrosis, which causes a "second hit" on the pancreas with activation of the enzyme cascade.[44] Hemoconcentration, a marker of fluid losses, is associated with an increased risk of pancreatic necrosis and organ failure.[45] Aggressive early hydration is therefore thought to augment circulatory support to prevent complications of AP, such as necrosis or organ failure.[46]

Two well-conducted randomized controlled trials (RCTs) demonstrated lactated Ringer solution (LR) to be beneficial over normal saline and one RCT demonstrated aggressive or goal-directed hydration with LR to be more beneficial compared with standard hydration with LR among patients with mild AP.[47–49] In the setting of AP, LR has additional benefits because of a direct inhibitory effect on macrophage-mediated inflammation when compared with normal saline.[49,50]

Based on the pathophysiology of AP, fluid therapy is thought to play the most crucial role during the first 12 to 24 hours and early hydration in the emergency room is of utmost importance.[46] The rate and volume of fluid therapy is based on conflicting guidelines and data from two RCTs (**Table 4**). Furthermore, few of the previously conducted studies suggested increased morbidities, such as respiratory complications, compartment syndrome, and even mortality from aggressive early hydration in the first 48 hours, but these studies included much sicker patients and could be caused by reverse causation.[51,52] Aggressive hydration requires additional caution among elderly patients and those with cardiopulmonary and renal comorbidities who are more susceptible to complications from volume overload.

Table 4
Fluid type and rate in recent guidelines and RCT

	Initial Fluid Administration	Maintenance Fluid Administration
Guideline		
AGA guidelines, 2018	Goal directed	Goal-directed maintenance
ACG guidelines, 2013	Goal directed	Goal-directed maintenance
	Aggressive 250–500 mL/h crystalloid	
IAP/APA guidelines, 2013	Goal directed 5–10 mL/kg/h	Goal-directed maintenance
RCT author		
de-Madaria et al,[49] 2018	Goal directed	Aggressive LR/NS 1.2 mL/kg/h
	Aggressive LR/NS 15 mL/kg bolus	Standard LR/NS 1 mL/kg/h
	Standard LR/NS 10 mL/kg bolus	
Buxbaum et al,[48] 2017	Goal directed	Aggressive LR 3 mL/kg/h
	Aggressive LR 20 mL/kg bolus	Standard LR 1.5 mL/kg/h
	Standard LR 10 mL/kg bolus	
Wu et al,[47] 2011	Goal directed	Goal directed LR/NS
	LR/NS 20 mL/kg bolus	3 mL/kg/h or 1.5 mL/kg/h
	Standard physician directed LR/NS	

Abbreviations: ACG, American College of Gastroenterology; AGA, American Gastroenterological Association; APA, American Pancreatic Association; IAP, International Association of Pancreatology; NJ, nasojejunal; NS, normal saline.

Pain Control in Acute Pancreatitis

Pain is a key symptom of AP with diagnostic and prognostic value. It was noted that the duration of pain before hospitalization impacts the severity of AP among patients with hemoconcentration at the time of admission.[53] Hypovolemia and fluid losses associated with AP can result in pain from visceral ischemia; therefore, adequate fluid therapy as discussed previously is important. A mild episode of AP might be adequately treated with nonsteroidal anti-inflammatory drugs alone[54] and for appropriate pain control for more severe episode, more potent opioid analgesics are typically used.[55] A Cochrane review of trials of nonopioids and opioids analgesics found similar improvements in pain at 2 days for all analgesics.[56] A prospective cohort study reported an increased risk of gastrointestinal dysmotility among patients with AP receiving opioid analgesics compared with those receiving nonopioid analgesics and this results in delays in oral refeeding and impacts quality of life.[57] Nonopioid analgesics should therefore be considered for pain control in patients with AP.

Role of Endoscopy in Biliary Acute Pancreatitis

Biliary pancreatitis is caused by obstruction of the ampulla of Vater by a stone, which results in increased pancreatic ductal pressure and reflux of bile into the pancreatic duct that activates pancreatic enzymes and the inflammatory cascade. Most stones pass spontaneously into the duodenum but a minority of these result in obstruction and thus require removal.[58] Endoscopic retrograde cholangiopancreatography (ERCP) is a therapeutic modality to relieve persistent ductal obstruction from a biliary stone. However, it must be noted that cholestasis can also be caused by ampullary edema from a previously passed stone or from edema causing compression of the duct in the head of pancreas and, therefore, appropriate patient selection is needed to identify those who require ERCP.[59] A meta-analysis of eight RCTs comparing early ERCP versus conservative management in biliary AP showed that urgent ERCP does not impact important clinical outcomes, such as mortality, organ failure, and pancreatic necrosis.[60] Urgent ERCP is therefore not recommended in the setting of cholestasis alone without cholangitis. The impact of endoscopic sphincterotomy on complications in these patients is the subject of an ongoing trial in the Netherlands.[61]

Cholecystectomy in Biliary Acute Pancreatitis

If cholecystectomy is delayed after an initial hospitalization for biliary AP, several cohort studies have demonstrated that the risk of recurrent biliary complications, including recurrent AP, acute cholecystitis, or choledocholithiasis is around 17% at 6 months.[62] Biliary sphincterotomy alone has been shown to reduce the risk of recurrent AP but no other biliary complications in those with a gallbladder.[63] Cholecystectomy after an episode of biliary AP is recommended by current guidelines with high degree of adherence but the timing of cholecystectomy has been much debated.[64] Three RCTs[62,65,66] have evaluated the timing of cholecystectomy after biliary AP and suggested that cholecystectomy is safely performed during the index hospitalization for mild AP. In the setting of moderate to severe AP, especially with fluid collections, surgery should be delayed until the acute inflammation/fluid collections have resolved or stabilized.[67] Delaying surgery in the setting of pancreatic necrosis or severe AP reduces the risk of surgical complications. The timing of surgery in these situations should be delayed to around 6 weeks.[68]

Nutrition in Acute Pancreatitis

Nutrition therapy in AP pertains to the timing of reinitiating oral feeding or other mode of enteral feeding, composition of feeding, and/or need for parenteral nutrition.

Timing of reinitiating oral feeding

Clinical practice has historically focused on the tolerance of oral feeding as a criterion for discharge and maintaining strict nothing by mouth status until the resolution of abdominal pain.[69] Nothing by mouth status is initiated to reduce the stimulation of pancreatic secretion and prevent further activation of the pancreatic enzymes and resulting inflammatory response. However, there is little evidence to support this concept.[70] There is also increased concern regarding intestinal mucosal atrophy with nothing by mouth status thereby affecting the gut-mucosal barrier, which increases the risk of transmigration of gut flora. Early initiation of oral feeding has been shown in multiple studies to reduce the risk of infectious complications of AP and overall morbidity and mortality associated with severe AP.[12] However, AP can result in gastrointestinal dysmotility and ileus leading to nausea and vomiting, which limits the tolerance of oral intake.

A recent systematic review of 11 RCTs comparing early with delayed feeding in patients with mild to moderate AP[71] demonstrated that early feeding reduces length of hospital stay and with no increased risk of adverse events. A soft low-fat, low-residue diet was noted to provide more calories compared with clear liquid diet, without any increase in pain recurrence rates.[72] Patient-reported resolution of nausea, emesis, and abdominal pain should determine the timing of oral feeding reinitiation.

Nonoral enteral feeding and parenteral feeding

Patients who cannot tolerate oral intake in 48 to 72 hours, especially those with severe AP and with ileus, require an alternate method of nutritional support. Total parenteral nutrition has been compared with enteral nutrition administered through a nasogastric (NG) or nasojejunal (NJ) tube in 12 RCTs.[60] The cumulative evidence from these RCTs has suggested a lower length of stay, organ failure, and pancreatic infection among the NG/NJ compared with total parenteral nutrition group. Dysfunction of the gut barrier in the absence of enteral nutrition and transmigration of the gut flora has been suggested to increase the risk of infected pancreatic necrosis.[73] Based on this evidence, enteral nutrition is recommended even among patients with severe AP, through the NG/NJ if the oral route is not tolerated. Total parenteral nutrition or peripheral parenteral nutrition is not the preferred route for nutrition unless the enteral access is not available, is not tolerated (including trophic feeds), or is not able to meet adequate caloric requirements. Bakker and colleagues[74] compared NJ feed initiation in 24 hours with an oral diet after 72 hours with insertion of an NJ tube if not tolerated in an RCT of patients with predicted severe AP and demonstrated no difference in a composite outcome that included mortality or infectious complications.

Comparison of nasogastric or nasojejunal routes and formulations

NJ route was conventionally preferred over NG route to avoid the gastroduodenal phase of pancreatic stimulation. However, four RCTs have compared NJ and NG routes in patients with severe AP, in a meta-analysis[75] and have shown no difference in mortality, infectious complications, or length of hospital stay among the two groups. There were few reports suggesting reduced risk of aspiration pneumonitis in the NJ group but this was not conclusively demonstrated in the meta-analysis. The risk of pneumonitis is reduced by maintaining aspiration precautions, such as elevation of the head of the bed and monitoring for residuals in the stomach. NG tube placement is simpler, avoiding the need for endoscopic or interventional radiology services.

Role of Prophylactic Antibiotics in Acute Pancreatitis

AP, especially in moderate-severe form, is associated with local and systemic infectious complications. A recent systematic review has reported a two-fold increase in mortality in patients with infected pancreatic necrosis and organ failure (35.2%) when compared with sterile pancreatic necrosis and organ failure (19.8%).[76] SIRS caused by AP and nonpancreatic infections cannot be differentiated. Although antibiotics are clearly indicated in the setting of confirmed presence of infection, the use of antibiotics prophylactically in the setting of severe AP or sterile pancreatic necrosis to prevent infected pancreatic necrosis is controversial. Infected pancreatic necrosis was previously suspected to be a late complication of AP, but recent evidence has suggested otherwise, with nearly 50% of cases occurring within the first 7 days of hospitalization.[77] Multiple meta-analyses over the past few decades have provided contradictory recommendations regarding the use of prophylactic antibiotics in the setting of AP, because of underpowered RCTs lack of double blinding and with heterogeneity in patient population or antibiotic choice.[78] A recent Cochrane review[79] and an updated meta-analysis[60] summarized results from 10 RCTs and showed no mortality benefit or reduction in rate of infected pancreatic necrosis or persistent organ failure with the use of prophylactic antibiotics.

REFERENCES

1. Yadav D, Lowenfels AB. The epidemiology of pancreatitis and pancreatic cancer. Gastroenterology 2013;144(6):1252–61.
2. Peery AF, Crockett SD, Barritt AS, et al. Burden of gastrointestinal, liver, and pancreatic diseases in the United States. Gastroenterology 2015;149(7): 1731–41.e3.
3. Peery AF, Dellon ES, Lund J, et al. Burden of gastrointestinal disease in the United States: 2012 update. Gastroenterology 2012;143(5):1179–87.e1-3.

4. Banks PA, Bollen TL, Dervenis C, et al. Classification of acute pancreatitis–2012: revision of the Atlanta classification and definitions by international consensus. Gut 2013;62(1):102–11.
5. Muniraj T, Dang S, Pitchumoni CS. PANCREATITIS OR NOT?–Elevated lipase and amylase in ICU patients. J Crit Care 2015;30(6):1370–5.
6. Hameed AM, Lam VW, Pleass HC. Significant elevations of serum lipase not caused by pancreatitis: a systematic review. HPB 2015;17(2):99–112.
7. Forsmark CE, Baillie J. AGA Institute technical review on acute pancreatitis. Gastroenterology 2007;132(5):2022–44.
8. Newell AL. Editorial. Attitudes hinder communications. NACDL J 1970;17(10):15.
9. Lowenfels AB, Maisonneuve P, Sullivan T. The changing character of acute pancreatitis: epidemiology, etiology, and prognosis. Curr Gastroenterol Rep 2009;11(2):97–103.
10. Everhart JE, Khare M, Hill M, et al. Prevalence and ethnic differences in gallbladder disease in the United States. Gastroenterology 1999;117(3):632–9.
11. Friedman GD. Natural history of asymptomatic and symptomatic gallstones. Am J Surg 1993;165(4):399–404.
12. Tenner S, Baillie J, DeWitt J, et al. American College of Gastroenterology guideline: management of acute pancreatitis. Am J Gastroenterol 2013;108(9): 1400–15, 1416.
13. Tenner S, Dubner H, Steinberg W. Predicting gallstone pancreatitis with laboratory parameters: a meta-analysis. Am J Gastroenterol 1994;89(10):1863–6.
14. Trna J, Vege SS, Pribramska V, et al. Lack of significant liver enzyme elevation and gallstones and/or sludge on ultrasound on day 1 of acute pancreatitis is associated with recurrence after cholecystectomy: a population-based study. Surgery 2012;151(2):199–205.
15. Lankisch PG, Lowenfels AB, Maisonneuve P. What is the risk of alcoholic pancreatitis in heavy drinkers? Pancreas 2002;25(4):411–2.
16. Kristiansen L, Gronbaek M, Becker U, et al. Risk of pancreatitis according to alcohol drinking habits: a population-based cohort study. Am J Epidemiol 2008;168(8):932–7.
17. Sadr Azodi O, Orsini N, Andren-Sandberg A, et al. Effect of type of alcoholic beverage in causing acute pancreatitis. Br J Surg 2011;98(11):1609–16.
18. Yuhara H, Ogawa M, Kawaguchi Y, et al. Smoking and risk for acute pancreatitis: a systematic review and meta-analysis. Pancreas 2014;43(8):1201–7.
19. Sasco AJ, Secretan MB, Straif K. Tobacco smoking and cancer: a brief review of recent epidemiological evidence. Lung Cancer 2004;45(Suppl 2):S3–9.
20. Chang CC, Hsieh YY, Tsai HD, et al. Acute pancreatitis in pregnancy. Zhonghua Yi Xue Za Zhi (Taipei) 1998;61(2):85–92.
21. Koutroumpakis E, Slivka A, Furlan A, et al. Management and outcomes of acute pancreatitis patients over the last decade: a US tertiary-center experience. Pancreatology 2017;17(1):32–40.
22. Scherer J, Singh VP, Pitchumoni CS, et al. Issues in hypertriglyceridemic pancreatitis: an update. J Clin Gastroenterol 2014;48(3):195–203.
23. Pedersen SB, Langsted A, Nordestgaard BG. Nonfasting mild-to-moderate hypertriglyceridemia and risk of acute pancreatitis. JAMA Intern Med 2016; 176(12):1834–42.
24. Berglund L, Brunzell JD, Goldberg AC, et al. Evaluation and treatment of hypertriglyceridemia: an Endocrine Society clinical practice guideline. J Clin Endocrinol Metab 2012;97(9):2969–89.

25. Christian JB, Bourgeois N, Snipes R, et al. Prevalence of severe (500 to 2,000 mg/dl) hypertriglyceridemia in United States adults. Am J Cardiol 2011;107(6):891–7.
26. Christian JB, Arondekar B, Buysman EK, et al. Determining triglyceride reductions needed for clinical impact in severe hypertriglyceridemia. Am J Med 2014;127(1):36–44.e1.
27. Tsuang W, Navaneethan U, Ruiz L, et al. Hypertriglyceridemic pancreatitis: presentation and management. Am J Gastroenterol 2009;104(4):984–91.
28. Stimec B, Bulajic M, Korneti V, et al. Ductal morphometry of ventral pancreas in pancreas divisum. Comparison between clinical and anatomical results. Ital J Gastroenterol 1996;28(2):76–80.
29. DiMagno MJ, Wamsteker EJ. Pancreas divisum. Curr Gastroenterol Rep 2011; 13(2):150–6.
30. Bertin C, Pelletier AL, Vullierme MP, et al. Pancreas divisum is not a cause of pancreatitis by itself but acts as a partner of genetic mutations. Am J Gastroenterol 2012;107(2):311–7.
31. Alexakis N, Lombard M, Raraty M, et al. When is pancreatitis considered to be of biliary origin and what are the implications for management? Pancreatology 2007; 7(2–3):131–41.
32. Whitcomb DC. Genetic risk factors for pancreatic disorders. Gastroenterology 2013;144(6):1292–302.
33. Banks PA, Freeman ML. Practice guidelines in acute pancreatitis. Am J Gastroenterol 2006;101(10):2379–400.
34. Dellinger EP, Forsmark CE, Layer P, et al. Determinant-based classification of acute pancreatitis severity: an international multidisciplinary consultation. Ann Surg 2012;256(6):875–80.
35. Bradley EL 3rd. A clinically based classification system for acute pancreatitis. Summary of the International Symposium on Acute Pancreatitis, Atlanta, Ga, September 11 through 13, 1992. Arch Surg 1993;128(5):586–90.
36. Tenner S. Initial management of acute pancreatitis: critical issues during the first 72 hours. Am J Gastroenterol 2004;99(12):2489–94.
37. Balthazar EJ, Robinson DL, Megibow AJ, et al. Acute pancreatitis: value of CT in establishing prognosis. Radiology 1990;174(2):331–6.
38. Wu BU, Johannes RS, Sun X, et al. The early prediction of mortality in acute pancreatitis: a large population-based study. Gut 2008;57(12):1698–703.
39. Papachristou GI, Muddana V, Yadav D, et al. Comparison of BISAP, Ranson's, APACHE-II, and CTSI scores in predicting organ failure, complications, and mortality in acute pancreatitis. Am J Gastroenterol 2010;105(2):435–41 [quiz: 442].
40. Mounzer R, Langmead CJ, Wu BU, et al. Comparison of existing clinical scoring systems to predict persistent organ failure in patients with acute pancreatitis. Gastroenterology 2012;142(7):1476–82 [quiz: e1415–76].
41. Singh VK, Wu BU, Bollen TL, et al. Early systemic inflammatory response syndrome is associated with severe acute pancreatitis. Clin Gastroenterol Hepatol 2009;7(11):1247–51.
42. Buxbaum J, Quezada M, Chong B, et al. The Pancreatitis Activity Scoring System predicts clinical outcomes in acute pancreatitis: findings from a prospective cohort study. Am J Gastroenterol 2018;113(5):755–64.
43. Whitlock TL, Repas K, Tignor A, et al. Early readmission in acute pancreatitis: incidence and risk factors. Am J Gastroenterol 2010;105(11):2492–7.

44. Takeda K, Mikami Y, Fukuyama S, et al. Pancreatic ischemia associated with vasospasm in the early phase of human acute necrotizing pancreatitis. Pancreas 2005;30(1):40–9.

45. Brown A, Orav J, Banks PA. Hemoconcentration is an early marker for organ failure and necrotizing pancreatitis. Pancreas 2000;20(4):367–72.

46. Singh VK, Gardner TB, Papachristou GI, et al. An international multicenter study of early intravenous fluid administration and outcome in acute pancreatitis. United European Gastroenterol J 2017;5(4):491–8.

47. Wu BU, Hwang JQ, Gardner TH, et al. Lactated Ringer's solution reduces systemic inflammation compared with saline in patients with acute pancreatitis. Clin Gastroenterol Hepatol 2011;9(8):710–7.e1.

48. Buxbaum JL, Quezada M, Da B, et al. Early aggressive hydration hastens clinical improvement in mild acute pancreatitis. Am J Gastroenterol 2017;112(5): 797–803.

49. de-Madaria E, Herrera-Marante I, Gonzalez-Camacho V, et al. Fluid resuscitation with lactated Ringer's solution vs normal saline in acute pancreatitis: a triple-blind, randomized, controlled trial. United European Gastroenterol J 2018;6(1): 63–72.

50. Lerch MM, Conwell DL, Mayerle J. The anti-inflammasome effect of lactate and the lactate GPR81-receptor in pancreatic and liver inflammation. Gastroenterology 2014;146(7):1602–5.

51. Mao EQ, Fei J, Peng YB, et al. Rapid hemodilution is associated with increased sepsis and mortality among patients with severe acute pancreatitis. Chin Med J 2010;123(13):1639–44.

52. de-Madaria E, Soler-Sala G, Sanchez-Paya J, et al. Influence of fluid therapy on the prognosis of acute pancreatitis: a prospective cohort study. Am J Gastroenterol 2011;106(10):1843–50.

53. Kapoor K, Repas K, Singh VK, et al. Does the duration of abdominal pain prior to admission influence the severity of acute pancreatitis? JOP 2013;14(2):171–5.

54. Pezzilli R, Uomo G, Gabbrielli A, et al. A prospective multicentre survey on the treatment of acute pancreatitis in Italy. Dig Liver Dis 2007;39(9):838–46.

55. Vargas-Schaffer G. Is the WHO analgesic ladder still valid? Twenty-four years of experience. Can Fam Physician 2010;56(6):514–7, e202-515.

56. Basurto Ona X, Rigau Comas D, Urrutia G. Opioids for acute pancreatitis pain. Cochrane Database Syst Rev 2013;(7):CD009179.

57. Wu LM, Pendharkar SA, Asrani VM, et al. Effect of intravenous fluids and analgesia on dysmotility in patients with acute pancreatitis: a prospective cohort study. Pancreas 2017;46(7):858–66.

58. Acosta JM, Ledesma CL. Gallstone migration as a cause of acute pancreatitis. N Engl J Med 1974;290(9):484–7.

59. van Santvoort HC, Bakker OJ, Besselink MG, et al. Prediction of common bile duct stones in the earliest stages of acute biliary pancreatitis. Endoscopy 2011;43(1):8–13.

60. Vege SS, DiMagno MJ, Forsmark CE, et al. Initial medical treatment of acute pancreatitis: American Gastroenterological Association Institute Technical Review. Gastroenterology 2018;154(4):1103–39.

61. Schepers NJ, Bakker OJ, Besselink MG, et al. Early biliary decompression versus conservative treatment in acute biliary pancreatitis (APEC trial): study protocol for a randomized controlled trial. Trials 2016;17:5.

62. da Costa DW, Bouwense SA, Schepers NJ, et al. Same-admission versus interval cholecystectomy for mild gallstone pancreatitis (PONCHO): a multicentre randomised controlled trial. Lancet 2015;386(10000):1261–8.

63. Welbourn CR, Beckly DE, Eyre-Brook IA. Endoscopic sphincterotomy without cholecystectomy for gall stone pancreatitis. Gut 1995;37(1):119–20.

64. Kamal A, Akhuemonkhan E, Akshintala VS, et al. Effectiveness of guideline-recommended cholecystectomy to prevent recurrent pancreatitis. Am J Gastroenterol 2017;112(3):503–10.

65. Kelly TR, Wagner DS. Gallstone pancreatitis: a prospective randomized trial of the timing of surgery. Surgery 1988;104(4):600–5.

66. Aboulian A, Chan T, Yaghoubian A, et al. Early cholecystectomy safely decreases hospital stay in patients with mild gallstone pancreatitis: a randomized prospective study. Ann Surg 2010;251(4):615–9.

67. van Baal MC, Besselink MG, Bakker OJ, et al. Timing of cholecystectomy after mild biliary pancreatitis: a systematic review. Ann Surg 2012;255(5):860–6.

68. Working Group IAP/APA Acute Pancreatitis Guidelines. IAP/APA evidence-based guidelines for the management of acute pancreatitis. Pancreatology 2013;13(4 Suppl 2):e1–15.

69. Steinberg WM. Controversies in clinical pancreatology: should the sphincter of Oddi be measured in patients with idiopathic recurrent acute pancreatitis, and should sphincterotomy be performed if the pressure is high? Pancreas 2003; 27(2):118–21.

70. Petrov MS. Moving beyond the 'pancreatic rest' in severe and critical acute pancreatitis. Crit Care 2013;17(4):161.

71. Vaughn VM, Shuster D, Rogers MAM, et al. Early versus delayed feeding in patients with acute pancreatitis: a systematic review. Ann Intern Med 2017;166(12): 883–92.

72. Moraes JM, Felga GE, Chebli LA, et al. A full solid diet as the initial meal in mild acute pancreatitis is safe and result in a shorter length of hospitalization: results from a prospective, randomized, controlled, double-blind clinical trial. J Clin Gastroenterol 2010;44(7):517–22.

73. Moran RA, Jalaly NY, Kamal A, et al. Ileus is a predictor of local infection in patients with acute necrotizing pancreatitis. Pancreatology 2016;16(6):966–72.

74. Bakker OJ, van Brunschot S, van Santvoort HC, et al. Early versus on-demand nasoenteric tube feeding in acute pancreatitis. N Engl J Med 2014;371(21): 1983–93.

75. Zhu Y, Yin H, Zhang R, et al. Nasogastric nutrition versus nasojejunal nutrition in patients with severe acute pancreatitis: a meta-analysis of randomized controlled trials. Gastroenterol Res Pract 2016;2016:6430632.

76. Werge M, Novovic S, Schmidt PN, et al. Infection increases mortality in necrotizing pancreatitis: a systematic review and meta-analysis. Pancreatology 2016; 16(5):698–707.

77. Besselink MG, van Santvoort HC, Boermeester MA, et al. Timing and impact of infections in acute pancreatitis. Br J Surg 2009;96(3):267–73.

78. de Vries AC, Besselink MG, Buskens E, et al. Randomized controlled trials of antibiotic prophylaxis in severe acute pancreatitis: relationship between methodological quality and outcome. Pancreatology 2007;7(5–6):531–8.

79. Villatoro E, Mulla M, Larvin M. Antibiotic therapy for prophylaxis against infection of pancreatic necrosis in acute pancreatitis. Cochrane Database Syst Rev 2010;(5):CD002941.

80. Rompianesi G, Hann A, Komolafe O, et al. Serum amylase and lipase and urinary trypsinogen and amylase for diagnosis of acute pancreatitis. Cochrane Database Syst Rev 2017;(4):CD012010.

81. American Society for Clinical Pathology: choosing wisely. Available at: https://www.ascp.org/content/docs/default-source/get-involved-pdfs/20-things-to-question.pdf?sfvrsn=4. Accessed March 24, 2018.

82. Reisman A, Cho HJ, Holzer H. Unnecessary repeat enzyme testing in acute pancreatitis: a teachable moment. JAMA Intern Med 2018;178(5):702–3.

83. Thoeni RF. Imaging of acute pancreatitis. Radiol Clin North Am 2015;53(6): 1189–208.

84. Stimac D, Miletic D, Radic M, et al. The role of nonenhanced magnetic resonance imaging in the early assessment of acute pancreatitis. Am J Gastroenterol 2007; 102(5):997–1004.

How to Avoid Post–Endoscopic Retrograde Cholangiopancreatography Pancreatitis

Bonna Leerhøy, MSc[a], B. Joseph Elmunzer, MD[b],*

KEYWORDS

- Endoscopic retrograde cholangiopancreatography • ERCP • Pancreatitis
- Post-ERCP pancreatitis • Complications

KEY POINTS

- The most effective strategy for avoiding post–endoscopic retrograde cholangiopancreatography (ERCP) pancreatitis remains thoughtful patient selection; in this era of highly accurate diagnostic alternatives, ERCP should be an almost exclusively therapeutic procedure.
- Risk stratification according to patient and procedure-related predictors should guide clinical decision-making and the implementation of prophylactic interventions.
- Sound procedural technique, which includes wire-guided cannulation, early use of alternative cannulation methods in challenging cases, and avoidance of aggressive/repeated pancreatic injections should be used in all cases.
- Prophylactic pancreatic stents should be placed in all high-risk cases.
- Rectal nonsteroidal anti-inflammatory drugs and aggressive lactated Ringer's solution should be considered in all patients undergoing ERCP.

INTRODUCTION

Despite recent advances in prevention, the incidence of pancreatitis after endoscopic retrograde cholangiopancreatography (ERCP) remains 3% to 15%, resulting in substantial morbidity and increased health care costs.[1–3] Approximately 5% of post-ERCP pancreatitis (PEP) will be severe in nature, requiring prolonged

The authors have no conflicts of interest to disclose.
[a] Digestive Disease Center, Bispebjerg Hospital, University of Copenhagen Nielsine Nielsens Vej 11, entrance 8, Copenhagen DK-2400, Denmark; [b] Division of Gastroenterology and Hepatology, Medical University of South Carolina, MSC 702, 114 Doughty Street, Suite 249, Charleston, SC 29425, USA
* Corresponding author.
E-mail address: Elmunzer@musc.edu

Gastrointest Endoscopy Clin N Am 28 (2018) 439–454
https://doi.org/10.1016/j.giec.2018.05.007
1052-5157/18/© 2018 Elsevier Inc. All rights reserved.

giendo.theclinics.com

hospitalization, intensive care unit admission, additional interventions to address local complications, and occasional death.[1] Moreover, post-ERCP pancreatitis (PEP) is a common reason for malpractice lawsuits related to ERCP and contributes significantly to endoscopist stress and burnout.[4,5] Recent advances in patient selection, risk stratification, procedural technique, and prophylactic interventions have improved our ability to avoid this potentially devastating complication and should be embraced by all who perform ERCP (**Fig. 1**). This review aims to provide an evidence-based approach to avoiding PEP and an overview of ongoing research initiatives in this highly relevant area.

DEFINITION

PEP is most commonly diagnosed according to 1 of 2 definitions:

1. Cotton's Consensus Criteria from 1991: new onset or increased upper abdominal pain; *and* pancreatic amylase elevation of 3 times greater than the upper limit of normal at 24 hours after ERCP (subsequently modified by convention to include lipase elevation); *and* resulting hospitalization or prolongation of ongoing hospitalization of 2 or more nights[6]; or,
2. The Atlanta classification of acute pancreatitis updated in 2012: 2 of the following 3 criteria: (1) abdominal pain consistent with acute pancreatitis (acute onset of a persistent, severe, epigastric pain often radiating to the back); (2) serum lipase (or amylase) level at least 3 times greater than the upper limit of normal; (3) characteristic findings of acute pancreatitis on contrast-enhanced computed tomography (CECT) or less commonly MRI or transabdominal ultrasonography.[7]

The Atlanta classification is more objective and appears to be more sensitive than Cotton's definition[8]; however, the clinical impact of this increased diagnostic sensitivity, which may only capture additional mild (self-limited) cases, is unclear. Further, the radiation exposure and costs of systematic computed tomography (CT) scan in all patients with post-ERCP pain are not justified. Both definitions are limited by the

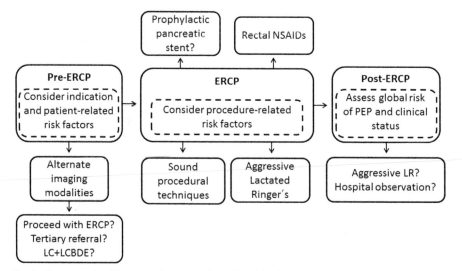

Fig. 1. Framework of interventions to reduce the risk of post-ERCP pancreatitis. LC, laparoscopic cholecystectomy; LCBDE, laparoscopic common bile duct exploration.

subjective nature of pain interpretation and varying practice styles surrounding hospitalization and the use of CECT. Thus, between-study and between-center comparisons of PEP incidence rates must be interpreted with caution, and blinding to treatment allocation is critical in PEP prevention trials.

Given the limitations of existing definitions, additional research aiming to elucidate a practical and accurate diagnostic tool for PEP is of substantial importance. For example, a biomarker that can be obtained in the immediate postprocedural setting and correlates strongly with the development of clinically important pancreatic inflammation would be of major value by helping guide clinical decision-making and serving as a surrogate marker for PEP in prevention studies.

PATIENT SELECTION

Thoughtful patient selection, which focuses on minimizing (ideally eliminating) avoidable ERCP, remains the most effective strategy for reducing the incidence of PEP. Endoscopic ultrasound (EUS) and magnetic resonance cholangiopancreatography (MRCP) have largely replaced ERCP in the diagnosis of pancreaticobiliary disease because they provide highly accurate anatomic information without the risk of pancreatitis or other serious complications. Indeed, meta-analyses have demonstrated both modalities to be highly accurate in the detection of choledocholithiasis, although MRI may be less sensitive than EUS for stones smaller than 6 mm.[9–11] Along these lines, among patients with concomitant gallbladder and bile duct stones, randomized trials have demonstrated that single-setting laparoscopic common bile duct exploration and cholecystectomy is associated with improved outcomes relative to the sequence of ERCP followed by cholecystectomy and virtually eliminates the risk of PEP.[12,13] Thus, despite a marked decrease in utilization,[14] this combined surgical approach remains a viable option to reduce risk in which expertise is available. EUS, MRCP, and other noninvasive modalities (eg, radionucleotide-labeled scan and percutaneous drain fluid analysis) are also accurate in diagnosing a multitude of other pancreaticobiliary processes, such as chronic pancreatitis, malignancy, and leaks, often obviating the need for diagnostic ERCP.

An exception to the growing practice of reserving ERCP for patients with a high likelihood of therapeutic intervention has been the evaluation of patients with suspected sphincter of Oddi dysfunction (SOD), for which the preferred diagnostic approach has become an empiric sphincterotomy when the condition is strongly suspected. When suspecting SOD, however, thoughtful clinical judgment is necessary to select those who are most likely to benefit from the procedure. The EPISOD study, a randomized trial of ERCP, manometry, and sphincterotomy for patients with unexplained pancreaticobiliary pain (formerly type 3 SOD), has largely eliminated the use of ERCP in the evaluation and treatment of this challenging and complication-prone patient population.[15] However, additional studies are necessary to determine whether ERCP is truly beneficial in cases of suspected type 2 biliary SOD or recurrent unexplained pancreatitis (possible pancreatic SOD). Pending such studies, many experts believe ERCP remains reasonable in these scenarios after careful assessment of the risk-benefit ratio and detailed informed consent. Another possible exception to the therapeutic ERCP trend may be the evaluation of biliary complications in liver transplant recipients, for whom a recent retrospective study suggested that diagnostic ERCP is a reasonable and efficient clinical approach in this patient population based on a high likelihood of therapeutic intervention and a very low rate of complications, in particular PEP.[16]

RISK STRATIFICATION

Risk stratification of patients on the basis of well-established clinical characteristics can inform the decision-making process that surrounds (1) proceeding with ERCP, (2) referral to a tertiary center, (3) fluid resuscitation, (4) prophylactic stent placement, (5) pharmacoprevention, and (6) postprocedural hospital observation. The independent predictors of PEP can be divided into patient-related and procedure-related characteristics (**Table 1**). The definite and probable patient-related factors that predispose to PEP are a clinical suspicion of SOD, a history of prior PEP, a history of recurrent pancreatitis, normal bilirubin, younger age, and female sex. The definite and probable procedure-related risk factors for PEP are difficult cannulation, pancreatic duct wire passages (see later in this article), pancreatic sphincterotomy, ampullectomy, repeated or aggressive pancreatography, and short-duration balloon dilation of an intact biliary sphincter. Two recent systematic reviews have affirmed the association of most of these factors with PEP.[17,18] Additional risk factors that have been implicated, but are not definitively accepted as independent predictors of PEP are precut (access) sphincterotomy, pancreatic acinarization, long-duration balloon dilation of an intact papilla, biliary sphincterotomy, self-expanding metal stent placement, nondilated bile duct, intraductal papillary mucinous neoplasm, intraductal ultrasound, and Billroth 2 anatomy.

It is important to consider that predictors of PEP appear to be multiplicative in nature. For example, a widely referenced multicenter study by Freeman and colleagues,[19] predating mechanical and pharmacologic prophylaxis, showed that a young woman with a clinical suspicion of SOD, normal bilirubin, and a difficult cannulation has a risk of PEP in excess of 40%. A more recent randomized controlled trial (RCT) confirmed this nonlinear relationship, even with the use of nonsteroidal anti-inflammatory drugs (NSAIDs) and stents.[20] In addition, patients with a clinical suspicion of SOD, particularly women, are not only at increased risk for PEP in general, but are also more likely to develop severe pancreatitis and death.[19,21] When considering the risk-benefit ratio of ERCP in this patient population, not only should the patient's overall risk of PEP be assessed, but their probability of experiencing a more catastrophic clinical course also should be considered and discussed.

Conversely, several characteristics are thought to reduce the risk of PEP. First, biliary interventions in patients with a preexisting biliary sphincterotomy probably confer a very low risk of PEP. Prior sphincterotomy will have generally separated the biliary and pancreatic orifices, allowing avoidance of the pancreas, and rendering

Table 1	
Definite and probable predictors of post–endoscopic retrograde cholangiopancreatography pancreatitis	
Patient-Related Factors	**Procedure-Related Factors**
Suspected sphincter of Oddi dysfunction	Difficult cannulation
Prior post–endoscopic retrograde cholangiopancreatography pancreatitis	Ampullectomy
History of recurrent pancreatitis	Pancreatic sphincterotomy
Younger age	Pancreatic wire passages
Female sex	Repeated or aggressive pancreatography
Normal bilirubin	Short-duration balloon dilation of an intact biliary sphincter
Absence of chronic pancreatitis	

pancreatic sphincter or duct trauma unlikely. Further, patients with significant chronic pancreatitis, in particular those with calcifications, are at lower risk for PEP because of gland atrophy, fibrosis, and consequent decrease in exocrine enzymatic activity.[19] Similarly, the progressive decline in pancreatic exocrine function associated with aging may protect older patients from pancreatic injury.[22] Last, perhaps due to postobstructive parenchymal atrophy, patients with pancreatic head malignancy appear to be relatively protected as well.[23]

Operator (endoscopist)-dependent characteristics have also been implicated in risk. Endoscopist procedure volume is suggested to be a risk factor for PEP, although multicenter studies have not confirmed this observation, presumably because low-volume endoscopists tend to perform lower-risk cases.[24–26] Nevertheless, potentially dangerous cases (based on either patient-related factors or anticipated high-risk interventions) are best referred to expert medical centers where a high-volume endoscopist with expertise in prophylactic pancreatic stent placement can perform the case, and where more experience with rescue from serious complications may improve clinical outcomes.[27] Similarly, trainee involvement in ERCP is a possible independent risk factor for PEP, although results of existing multivariable analyses are conflicting.[19,28] Inexperienced trainees may augment procedure-related risk factors, such as prolonging a difficult cannulation or delivering excess diathermy during an inefficient pancreatic sphincterotomy. Therefore, additional research focused on improving the process of ERCP training is necessary to minimize the contribution of trainee involvement to the development of PEP.

PROCEDURAL TECHNIQUE

Efficient and atraumatic procedural technique during ERCP is believed to be important in minimizing the risk of pancreatitis. Many of the procedure-related risk factors listed previously, although predisposing to PEP, are mandatory elements of a successful case. Even though these high-risk interventions (such as ampullectomy) are unavoidable for execution of the clinical objective, certain procedural strategies can be used to minimize risk.

Because difficult cannulation and pancreatic duct injection are independent risk factors for PEP, interventions that improve the efficiency of cannulation and limit injection of contrast into the pancreas are likely to improve outcomes. Guidewire-assisted cannulation accomplishes both by using a small-caliber wire with a hydrophilic tip to negotiate the papilla, subsequently guiding passage of the catheter into the intended duct. Because the wire is thinner, softer, and more maneuverable than the cannula, it is easier to advance across a potentially narrow and off-angle orifice. Moreover, this process limits the likelihood of an inadvertent pancreatic or intramural papillary injection. Indeed, a meta-analysis of RCTs enrolling 3450 subjects demonstrates that guidewire-assisted cannulation reduces the risk of PEP by approximately 50% (Relative Risk 0.51, 95% confidence interval [CI] 0.32–0.82).[29] Two subsequent RCTs that were underpowered to detect medium or small differences in PEP have not confirmed the protective benefit of wire-guided cannulation, but one of these studies did show benefit in terms of efficiency of cannulation.[30,31] Overall, the literature in aggregate does suggest that wire-guided cannulation is the preferred approach, although gentle injection of contrast to better define anatomy is often used when the wire does not advance seamlessly into either duct.

The most significant risk of wire-guided cannulation is pancreatic duct perforation, which may occur during intended biliary cannulation if the wire is actually in the pancreatic duct, where forceful advancement may result in sidebranch penetration.

Similarly, excess force during intended pancreatic cannulation may result in perforation due to variations in pancreatic ductal anatomy. Thus cautious wire advancement is critical and gentle injection of contrast is advisable if the wire does not travel seamlessly in its intended direction. A recent randomized trial demonstrated that control of the guidewire by the endoscopist, using the so-called short-wire technique, results in fewer complications (including PEP) than assistant control.[32] This finding is mechanistically plausible because the controlling endoscopist is best suited to sense and quickly adjust to tactile feedback from the wire, reducing the likelihood of pancreatic injury. It is nevertheless important to consider that the results of this study may have been influenced by its unblinded nature, given the aforementioned subjectivity in the definition of PEP, unmasking of clinicians caring for study subjects and those adjudicating the outcomes could have biased in favor of the endoscopist-control group. Additional data are needed before ERCP teams are expected to change their approach on this fundamental issue.

When initial cannulation attempts are unsuccessful, several alternative techniques are available to facilitate biliary access. The double-wire technique is a common second-line approach when initial cannulation attempts result in unintentional passage of the wire into the pancreas. The wire is left in the pancreatic duct, thereby straightening the common channel, partially occluding the pancreatic orifice, and providing a fluoroscopic reference vector, allowing subsequent biliary access alongside the existing pancreatic wire. This technique appears particularly helpful when cannulation is impeded by difficult anatomy, such as when there is a malignant biliary stricture or the ampulla is intradiverticular.[33] Although those who frequently use this technique advocate its benefits, a recent Cochrane Collaboration review suggests that the double-wire technique does not improve cannulation success but increases the risk of PEP compared with alternative techniques including precut sphincterotomy and cannulation alongside a pancreatic stent.[34] However, all component studies in this meta-analysis were unblinded, the experience and comfort level of participating endoscopists with the double-wire technique in these studies is unclear, and most included patients did not receive rectal NSAIDs or a prophylactic stent. Thus, as we await additional data, double-wire cannulation remains a viable option for endoscopists experienced in this technique.

If using the double-wire cannulation technique, it is important to consider that there is mounting evidence that pancreatic wire passage increases the risk of pancreatitis.[35–37] Along these lines, an RCT of difficult cannulation cases requiring this technique demonstrated that prophylactic pancreatic stent placement reduced the incidence of PEP in this patient population.[38] On this basis, some experts believe that a prophylactic pancreatic stent should be placed in all patients requiring double-wire cannulation. Others, however, believe that passage of a wire in the pancreas does not always predispose to PEP, and that pancreatitis in this context may be related to the preceding difficult cannulation. Thus, if the double-wire technique is used early (within 2–3 cannulation attempts) in a low-risk patient, and the wire advances seamlessly in a typical pancreatic trajectory, stent placement may not be necessary if rectal indomethacin is given.

Additional alternative cannulation techniques include wire cannulation alongside a pancreatic stent, needle knife precut sphincterotomy, transpancreatic septotomy, and fistulotomy. Although RCTs have attempted to determine the optimal rescue technique, it is likely that each of these methods is most appropriate in certain circumstances, depending on anatomic factors and operator experience. Based on existing evidence, the specific cannulation technique appears to be less important than implementing these techniques early in a challenging case. This principle is best demonstrated by a meta-analysis of 6 randomized trials that showed that early precut sphincterotomy significantly reduced the risk of PEP when compared with repeated standard cannulation attempts (2.5% vs 5.3%, odds ratio [OR] 0.47).[39] Additional observational and randomized data have also suggested that precut sphincterotomy, especially if successful, is not an independent risk factor for PEP as previously considered[40–42]; however, the technique should be performed by endoscopists with adequate expertise to limit serious complications; the European Society of Gastrointestinal Endoscopy (ESGE) recommends that it be used only by practitioners with greater than 80% cannulation success using standard techniques.[21,43] A recent study has reported that early precut sphincterotomy without a prophylactic pancreatic stent is equivalent to, but more cost-effective than ongoing cannulation attempts alongside a prophylactic stent (with late precut if necessary).[44] Although these findings support the concept that early implementation of alternative techniques is advantageous, this study was profoundly underpowered (N = 100; 4 outcome events) to detect a difference in PEP. Based on existing evidence, withholding a prophylactic stent after a difficult cannulation that is followed by precut sphincterotomy should be strongly discouraged (see later in this article).

Other technical strategies that reduce the risk of PEP include minimizing the frequency and vigor of pancreatic duct injection and avoiding balloon dilation of an intact sphincter. In coagulopathic patients with choledocholithiasis and native papillae, balloon dilation can be avoided by providing real-time decompression with a bile duct stent and repeating the ERCP with sphincterotomy and stone extraction when coagulation parameters have been restored. If this is not possible, and balloon dilation is mandatory, longer duration dilation (2–5 minutes) appears to result in lower rates of pancreatitis compared with 1-minute dilation.[45] Of note is that balloon dilation after biliary sphincterotomy to facilitate large stone extraction does not appear to increase the risk of PEP.[46]

PANCREATIC STENT PLACEMENT

Prophylactic pancreatic stent placement (PSP) was the first intervention to successfully prevent PEP and remains a mainstay of the prophylactic armamentarium. PSP is believed to reduce the risk of PEP by decreasing pancreatic ductal hypertension due to poor drainage as a result of procedure-related inflammation and transient stenosis of the pancreatic orifice. More than a dozen published RCTs and as at least as many nonrandomized studies have consistently demonstrated that PSP reduces the risk of PEP by approximately 60% to 70%.[47–49] Importantly, prophylactic pancreatic stents appear to profoundly reduce the likelihood of severe and necrotizing pancreatitis.[47,48]

The demonstrated benefits of PSP must be weighed against several possible disadvantages. First, attempted but failed PSP substantially increases the risk of PEP by inducing additional injury to the pancreatic orifice without subsequent ductal compression.[50] Second, PSP can be complicated by stent migration and duct perforation in approximately 4% to 5% of cases.[51] Finally, PSP is associated with patient inconvenience and increased costs related to routine radiography to ensure spontaneous stent passage and repeat endoscopy to retrieve retained stents in 5% to 10% of cases.[52–54] PSP is nevertheless commonly used across the United States and Europe, and is recommended in multiple society guidelines.[55,56] Given the aforementioned risks and costs, PSP should however be limited to high-risk patients based on independent patient and procedure-related risk factors, such as (1) clinical suspicion of SOD, (2) prior PEP, (3) difficult cannulation, (4) precut sphincterotomy,

(5) pancreatic sphincterotomy, (6) ampullectomy, (7) excessive or repeated pancreatic duct injection, and (8) short-duration balloon dilation of intact biliary sphincter.[43,57,58]

Several questions surrounding PSP remain. First, the true magnitude of benefit of PSP remains unclear, as none of the RCTs evaluating this intervention were blinded in nature. Studies without treatment allocation blinding are often biased in favor of the intervention and exaggerate perceived effects. Second, there is limited consensus regarding the optimal stent length and caliber.[58] An early study suggested improved outcomes with 3-Fr or 4-Fr stents,[59] a subsequent RCT showed no difference in PEP rates but a higher insertion success rate with the 5-Fr stents,[54] and a recent network meta-analysis comprising the broader prophylaxis literature suggests that 5-Fr stents are most effective.[60] Similarly, there is little consensus regarding optimal stent length. Most experts agree that the intrapancreatic tip of the stent should not rest at the pancreatic genu or in a side-branch[57]; however, whether short stents (ending in the pancreatic head) or longer stents (ending in the body or tail) are preferable is unknown, and comparative effectiveness studies in this area are needed.

Finally, the acceptable amount of time that can be spent on the insertion process in cases of difficult pancreatic access remains unknown. Although the merits of PSP have been clearly presented previously, if achieving pancreatic access proves difficult, there is presumably a point of diminishing returns beyond which the risk of additional attempts outweighs the benefit of stent placement, especially if insertion eventually proves unsuccessful. Future clinical studies are unlikely to answer this question in a methodologically rigorous fashion; therefore, endoscopists should be aware of this important clinical balance, and use their best judgment regarding the acceptable duration of time for stent insertion. One potential approach to circumvent this problem in cases of anticipated stent placement (for example, ampullectomy or SOD cases) is to place and maintain a guidewire in the pancreatic duct early in the case to guarantee pancreatic duct access later on, avoiding the occasional phenomenon of failing to identify the pancreatic orifice due to the anatomic distortion that develops as a consequence of trauma, edema, or bleeding. Another approach is to place the prophylactic pancreatic stent before therapeutic intervention.

PHARMACOPREVENTION

Pharmacologic prevention of PEP has been the subject of extensive research efforts with largely disappointing results. Recently, however, rectally administered NSAIDs and aggressive hydration with lactated Ringer solution (LR) have reinvigorated the field of pharmacoprevention. Other mechanistically promising agents that are currently under investigation include sublingual nitroglycerin, nafamostat, magnesium, calcineurin inhibitors, and hemin.[61] Although a discussion of these agents is outside the scope of this review, combination therapy including 1 or more of these medications in addition to rectal NSAIDs and LR is likely to represent the future of pharmacoprevention.

Rectal Nonsteroidal Anti-inflammatory Drugs

The exact mechanism of action of rectal NSAIDs in preventing PEP remains unclear. The most popular hypothesis is that indomethacin and diclofenac are specifically protective because they are particularly potent inhibitors of phospholipase A2, which appears important in initiating the inflammatory cascade that leads to pancreatitis,[62] although a more complex mechanism that also involves cyclooxygenase is likely the case. Nevertheless, at least 15 RCTs evaluating the efficacy of rectal NSAIDs have been published; recent meta-analyses have consistently demonstrated an associated reduction in PEP in the range of 40% to 60%.[63–67] Two recent observational studies comparing clinical practice eras before and after the routine administration of rectal NSAIDs have confirmed this benefit, providing some evidence of real-world clinical effectiveness.[68,69]

Because the most high profile of the published RCTs supporting the use of rectal NSAIDs was conducted in high-risk subjects,[20] controversy has remained regarding the role of NSAIDs in average-risk cases. This controversy was further fueled by a recent single-center RCT enrolling consecutive (mostly average and low-risk) patients, which showed no benefit associated with rectal indomethacin.[70] However, subsequent meta-analyses restricted to studies enrolling average-risk cases highlight that this study is an outlier relative to the existing literature, and that despite its inclusion, rectal NSAIDs appear effective in the average-risk patient population.[65,67,71] Most recently, the largest RCT in PEP pharmacoprevention history showed a 54% relative risk reduction associated with administration of rectal indomethacin compared with no intervention among 2014 average-risk subjects.[72] Although this study was not exclusively designed to assess the impact of rectal NSAIDs in average-risk cases, and subjects were not blinded to study group assignment, the findings do support the universal use of indomethacin. The 2 aforementioned real-world effectiveness studies seem to confirm benefit in unselected patients.[68,69] In light of these data, the very low cost of NSAIDs, and their highly favorable safety profile, it is reasonable to administer these medications in all patients undergoing ERCP, as recommended by the ESGE.[56]

Recent investigation has explored the timing of administration of rectal NSAIDs. Most RCTs administered the drug before ERCP, whereas at least 4 studies administered the drug following the procedure. Existing meta-analyses suggest that the timing of administration does not impact efficacy.[63,64,67,73] However, the aforementioned large-scale RCT evaluating the effect of indomethacin in more than 2000 average-risk patients also compared preadministration (30 minutes before ERCP) versus postadministration (immediately after ERCP) among 586 high-risk subjects. In this subgroup, administration before ERCP reduced the risk of PEP by more than 50%.[72] To reconcile the findings of this study with those of other trials in which NSAIDs were given after ERCP, we recommend that the medication be administered at the beginning of cannulation, ensuring that it is not delivered too late in the event of a very long case (if delivered after ERCP) or too early (when delivered before ERCP) in the event cannulation is delayed (eg, case delay or difficulty advancing scope to papilla). This approach seems to integrate well into real-world clinical practice, wherein accurately predicting 30 minutes before the next ERCP is challenging.

The terminal half-life of rectal indomethacin and diclofenac (1–2 hours) and their active metabolites (1–4 hours) is short, highlighting the challenge in maximizing plasma concentrations at the exact time at which the drug is most likely to impact the disease. Complicating matters is that indomethacin and diclofenac are mainly metabolized by hydroxylation by the cytochrome P450 (CYP) 2C9 enzyme (CYP2C9),[74] which is highly polymorphic, resulting in variable metabolism rates. Population data have confirmed significant variability in mutation prevalence of CYP2C9 between African American, White, and Asian individuals.[74,75] Genetic differences at the CYP2C9 level or in other areas (such as the microbiome) might explain some of the heterogeneity in outcomes observed in NSAID trials and may serve as the basis for future personalized approaches to pharmacoprevention with NSAIDs and other agents. The results of an ongoing case-control study evaluating the effect of CYP2C9 gene polymorphisms on PEP risk in patients receiving prophylactic diclofenac will provide valuable information to this end. It is conceivable that rectal NSAIDs at the standard dose and timing will prove effective in only a subset of patients, whereas alternative administration approaches will be required to achieve adequate plasma concentrations in patients with varying enzyme activity.

As we await such data, there remains interest in the utility of higher doses of NSAIDs because they are generally safe medications. Indeed, an observational study from Denmark suggested that the standard dose of rectal NSAIDs may not be as effective in patients with increased body weight.[76] An ongoing RCT comparing indomethacin at standard versus high dose (150 mg immediately after ERCP followed by a 50-mg dose 4 hours later) will help answer this question. RCTs evaluating NSAIDs administered via nonrectal routes have demonstrated lack of efficacy in preventing PEP, and thus non-rectal delivery is not recommended.

Available data indicate that rectal NSAIDs are effective *in addition* to PSP in high-risk cases, but to date, there are no clinical trial data examining whether indomethacin is effective when administered *instead* of PSP. Because PSP is technically challenging, potentially dangerous, time-consuming, and costly,[52,77–79] major clinical and cost benefits in ERCP practice could be realized if rectal NSAIDs were to obviate the need for pancreatic stent placement. Two hypothesis-generating analyses suggest that the combination of NSAIDs and PSP is not superior to rectal NSAIDs alone.[80,81] An ongoing multicenter randomized noninferiority trial comparing rectal indomethacin alone versus the combination of indomethacin and prophylactic stent placement will hopefully provide concrete guidance for this critical management issue.[82] Until the results of this trial are available, however, the combination of rectal indomethacin and prophylactic stent placement should remain the standard approach to preventing PEP in high-risk patients.

Aggressive Lactated Ringer Infusion

The most recent progress within the field of pharmacoprevention has focused on aggressive LR infusion, which is believed to protective by maintaining pancreatic perfusion and attenuating the acidosis that promotes zymogen activation and resultant pancreatic inflammation. Preclinical models have demonstrated the potent anti-inflammatory effect of lactate through immunomodulatory mechanisms and a small RCT in non-ERCP pancreatitis observed less systemic inflammation in subjects who received LR compared with those who received saline.[83,84] Thus far, several RCTs[85–88] have shown lower PEP rates associated with LR administration and a recent meta-analyses of these trials demonstrated an approximately 50% risk reduction (OR 0.47, 95% CI 0.25–0.59).[89] Three of these studies administered a prolonged infusion, whereas the fourth evaluated the effect of a 1-L bolus in conjunction with rectal indomethacin.[88] Additional large-scale studies are necessary to define the optimal dose and infusion regimen of aggressive hydration, ideally being a bolus that can be delivered over a reasonable time frame in the periprocedural setting. Awaiting such data, a partly evidence-based approach is to infuse approximately 3 L of LR in the periprocedural setting to younger healthy patients. If they are admitted to the hospital with pain, LR is continued at a rate of 250 to 350 mL per hour overnight with close volume status assessment.

REFERENCES

1. Kochar B, Akshintala VS, Afghani E, et al. Incidence, severity, and mortality of post-ERCP pancreatitis: a systematic review by using randomized, controlled trials. Gastrointest Endosc 2015;81:143–9.e9.

2. Freeman ML, Guda NM. Prevention of post-ERCP pancreatitis: a comprehensive review. Gastrointest Endosc 2004;59:845–64.

3. Healthcare cost and utilization project 2012. Available at: http://hcupnet.ahrq.gov. Accessed March 22, 2015.

4. Cotton PB. Analysis of 59 ERCP lawsuits; mainly about indications. Gastrointest Endosc 2006;63:378–82 [quiz: 464].

5. Keswani RN, Taft TH, Cote GA, et al. Increased levels of stress and burnout are related to decreased physician experience and to interventional gastroenterology career choice: findings from a US survey of endoscopists. Am J Gastroenterol 2011;106:1734–40.

6. Cotton PB, Lehman G, Vennes J, et al. Endoscopic sphincterotomy complications and their management: an attempt at consensus. Gastrointest Endosc 1991;37: 383–93.

7. Banks PA, Bollen TL, Dervenis C, et al. Classification of acute pancreatitis–2012: revision of the Atlanta classification and definitions by international consensus. Gut 2013;62:102–11.

8. Artifon EL, Chu A, Freeman M, et al. A comparison of the consensus and clinical definitions of pancreatitis with a proposal to redefine post-endoscopic retrograde cholangiopancreatography pancreatitis. Pancreas 2010;39:530–5.

9. Tse F, Liu L, Barkun AN, et al. EUS: a meta-analysis of test performance in suspected choledocholithiasis. Gastrointest Endosc 2008;67:235–44.

10. Romagnuolo J, Bardou M, Rahme E, et al. Magnetic resonance cholangiopancreatography: a meta-analysis of test performance in suspected biliary disease. Ann Intern Med 2003;139:547–57.

11. Giljaca V, Gurusamy KS, Takwoingi Y, et al. Endoscopic ultrasound versus magnetic resonance cholangiopancreatography for common bile duct stones. Cochrane Database Syst Rev 2015;(2):CD011549.

12. Ding G, Cai W, Qin M. Single-stage vs. two-stage management for concomitant gallstones and common bile duct stones: a prospective randomized trial with long-term follow-up. J Gastrointest Surg 2014;18:947–51.

13. Bansal VK, Misra MC, Rajan K, et al. Single-stage laparoscopic common bile duct exploration and cholecystectomy versus two-stage endoscopic stone extraction followed by laparoscopic cholecystectomy for patients with concomitant gallbladder stones and common bile duct stones: a randomized controlled trial. Surg Endosc 2014;28:875–85.

14. Wandling MW, Hungness ES, Pavey ES, et al. Nationwide assessment of trends in choledocholithiasis management in the United States From 1998 to 2013. JAMA Surg 2016;151:1125–30.

15. Cotton PB, Durkalski V, Romagnuolo J, et al. Effect of endoscopic sphincterotomy for suspected sphincter of Oddi dysfunction on pain-related disability following cholecystectomy: the EPISOD randomized clinical trial. JAMA 2014;311:2101–9.

16. Elmunzer BJ, Debenedet AT, Volk ML, et al. Clinical yield of diagnostic endoscopic retrograde cholangiopancreatography in orthotopic liver transplant recipients with suspected biliary complications. Liver Transpl 2012;18:1479–84.

17. Chen JJ, Wang XM, Liu XQ, et al. Risk factors for post-ERCP pancreatitis: a systematic review of clinical trials with a large sample size in the past 10 years. Eur J Med Res 2014;19:26.

18. Ding X, Zhang F, Wang Y. Risk factors for post-ERCP pancreatitis: a systematic review and meta-analysis. Surgeon 2015;13:218–29.

19. Freeman ML, DiSario JA, Nelson DB, et al. Risk factors for post-ERCP pancreatitis: a prospective, multicenter study. Gastrointest Endosc 2001;54:425–34.

20. Elmunzer BJ, Scheiman JM, Lehman GA, et al. A randomized trial of rectal indomethacin to prevent post-ERCP pancreatitis. N Engl J Med 2012;366:1414–22.

21. Freeman ML, Nelson DB, Sherman S, et al. Complications of endoscopic biliary sphincterotomy. N Engl J Med 1996;335:909–18.

22. Laugier R, Bernard JP, Berthezene P, et al. Changes in pancreatic exocrine secretion with age: pancreatic exocrine secretion does decrease in the elderly. Digestion 1991;50:202–11.

23. Banerjee N, Hilden K, Baron TH, et al. Endoscopic biliary sphincterotomy is not required for transpapillary SEMS placement for biliary obstruction. Dig Dis Sci 2011;56:591–5.

24. Loperfido S, Angelini G, Benedetti G, et al. Major early complications from diagnostic and therapeutic ERCP: a prospective multicenter study. Gastrointest Endosc 1998;48:1–10.

25. Rabenstein T, Schneider HT, Bulling D, et al. Analysis of the risk factors associated with endoscopic sphincterotomy techniques: preliminary results of a prospective study, with emphasis on the reduced risk of acute pancreatitis with low-dose anticoagulation treatment. Endoscopy 2000;32:10–9.

26. Masci E, Mariani A, Curioni S, et al. Risk factors for pancreatitis following endoscopic retrograde cholangiopancreatography: a meta-analysis. Endoscopy 2003;35:830–4.

27. Ghaferi AA, Birkmeyer JD, Dimick JB. Variation in hospital mortality associated with inpatient surgery. N Engl J Med 2009;361:1368–75.

28. Cheng CL, Sherman S, Watkins JL, et al. Risk factors for post-ERCP pancreatitis: a prospective multicenter study. Am J Gastroenterol 2006;101:139–47.

29. Tse F, Yuan Y, Moayyedi P, et al. Guidewire-assisted cannulation of the common bile duct for the prevention of post-endoscopic retrograde cholangiopancreatography (ERCP) pancreatitis. Cochrane Database Syst Rev 2012;12:CD009662.

30. Kawakami H, Maguchi H, Mukai T, et al. A multicenter, prospective, randomized study of selective bile duct cannulation performed by multiple endoscopists: the BIDMEN study. Gastrointest Endosc 2012;75:362–72, 372.e1.

31. Kobayashi G, Fujita N, Imaizumi K, et al. Wire-guided biliary cannulation technique does not reduce the risk of post-ERCP pancreatitis: multicenter randomized controlled trial. Dig Endosc 2013;25:295–302.

32. Buxbaum J, Leonor P, Tung J, et al. Randomized trial of endoscopist-controlled vs. assistant-controlled wire-guided cannulation of the bile duct. Am J Gastroenterol 2016;111:1841–7.

33. Sasahira N, Kawakami H, Isayama H, et al. Early use of double-guidewire technique to facilitate selective bile duct cannulation: the multicenter randomized controlled EDUCATION trial. Endoscopy 2015;47:421–9.

34. Tse F, Yuan Y, Bukhari M, et al. Pancreatic duct guidewire placement for biliary cannulation for the prevention of post-endoscopic retrograde cholangiopancreatography (ERCP) pancreatitis. Cochrane Database Syst Rev 2016;(5):CD010571.

35. Herreros de Tejada A, Calleja JL, Diaz G, et al. Double-guidewire technique for difficult bile duct cannulation: a multicenter randomized, controlled trial. Gastrointest Endosc 2009;70:700–9.

36. Nakai Y, Isayama H, Sasahira N, et al. Risk factors for post-ERCP pancreatitis in wire-guided cannulation for therapeutic biliary ERCP. Gastrointest Endosc 2015; 81:119–26.

37. Wang P, Li ZS, Liu F, et al. Risk factors for ERCP-related complications: a prospective multicenter study. Am J Gastroenterol 2009;104:31–40.

38. Ito K, Fujita N, Noda Y, et al. Can pancreatic duct stenting prevent post-ERCP pancreatitis in patients who undergo pancreatic duct guidewire placement for

achieving selective biliary cannulation? A prospective randomized controlled trial. J Gastroenterol 2010;45:1183–91.

39. Cennamo V, Fuccio L, Zagari RM, et al. Can early precut implementation reduce endoscopic retrograde cholangiopancreatography-related complication risk? Meta-analysis of randomized controlled trials. Endoscopy 2010;42:381–8.

40. Navaneethan U, Konjeti R, Lourdusamy V, et al. Precut sphincterotomy: efficacy for ductal access and the risk of adverse events. Gastrointest Endosc 2015;81(4): 924–31.

41. Swan MP, Alexander S, Moss A, et al. Needle knife sphincterotomy does not increase the risk of pancreatitis in patients with difficult biliary cannulation. Clin Gastroenterol Hepatol 2013;11:430–6.e1.

42. Mariani A, Di Leo M, Giardullo N, et al. Early precut sphincterotomy for difficult biliary access to reduce post-ERCP pancreatitis: a randomized trial. Endoscopy 2016;48:530–5.

43. Testoni PA, Mariani A, Aabakken L, et al. Papillary cannulation and sphincterotomy techniques at ERCP: European Society of Gastrointestinal Endoscopy (ESGE) Clinical Guideline. Endoscopy 2016;48:657–83.

44. Hwang HJ, Guidi MA, Curvale C, et al. Post-ERCP pancreatitis: early precut or pancreatic duct stent? A multicenter, randomized-controlled trial and cost-effectiveness analysis. Rev Esp Enferm Dig 2017;109:174–9.

45. Liao WC, Tu YK, Wu MS, et al. Balloon dilation with adequate duration is safer than sphincterotomy for extracting bile duct stones: a systematic review and meta-analyses. Clin Gastroenterol Hepatol 2012;10:1101–9.

46. Misra SP, Dwivedi M. Large-diameter balloon dilation after endoscopic sphincterotomy for removal of difficult bile duct stones. Endoscopy 2008;40:209–13.

47. Mazaki T, Mado K, Masuda H, et al. Prophylactic pancreatic stent placement and post-ERCP pancreatitis: an updated meta-analysis. J Gastroenterol 2014;49: 343–55.

48. Choudhary A, Bechtold ML, Arif M, et al. Pancreatic stents for prophylaxis against post-ERCP pancreatitis: a meta-analysis and systematic review. Gastrointest Endosc 2011;73:275–82.

49. Vadala di Prampero SF, Faleschini G, Panic N, et al. Endoscopic and pharmacological treatment for prophylaxis against postendoscopic retrograde cholangiopancreatography pancreatitis: a meta-analysis and systematic review. Eur J Gastroenterol Hepatol 2016;28:1415–24.

50. Choksi NS, Fogel EL, Cote GA, et al. The risk of post-ERCP pancreatitis and the protective effect of rectal indomethacin in cases of attempted but unsuccessful prophylactic pancreatic stent placement. Gastrointest Endosc 2015;81:150–5.

51. Mazaki T, Masuda H, Takayama T. Prophylactic pancreatic stent placement and post-ERCP pancreatitis: a systematic review and meta-analysis. Endoscopy 2010;42:842–53.

52. Zolotarevsky E, Fehmi SM, Anderson MA, et al. Prophylactic 5-Fr pancreatic duct stents are superior to 3-Fr stents: a randomized controlled trial. Endoscopy 2011; 43:325–30.

53. Chahal P, Baron TH, Petersen BT, et al. Pancreatic stent prophylaxis of post endoscopic retrograde cholangiopancreatography pancreatitis: spontaneous migration rates and clinical outcomes. Minerva Gastroenterol Dietol 2007;53:225–30.

54. Chahal P, Tarnasky PR, Petersen BT, et al. Short 5Fr vs long 3Fr pancreatic stents in patients at risk for post-endoscopic retrograde cholangiopancreatography pancreatitis. Clin Gastroenterol Hepatol 2009;7:834–9.

55. ASGE Standards of Practice Committee, Chandrasekhara V, Khashab MA, Muthusamy VR, et al. Adverse events associated with ERCP. Gastrointest Endosc 2017;85:32–47.

56. Dumonceau JM, Andriulli A, Elmunzer BJ, et al. Prophylaxis of post-ERCP pancreatitis: European Society of Gastrointestinal Endoscopy (ESGE) Guideline - updated June 2014. Endoscopy 2014;46:799–815.

57. Freeman ML. Pancreatic stents for prevention of post-endoscopic retrograde cholangiopancreatography pancreatitis. Clin Gastroenterol Hepatol 2007;5: 1354–65.

58. Brackbill S, Young S, Schoenfeld P, et al. A survey of physician practices on prophylactic pancreatic stents. Gastrointest Endosc 2006;64:45–52.

59. Rashdan A, Fogel EL, McHenry L Jr, et al. Improved stent characteristics for prophylaxis of post-ERCP pancreatitis. Clin Gastroenterol Hepatol 2004;2:322–9.

60. Afghani E, Akshintala VS, Khashab MA, et al. 5-Fr vs. 3-Fr pancreatic stents for the prevention of post-ERCP pancreatitis in high-risk patients: a systematic review and network meta-analysis. Endoscopy 2014;46:573–80.

61. Kubiliun NM, Adams MA, Akshintala VS, et al. Evaluation of pharmacologic prevention of pancreatitis after endoscopic retrograde cholangiopancreatography: a systematic review. Clin Gastroenterol Hepatol 2015;13:1231–9 [quiz: e70–1].

62. Makela A, Kuusi T, Schroder T. Inhibition of serum phospholipase-A2 in acute pancreatitis by pharmacological agents in vitro. Scand J Clin Lab Invest 1997; 57:401–7.

63. Sun HL, Han B, Zhai HP, et al. Rectal NSAIDs for the prevention of post-ERCP pancreatitis: a meta-analysis of randomized controlled trials. Surgeon 2014;12: 141–7.

64. Sethi S, Sethi N, Wadhwa V, et al. A meta-analysis on the role of rectal diclofenac and indomethacin in the prevention of post-endoscopic retrograde cholangiopancreatography pancreatitis. Pancreas 2014;43:190–7.

65. Shen C, Shi Y, Liang T, et al. Rectal NSAIDs in the prevention of post-endoscopic retrograde cholangiopancreatography pancreatitis in unselected patients: systematic review and meta-analysis. Dig Endosc 2017;29:281–90.

66. Puig I, Calvet X, Baylina M, et al. How and when should NSAIDs be used for preventing post-ERCP pancreatitis? A systematic review and meta-analysis. PLoS One 2014;9:e92922.

67. Patai A, Solymosi N, Mohacsi L, et al. Indomethacin and diclofenac in the prevention of post-ERCP pancreatitis: a systematic review and meta-analysis of prospective controlled trials. Gastrointest Endosc 2017;85:1144–56.e1.

68. Leerhoy B, Nordholm-Carstensen A, Novovic S, et al. Diclofenac is associated with a reduced incidence of post-endoscopic retrograde cholangiopancreatography pancreatitis: results from a Danish cohort study. Pancreas 2014;43:1286–90.

69. Thiruvengadam NR, Forde KA, Ma GK, et al. Rectal indomethacin reduces pancreatitis in high- and low-risk patients undergoing endoscopic retrograde cholangiopancreatography. Gastroenterology 2016;151:288–97.e4.

70. Levenick JM, Gordon SR, Fadden LL, et al. Rectal indomethacin does not prevent post-ERCP pancreatitis in consecutive patients. Gastroenterology 2016;150: 911–7 [quiz: e19].

71. Elmunzer BJ, Foster LD, Durkalski V. Should we still administer prophylactic rectal NSAIDs to average-risk patients undergoing ERCP? Gastroenterology 2016;151: 566–7.

72. Luo H, Zhao L, Leung J, et al. Routine pre-procedural rectal indometacin versus selective post-procedural rectal indometacin to prevent pancreatitis in patients

undergoing endoscopic retrograde cholangiopancreatography: a multicentre, single-blinded, randomised controlled trial. Lancet 2016;387:2293–301.

73. Wan J, Ren Y, Zhu Z, et al. How to select patients and timing for rectal indomethacin to prevent post-ERCP pancreatitis: a systematic review and meta-analysis. BMC Gastroenterol 2017;17:43.

74. Bruno A, Tacconelli S, Patrignani P. Variability in the response to non-steroidal anti-inflammatory drugs: mechanisms and perspectives. Basic Clin Pharmacol Toxicol 2014;114:56–63.

75. Lee CR, Goldstein JA, Pieper JA. Cytochrome P450 2C9 polymorphisms: a comprehensive review of the in-vitro and human data. Pharmacogenetics 2002; 12:251–63.

76. Leerhoy B, Nordholm-Carstensen A, Novovic S, et al. Effect of body weight on fixed dose of diclofenac for the prevention of post-endoscopic retrograde cholangiopancreatography pancreatitis. Scand J Gastroenterol 2016;51:1007–12.

77. Das A, Singh P, Sivak MV Jr, et al. Pancreatic-stent placement for prevention of post-ERCP pancreatitis: a cost-effectiveness analysis. Gastrointest Endosc 2007;65:960–8.

78. Tarnasky PR, Palesch YY, Cunningham JT, et al. Pancreatic stenting prevents pancreatitis after biliary sphincterotomy in patients with sphincter of Oddi dysfunction. Gastroenterology 1998;115:1518–24.

79. Fazel A, Quadri A, Catalano MF, et al. Does a pancreatic duct stent prevent post-ERCP pancreatitis? A prospective randomized study. Gastrointest Endosc 2003; 57:291–4.

80. Elmunzer BJ, Higgins PD, Saini SD, et al. Does rectal indomethacin eliminate the need for prophylactic pancreatic stent placement in patients undergoing high-risk ERCP? Post hoc efficacy and cost-benefit analyses using prospective clinical trial data. Am J Gastroenterol 2013;108:410–5.

81. Akbar A, Abu Dayyeh BK, Baron TH, et al. Rectal nonsteroidal anti-inflammatory drugs are superior to pancreatic duct stents in preventing pancreatitis after endoscopic retrograde cholangiopancreatography: a network meta-analysis. Clin Gastroenterol Hepatol 2013;11:778–83.

82. Elmunzer BJ, Serrano J, Chak A, et al. Rectal indomethacin alone versus indomethacin and prophylactic pancreatic stent placement for preventing pancreatitis after ERCP: study protocol for a randomized controlled trial. Trials 2016;17: 120.

83. Hoque R, Farooq A, Ghani A, et al. Lactate reduces liver and pancreatic injury in Toll-like receptor- and inflammasome-mediated inflammation via GPR81-mediated suppression of innate immunity. Gastroenterology 2014;146:1763–74.

84. Wu BU, Hwang JQ, Gardner TH, et al. Lactated Ringer's solution reduces systemic inflammation compared with saline in patients with acute pancreatitis. Clin Gastroenterol Hepatol 2011;9:710–7.e1.

85. Buxbaum J, Yan A, Yeh K, et al. Aggressive hydration with lactated Ringer's solution reduces pancreatitis after endoscopic retrograde cholangiopancreatography. Clin Gastroenterol Hepatol 2014;12:303–7.e1.

86. Shaygan-Nejad A, Masjedizadeh AR, Ghavidel A, et al. Aggressive hydration with Lactated Ringer's solution as the prophylactic intervention for postendoscopic retrograde cholangiopancreatography pancreatitis: a randomized controlled double-blind clinical trial. J Res Med Sci 2015;20:838–43.

87. Choi JH, Kim HJ, Lee BU, et al. Vigorous periprocedural hydration with lactated ringer's solution reduces the risk of pancreatitis after retrograde

cholangiopancreatography in hospitalized patients. Clin Gastroenterol Hepatol 2017;15:86–92.e1.

88. Mok SRS, Ho HC, Shah P, et al. Lactated Ringer's solution in combination with rectal indomethacin for prevention of post-ERCP pancreatitis and readmission: a prospective randomized, double-blinded, placebo-controlled trial. Gastrointest Endosc 2017;85:1005–13.

89. Zhang ZF, Duan ZJ, Wang LX, et al. Aggressive hydration with lactated Ringer solution in prevention of postendoscopic retrograde cholangiopancreatography pancreatitis: a meta-analysis of randomized controlled trials. J Clin Gastroenterol 2017;51:e17–26.

The Role of Endotherapy in Recurrent Acute Pancreatitis

Averill Guo, MD, John M. Poneros, MD*

KEYWORDS

- Recurrent acute pancreatitis • Idiopathic pancreatitis
- Sphincter of Oddi dysfunction • Pancreas divisum • Endoscopic therapy
- Endoscopic sphincterotomy • Endoscopic stent placement

KEY POINTS

- Recurrent acute pancreatitis (RAP) is a significant cause of morbidity and mortality as well as a risk factor for the development of chronic pancreatitis.
- Endoscopic interventions have variable efficacies depending on the type of procedure and cause of RAP. To date, few long-term, prospective, randomized controlled trials assessing response rates to endotherapy have been conducted.
- Although endotherapy plays an important role in the management of RAP, whether or not endoscopic intervention truly alters the natural history of this disease remains unclear.

INTRODUCTION

Acute pancreatitis (AP) and chronic pancreatitis (CP) were originally described according to the Marseille Classification as 2 separate, well-defined clinical entities.[1] Mounting evidence now suggests that they can be opposite ends of a disease continuum with recurrent AP (RAP) being an intermediate transition stage.[2] AP is an acute inflammatory condition of the pancreas typified by epigastric pain, increased serum amylase or lipase level, and imaging consistent with pancreatitis. RAP is defined as 2 or more distinct episodes of AP with complete resolution of symptoms between episodes and no evidence of CP. AP has an incidence of 40 to 50 per 100,000 per year in the United States[3] and, among gastrointestinal diseases, is the most common indication for hospitalization, accounting for more than 250,000 annual admissions.[4] Although most cases of AP are self-limited and resolve without complication, a 2015 meta-analysis showed that, after a sentinel AP event, 22% of patients develop at least 1 episode of recurrence and 10% develop CP. Among those with RAP, 36% develop CP.[5] Given the significant morbidity and mortality associated with CP,

Disclosure: Dr J. Poneros is a consultant for Boston Scientific. No other disclosures.
Columbia University Medical Center, 161 Fort Washington Avenue, Suite 852, New York, NY 10032, USA
* Corresponding author.
E-mail address: jmp14@cumc.columbia.edu

interventions designed to eliminate recurrent episodes and prevent progression in these high-risk patients with RAP are critical to reducing health care costs and patient suffering. However, management options are limited. Although endoscopic therapy has provided a means to address biliary, obstructive, congenital, and functional causes of RAP via sphincterotomy and pancreatic stent placement, there is variable evidence supporting the efficacy of these interventions and their ability to alter the natural history of disease. This article discusses the current literature on the role of endotherapy in managing RAP with a focus on high-quality prospective randomized controlled studies.

RECURRENT ACUTE PANCREATITIS AND ITS NATURAL HISTORY

RAP is an incompletely understood and controversial clinical syndrome that is often misdiagnosed. By definition, patients must have 2 or more true episodes of pancreatitis in order to receive this diagnosis, which requires at least 2 of the following criteria: typical pancreatic pain, increased serum amylase and/or lipase level 3 times normal, and cross-sectional imaging findings supportive of inflammation. Patients with pain not severe enough to require hospitalization, those with only mild hyperenzymemia and no imaging findings, or those with only mild imaging abnormalities and normal laboratory tests may instead be more accurately classified as having abdominal pain without pancreatitis or sphincter of Oddi dysfunction (SOD) type 2 or 3. Symptom overlap between RAP and CP makes definitive diagnosis challenging. Patients presenting with an acute attack may either be having a true episode of recurrence or an acute-on-chronic flare with minimal imaging findings of CP. Alternatively, it is also possible for acute post pancreatitis changes to be mistaken for evidence of chronicity.

In addition to variable diagnosis, determining the cause of RAP remains challenging. Risk factors for RAP are numerous and are best summarized under the TIGAR-O (toxic-metabolic, idiopathic, genetic, autoimmune, recurrent and severe acute pancreatitis, obstructive) classification.[6] Failure to address any one of these factors after an initial AP episode may result in recurrence. Moreover, RAP is likely multifactorial and addressing one cause may not remediate another contributing factor, such as an underlying genetic mutation.[7] Preliminary testing in RAP reveals a cause in 70% to 80% of cases and advanced testing with endoscopic ultrasonography (EUS) and magnetic resonance cholangiopancreatography (MRCP) identifies another 10% to 15%, but in nearly 10% of cases no cause is discovered and these are termed idiopathic.[7] Patients with idiopathic RAP (IRAP) thus have no definite cause to intervene on and are left with few treatment options (**Table 1**).

The natural history of RAP is also poorly defined. In general, patients with RAP may cease to have recurrent episodes, continue to have symptom recurrence with no pathologic changes characteristic of CP, or continue to have attacks with progression to CP. Thirty-six percent of patients with at least 1 recurrence develop CP,[5] but not all of these patients have the same risk of progression. Subgroups within this high-risk group of patients may be stratified according to cause. Gallstone disease, which accounts for 10% to 30% of RAP cases,[3] is readily addressed after standard evaluation for an initial AP episode. Cholecystectomy dramatically reduces the risk of recurrence with delayed time to operation resulting in increased risk reduction in severe cases.[8,9] Alcohol abuse is the most common cause of RAP, with continued drinking at the same level tied to a 58% risk of recurrence and a 41% risk of progression to CP. Abstinence reduces this risk to a 20% and 13% risk of recurrence and progression, respectively.[10] A randomized controlled trial assessing the efficacy of abstinence programming on

Table 1 TIGAR-O classification	
TIGAR-O Classification, Risk Factors for RAP	
Toxic-metabolic	Alcohol consumption Smoking Hypercalcemia/hyperparathyroidism Hypertriglyceridemia Medications Toxins Organotin compounds (eg, di-n-butyltindichloride)
Idiopathic	Early onset Late onset Tropical
Genetic	Autosomal recessive/modifier genes CFTR mutations SPINK1 mutations Cationic trypsinogen (codon 16, 22, 23 mutations) Anionic trypsinogen PRSS2 α1-antitrypsin deficiency MCP-1
Autoimmune	Isolated Associated with other autoimmune disorders
Obstructive	Pancreatic divisum Sphincter of Oddi disorders Duct obstruction (eg, tumor, parasite) Choledochal cysts Abnormal pancreatobiliary union Inflammatory bowel disease/celiac sprue

Abbreviations: CFTR, cystic fibrosis transmembrane conductance regulator; MCP-1, monocyte chemoprotectant protein; SPINK-1, serine protease inhibitor Kazal-type 1.

Adapted from Guda NM, Romagnuolo J, Freeman ML. Recurrent and relapsing pancreatitis. Curr Gastroenterol Rep 2011;13:142; with permission.

reducing rates of recurrence support these findings.[11] Smoking is a significant dose-dependent risk factor for recurrence, but outcome benefits of smoking cessation have yet to be fully delineated.[12] Hereditary pancreatitis secondary to the *PRSS1* mutation carries the greatest risk of progression to CP, with about 80% of carriers having at least 1 AP episode and about 50% developing CP.[13] Hypertriglyceridemia has been found to have a 33% risk of progression from RAP to CP, with improved triglyceride control resulting in less frequent recurrent attacks.[14,15] In addition, between 20% and 50% of patients with IRAP progress to CP with no appreciable benefit from endoscopic intervention.[16–18]

Long-term data on the survival and causes of death in patients with RAP are not currently available. However, a Danish population study with 30-year follow-up after a sentinel AP episode showed that patients with progressive AP had a mortality 2.7 times higher than those with nonprogressive AP, which was 5.3 to 6.5 times the mortality of the background population.[19] This finding suggests that the mortality for patients with RAP is at the least appreciably higher than that of the background population. There are also no available data on the quality-of-life (QOL) effects of RAP, although it is known that CP significantly affects both physical and mental QOL, likely resulting in high rates of unemployment, work absenteeism, and low annual personal income.[20,21]

Given these findings, the need for appropriate interventions to reduce rates of recurrence and prevent progression to CP is clear. Strategies for managing the causes of RAP that are amenable to endoscopic therapy are reviewed here.

IDIOPATHIC RECURRENT ACUTE PANCREATITIS

As discussed earlier, 10% to 30% of cases of RAP are idiopathic with no identifiable underlying cause on routine laboratory and imaging investigations. With no clear cause to intervene on, these patients are left with few treatment options, of questionable benefit, and are typically offered endoscopic sphincterotomy (ES) with or without pancreatic duct stent (PSt) placement. The impact of endoscopic intervention on the long-term outcomes and natural history of IRAP have yet to be fully elucidated. Studies on this are often limited by their retrospective design; small sample size; lack of control group; short follow-up period; inconsistent definitions of IRAP; and inadequate quantifications of AP episode severity, rate, and progression to CP.

A recent retrospective controlled study was conducted by Das and colleagues[17] examining the impact of ES with or without stent placement on the natural history of IRAP compared with medical management. Data were extracted from the North American Pancreatitis Study 2 (NAPS2) cohort, a multicenter prospective study that enrolled 460 patients with RAP and 540 patients with CP from 2000 to 2006. Fifty with IRAP and 15 with alcoholic RAP from this cohort were included in the study described here. The alcoholic patients with RAP were included to provide a context for studying IRAP, acting as a kind of control group. Patients with IRAP were evaluated with metabolic bloodwork, diagnostic imaging, genetic testing, Sphincter of Oddi manometry (SOM) (discontinued in 2004 at University of Pittsburgh Medical Center), and biliary crystal analysis to rule out identifiable causes. Patients with no evidence of CP on initial evaluation were eligible for inclusion regardless of whether they were eventually enrolled in the NAPS2 study. Patients with IRAP received ES (26 out of 50) or medical management (24 out of 50) and alcoholic patients with RAP received medical management. The IRAP with ES group included both those who received SOM and those who were empirically treated with ES. Successful ES was defined as cannulation and biliary and/or pancreatic sphincterotomy with or without stent placement into the main pancreatic duct. The decision not to proceed with ES was made at initial evaluation. Medically managed patients received counseling on risk factors and diet. Data were collected from the initial evaluation as well as from medical records before and during follow-up, which was a median of 7 years (interquartile range, 4.4, 10.0). Measured outcomes included number of AP episodes before intervention, rate of AP in attacks per year postintervention excluding post–endoscopic retrograde cholangiopancreatography (ERCP) pancreatitis and patients with an unclear number of attacks, severity of AP rated by duration of hospital stay, and progression to CP. Patients with IRAP had similar baseline characteristics except for total number of prior AP episodes, which was significantly higher in the ES than the medically managed group (median 3 vs 2, $P = .039$). They also differed in duration of follow-up, with ES patients having a significantly longer follow-up period (median 11.6 vs 6.8 years, $P = .003$). The investigators found the overall absolute risk of AP in follow-up to be 46% with a median time to subsequent attack of 10.6 months. The risk of any RAP was higher in the ES compared with the medically managed group (58% vs 33%, $P = .08$), but this difference was not statistically significant. Time to RAP was similar in both groups (log rank test, 0.20). Although both ES and medically managed patients experienced a significant decrease ($P<.0001$) in the rate of RAP postintervention compared with preintervention, no significant difference in rates of

RAP in follow-up was noted between the two groups (median 0.16/y vs 0/y, P = .29). Poisson regression analysis revealed baseline burden of disease and gender to be independent factors significantly affecting the rate of AP in follow-up. A 1.2× increase in rate is seen for each doubling of AP before intervention, and women have about half the rate seen in men. Endoscopic therapy did not significantly affect the rate of RAP. An 18% progression to CP was seen in patients with IRAP overall, with a greater incidence in ES patients (27% vs 8%, P = .09) that was not statistically significant.

Compared with the IRAP group, alcoholic patients with RAP were more likely to be male with a lower rate of AP before evaluation and longer duration between first AP and evaluation. They were also noted to have a more aggressive disease course with a higher risk of any subsequent AP (80% vs 46%, P = .021), a higher number of attacks after evaluation (median 1 vs 0, P = .04), shorter time to first AP after evaluation (median 1.4 vs 6.4 y, P = .008), and a higher rate of AP during follow-up (median 0.25/y vs 0/y, P = .016). There was 27% risk of progression to CP, which was not significantly different from the risk of progression in patients with IRAP overall (27% vs 18%, P = .46). Note that risk of progression to CP in alcoholic RAP is very similar to that of the IRAP ES group (27%) and higher than that of the medically managed group (8%). This finding is likely related to the higher baseline rate of AP or longer duration of follow-up in the ES patients. Regression analysis showed that the rate of AP in follow-up increased 1.52 times for each doubling of AP attacks before intervention and that those with a history of severe AP had lower rates of AP in follow-up.

This retrospective study concludes that ES does not seem to alter the natural history of IRAP. Regardless of cause, RAP postprocedure is affected only by rate of AP before intervention. However, this study is methodologically flawed and limited by its retrospective design, small sample size, definition of IRAP, and statistically significant difference in follow-up times. Limited to a single tertiary academic center, the study population may not be representative of community patients. Furthermore, the IRAP group included patients with SOD and thus was not truly idiopathic. Although it provides valuable preliminary data, a prospective randomized clinical trial is needed to definitely assess the role of endoscopy in IRAP. Importantly, this study also makes several contributions to the understanding of the natural history of IRAP. The findings suggest that prior AP burden predicts severity of disease postintervention and also that number of attacks decreases over time. The latter is perhaps related to an increase in progression to CP and loss of pancreatic parenchyma. Compared with alcoholic RAP, patients with IRAP have a shorter duration of disease, a higher rate of AP, and a higher baseline rate of AP, which may be related to referral bias. The more aggressive disease course of alcoholic RAP may be related to continued tobacco and alcohol exposure.

In 2012, a large prospective randomized controlled trial evaluated the diagnostic and therapeutic utility of ES and SOM in the reduction of AP episodes in IRAP.[16] This study is described more fully in relation to SOD-associated RAP later, but the major findings pertaining to endotherapy in IRAP are summarized here. The investigators divided a cohort of patients with IRAP into 2 groups based on ERCP and SOM findings on initial evaluation. Patients with pancreatic SOD (pSOD) were randomly assigned to undergo biliary ES (BES) or dual ES (DES), and those with normal findings on SOM were randomly assigned to received BES or sham. Idiopathic was defined as absence of identifiable cause for RAP on history, physical, and routine laboratory tests and imaging. Genetic testing, EUS, MRCP, and empiric cholecystectomy were pursued at the discretion of the treating physician, but no further invasive testing was pursued before study enrollment. Patients with a history of prior ERCP or found to have an alternative cause for RAP on index ERCP were excluded. Those in whom cannulation and manometry were unsuccessful were also excluded. In follow-up, BES and DES were found to have similar effects on preventing RAP, with 48.5% and 47.2% recurrence ($P = 1.0$), respectively. The rate of early RAP (<12 months post–index ERCP) was higher with DES compared with BES but the difference was not statistically significant (41.7% vs 24.2%, $P = .20$). In the normal-SOM group, BES and sham patients had a similar incidence of RAP (27.3% vs 11.1%, $P = .59$).

These findings suggest that increased pancreatobiliary sphincter pressure may be an effect rather than a cause of RAP. Given that pancreatic ES (PES) did not lead to complete elimination of recurrent AP episodes, pSOD may not represent a definitive cause for RAP. It may instead be a marker of disease severity. Alternatively, this may indicate that a single endoscopic intervention is insufficient to normalize basal pancreatic sphincter pressure. Most of the patients who underwent repeat ERCP had persistent pSOD and required repeat PES. Despite this second intervention, most refractory patients had at least 1 additional subsequent AP attack. More than 2 procedures may be required to completely normalize pressures. Furthermore, based on these results, PES alone cannot be recommended as a curative therapy for IRAP. Given that PES provided no additional benefit compared with BES alone and did not reduce the risk of having at least 1 AP during follow-up, the additional risks of post-ERCP pancreatitis, bleeding, perforation, and sphincter restenosis cannot be accepted.

The study conducted by Jacob and colleagues[22] in 2001 is one of 2 randomized controlled trials assessing endoscopic therapy in IRAP and the only study to include a truly idiopathic group of patients with RAP. Study participants were evaluated with pancreatogram for CP, SOM for SOD, and bile microscopy post–intravenous cholecystokinin (CCK) for microlithiasis in patients with intact gallbladders. Thirty-four patients with IRAP were enrolled over 5 years and randomized to treatment (19 out of 34) or control (15 out of 34) groups. Patients in the treatment group received 3 pancreatic stents over 9 months, each stent left in place for 3 months. Four barbed 5-F or 7-F stents of varying length (3 and 5 cm) were placed over a 0.18-mm guidewire. Out of 57 total stents placed, 17 (sized 5-F in 9 out of 17 and 7-F in 8 out of 17) occluded and 14 (sized 5-F in 8 out of 14 5F and 7-F in 6 out of 14) migrated out. Overall, 35 out of 57 stents were 5-F and 22 out of 57 stents were 7-F. Pancreatograms were obtained at each stent exchange and at end of study. The control group received selective pancreatograms with no stents. An average of 5.7 and 4.4 AP attacks were seen in the stent and control groups, respectively, during the 5-year enrollment period before intervention. After a mean follow-up period of 33 months (range 13–77) and 35 months (range 10–78) in the stent and control groups, respectively, a significantly lower incidence of RAP was observed in the stent group (11% vs 53%, $P<.02$). This incidence includes 2 crossovers from the control group who had no further recurrence. Similar rates of continued pancreatic-type pain were seen in both the treatment and control groups (32% vs 40%, $P<.61$). Five of the stented patients who continued to have pancreatic-type pain were found to have occluded stents, but the pain was unrelated to occlusion and stent removal was not required. Mild post-ERCP pancreatitis was seen in 2 stent group patients and 1 control group patient after 2 years of follow-up. Ductal changes indicating CP were seen in 5 patients in the stent group and 4 in the control group. Although ductal changes in response to polyethylene pancreatic stents have previously been described, these changes are typically located proximally near the stent. Here, ductal changes were located distal to the stent in the treatment group patients and are thus more likely to represent true CP. It is possible that such findings indicate the presence of previously occult idiopathic CP rather than true IRAP. This possibility cannot be ruled out despite negative secretin testing at enrollment given that pancreatic function tests are insensitive early in the CP disease course. Although limited by a small sample size and short follow-up period, this study provides compelling evidence that pancreatic duct stenting in true IRAP results in a significant reduction in incidence of RAP despite continued pancreatic-type pain. These results suggest that a relative pancreatic duct obstruction or intermittent pancreatic sphincter dysfunction is a potential cause of RAP.

In 2002, Kaw and Brodmerkel[23] conducted a prospective study assessing the role of ERCP, bile microcrystal analysis, and SOM in the management of IRAP. One-hundred and twenty-six consecutive patients with IRAP were enrolled over 4 years. Referring physicians were unable to find any identifiable cause on routine laboratory tests or imaging and all patients had 2 or more episodes of AP within 1 year with a mean of 3.2 attacks (range 2–7) and a mean interval of 3.8 months between attacks. Patients with identifiable causes or significant risk factors for pancreatitis ascertained by history, laboratory analysis, and imaging, including ultrasonography and/or computed tomography were excluded. All enrolled patients underwent diagnostic ERCP with major and minor papillae inspection as well as bile and pancreatic duct cannulation. Cannulation of minor papillae was pursued when pancreas divisum (PD) was suspected. In patients with an intact gallbladder, post-CCK bile aspiration was performed for microcrystal analysis with a positive result defined as 5 or more microcrystals per low-power field. Intraductal secretin testing with pancreatic juice collection for bicarbonate concentration measurement was used to assess for CP. A positive result was defined as total bicarbonate output less than 80 mEq/L. SOM was performed in both biliary and pancreatic sphincters, with sphincter hypertension defined as basal sphincter pressure greater than 40 mm Hg. The investigators defined papillary stenosis as the presence of dilated ducts (bile duct >10 mm with intact gall-bladder, bile duct >12 mm after cholecystectomy, and/or pancreatic duct >5 mm) with delayed drainage (bile duct >45 mm and/or pancreatic duct >10 mm). Intervention response was defined as absence of RAP in the follow-up period. Patients were followed for a mean of 29.6 months (range 18–33 months).

Overall 79% (100 out of 126) of the study population was found to have an identifiable cause of RAP. For 37.3% (47 out of 126) a cause was discovered on initial ERCP. Papillary stenosis was the most frequent diagnosis, accounting for 20.6% (26 out of 126) patients, 7.1% (9 out of 126) were found to have PD on minor papilla cannulation, and 4.8% (6 out of 126) were found to have bile duct stone with 5 out of 6 of these patient having intact gallbladders. Two cases of CP were identified along with 2 cases of intrapapillary choledochocele and 2 cases of malignancy. Bile microcrystal analysis was conducted in 105 patients, 79 with no identifiable cause after initial ERCP and 26 with papillary stenosis. Biliary microcrystals were found in 50% of the 54 patients with intact gallbladders. Fifteen patients were found to have multiple causes with RAP resulting from microcrystals and either papillary stenosis or SOD. SOM was performed in the 79 patients with no identifiable cause after initial ERCP, and 51.9% (41 out of 79) of these patients were found to have SOD. Seventy-five percent (95 out of 126) of study participants overall received endoscopic intervention. Ninety-three percent (93 out of 100) of the patients found to have an identifiable cause received ES. Minor papilla sphincterotomy was successful in 89% (8 out of 9) patients with PD. BES was performed in all cases of SOD, choledocholithiasis, choledochocele, and papillary stenosis as well as 25 out of 27 cases of either biliary microlithiasis alone or in combination with papillary stenosis or SOD. Persistent pancreatic sphincter hypertension was seen in 78% of patients with SOD treated with BES. These patients underwent PES during the same ERCP procedure. PES was also performed in 6 out of 26 of the patients with papillary stenosis. There were only 3 cases of patients receiving nonendoscopic therapy alone. Two received cholecystectomy for biliary microlithiasis and 1 received surgery for malignancy. The overall clinical response rate to endotherapy ranged from 67% to 100%.

Although limited by a short follow-up period and lack of a control group, this study does support the utility of adjunctive ERCP techniques in the management of RAP. Although ERCP alone is able to identify treatable morphologic abnormalities in a significant number of patients with IRAP, bile microcrystal analysis and SOM can help to identify a cause in still more patients. Microcrystal analysis and SOM together result in an additional 65% (35 out of 54) of identifiable causes in patients with intact gallbladders and 47% (24 out of 51) in patients who have had a cholecystectomy. This study also suggests that, in cases of biliary microlithiasis, cholecystectomy or biliary sphincterotomy alone is likely the most appropriate intervention. For papillary stenosis or manometrically diagnosed SOD, BES alone may be sufficient given its ability to reduce pancreatic and well as biliary sphincter pressures. In some cases, however, pancreatic sphincter hypertension persists and PES is required.

Testoni and colleagues[24] conducted a prospective study comparing the efficacy of ES with ursodeoxycholic acid (UDCA) in IRAP. Forty patients with RAP and intact gallbladders were enrolled after a 24-month period in which they were observed to have 2 or more AP episodes. Excluded patients included those with alcohol/drug abuse, metabolic disorders, documented or suspected gallbladder or bile duct microlithiasis, biliary type 1 SOD (common bile duct [CBD] dilation >12 mm with increased transaminase and/or alkaline phosphatase levels), CP, and other causes of RAP identifiable on routine laboratory tests and imaging. All study participants were evaluated by diagnostic ERCP with subsequent biliary or minor papilla sphincterotomy for those found to have bile duct microlithiasis or sludge, type 2 SOD, or PD with dilated dorsal duct. Those with no identifiable anatomic or functional abnormalities and those who refused endoscopic therapy were treated with long-term UDCA (10 mg/kg/d). ERCP identified a cause in 70% (28 out of 40) of cases. Patients were divided into 4 groups based on causes. Group A (11 out of 40) included patients with bile duct microlithiasis without ductal dilation. Group B (14 out of 40) included patients with SOD. Within this group, 11 out of 14 had biliary type 2 SOD with CBD and delayed drainage and 3 out of 14 had pancreatic type 1 or 2 SOD with PD diameter greater than 6 mm in head and greater than 5 mm in body and/or delayed drainage. Group C (3 out of 40) included patients with PD. Within this group, 2 out of 3 had complete PD, 1 of which also had BD microlithiasis, and 1 out of 3 had functional or incomplete PD. Group D (12 out of 40) included patients with no biliopancreatic anatomic or functional abnormalities. Patients were followed for greater than or equal to 27 months (range 27–73 months) for RAP, although follow-up time differed by group. Patients who underwent biliary sphincterotomy and developed recurrence in follow-up received a 7-F pancreatic duct stent (PSt), which was left in place for a mean of 4.6 months (range 3–6 months) or until recurrence. Those who continued to have RAP were treated with PES. Patients who developed recurrence after treatment with UDCA received BES and then PSt in the case of continued RAP. In group C, those with complete PD (2 out of 3) received minor papilla ES (MPES) and the remaining patient without dorsal duct dilatation received BES followed by dorsal duct stenting for persistent RAP.

In total, 55 diagnostic and therapeutic endoscopic procedures were performed. Five out of 55 (9.1%) were complicated by postprocedural mild pancreatitis. These results indicate that BES is beneficial even when the disorder is restricted to the pancreatic duct, which is most likely caused by the resultant reduced basal pancreatic duct pressures, and continued recurrence then likely stems from persistently high pressures. By this rationale, PSt sphincter ablation may allow for assessment of the potential response to PES and should be pursued after failed BES, as was done here. BES was effectively curative in 22 out of 28 (78.6%) cases. Of the 6 cases in which BES failed, 3 out of 6 subsequent interventions with PSt were justified, leading to definitive treatment with PES that effectively reduced RAP. This finding suggests that pancreatic segment SOD was truly causal in only 3 out of 40 (7.5%) cases. UDCA was effective in 9 out of 12 (75%) of the cases, suggesting that a large proportion of group D patients had underlying microlithiasis. Overall, 3 out of 40 (7.5%) patients continued to have RAP despite multiple interventions, likely indicating truly idiopathic cases. In all patients with cholangiographic evidence of microlithiasis or bile sludge, BES resulted in symptom remission for the duration of follow-up. In patients with type 2 SOD, BES or PES overall was effective in 12 out of 14 (85.7%), BES was effective in 9 out of 14 (64.3%), and UDCA alone was effective in 1 patient. Although not randomized, limited by a short follow-up period, and inclusive of patients without truly idiopathic disease, this study does offer convincing evidence supporting the efficacy of BES in RAP caused by occult bile duct microlithiasis, SOD, and PD.

Definitive evidence regarding the efficacy of endoscopic therapy in IRAP remains mixed. Although recent studies suggest ES may not alter the natural history of IRAP in the context of increased pancreatic sphincter pressures and that DES may provide no added benefit compared with BES alone, previous prospective studies indicate PES may have some utility following recurrence in patients treated with BES alone. There are also randomized data that support the use of PSt alone, although studies with larger sample sizes and longer follow-up periods are needed to corroborate these findings. As such, the benefits of ES, particularly PES and PSt, still remain unclear. Prospective, randomized controlled trials evaluating the efficacy of these therapies in true IRAP are needed to guide management. At present, routine use of PES and PSt in patients with IRAP cannot be recommended. They may be pursued in patients with a high disease burden as a last resort. Continued investigation into the natural history of IRAP and potential environmental and genetic risk factors will also help to guide therapy.

SPHINCTER OF ODDI DYSFUNCTION

SOD presents as either postcholecystectomy pain or IRAP. This article focuses on the latter, which is thought to result from pancreatic sphincter stenosis or dyskinesia. This condition is marked by pancreatic-type pain often radiating to the back associated with increased pancreatic enzyme levels and no identifiable cause of pancreatitis. The diagnosis is typically suspected after alternative causes for pain are ruled out. Further investigation may entail hepatobiliary scintigraphy (HBS), diagnostic ERCP assessing for structural abnormalities, or SOM for definitive diagnosis defined by an increased basal sphincter pressure.

After a diagnosis has been made, cases of pSOD may be categorized according to the Milwaukee classification system, which allows patients to be divided into 3 major groups and also provides a rough approximation of the potential benefit that may be expected from ES. Type I SOD is defined by typical pancreatic pain associated with abnormal serum chemistries, dilated pancreatic ducts, and delayed drainage. As such, this group represents true cases of RAP and is the focus of this article. Patients with type II SOD have typical pain and only 1 or 2 of the additional criteria. Patients with type III SOD only have typical pain. Patients with type I SOD are more likely to experience the greatest benefit from endoscopic intervention and often present with an observable sphincter stenosis. However, the benefits of endotherapy in patients with type II and III SOD are more uncertain, with patients with type III SOD experiencing the least benefit.[25,26] A 2012 systematic review described response to ES as 83.3% to 100% improvement in type I SOD, 79% in type II SOD, and only 8% in type III SOD regardless of SOM findings with a high 69.8% rate of spontaneous symptom resolution.[27] Attempts to improve this classification system to provide additional diagnostic and prognostic value have been pursued. For example, Gong[28] proposed the addition of a double duct type and biliary or pancreatic reflux type to create a more anatomically derived categorization, but it is unclear how this would improve management.

Several challenges remain in the diagnosis and management of SOD. The need to accurately quantify the role of sphincterotomy in treating biliary and/or pSOD persists. Furthermore, the use of SOM in the definitive diagnosis of SOD is controversial because these patients have an increased risk for post-ERCP pancreatitis. The risk of serious complications in pursuing SOM seem to outweigh the marginal benefits. Several attempts have been made to develop alternatives to SOM, including functional MRI, optical coherence tomography, functional lumen imaging probe, and a guidewire-type manometer. However, these techniques remain experimental and cannot be recommended as standard of practice. Adjunctive diagnostic techniques of more promising but still limited utility include secretin stimulated ultrasonography, secretin-stimulated MRCP (ss-MRCP), HBS, and EUS. It is also challenging to rule out alternative causes in cases of persistent SOD postendotherapy. Persistent pain may stem from irritable bowel syndrome, duodenal spasm, right colon spasm, or psychosocial distress.

Previous studies evaluating the efficacy of endotherapy in SOD are limited by variable and often short follow-up periods, a lack of control groups, ill-defined measures of success, concurrent interventions, and a poor understanding of the natural history of SOD. The role of SOD as a direct cause or instead an apparent effect of RAP is still actively debated.[16,29] Moreover, both the optimal treatment modality and appropriate follow-up period to claim a cure for SOD-associated RAP remains unclear. Few studies measure average time to first recurrence. Evaluating SOD studies is made more challenging by the variable documentation of not only which duct, biliary or pancreatic, was manometrically interrogated but also which duct was intervened on. Some studies are limited to only 1 duct, whereas others evaluate both. This article is primarily concerned with studies addressing pSOD and associated RAP.

The 2012 prospective randomized controlled trial conducted by Coté and colleagues[16] described briefly earlier, provides valuable insights into the efficacy of endoscopic intervention in patients with IRAP found to have SOD. After undergoing initial evaluation with ERCP and SOM, the 89 enrolled patients with IRAP were divided into 2 groups composed of 69 with pSOD and 20 with normal SOM. Patients with pSOD were randomly assigned to undergo BES (33 out of 69) and DES (36 out of 69). Sphincterotomy technique was left up to the discretion of the endoscopist and a prophylactic polyethylene PD stent was placed whenever possible. Endoscopists were also given discretion to repeat ERCP with SOM for recurrent or persistent SOD. Of note, the BES group had higher rates of increased basal biliary sphincter pressure compared with the DES group (74.1% vs 41.4%, $P \geq .01$). Patients with normal SOM were randomly assigned to undergo BES (11 out of 20) or a sham procedure (9 out of 20). However, comparisons between these two groups are limited by below-target enrollment into the normal-SOM subset leading to a small sample size and inadequate statistical power. This limitation was the result of a higher than expected prevalence of SOD in the study population. All patients were followed annually by telephone and evaluated at 10 years post–index procedure.

After a median follow-up period of 78 months (range 1–10 years), response rates in patients treated with BES and DES in the SOD group (48.5% vs 47.2% recurrence, $P = 1.0$) as well as patients treated with BES and sham in the normal-SOM group (27.3% vs 11.1% recurrence, $P = .59$) were similar. A nonsignificant difference in rate of early RAP (<12 months post–index ERCP) was seen in patients with SOD treated with DES compared with BES (41.7% vs 24.2%, $P = .20$). The 11.1% risk of subsequent RAP in the sham group may approximate the natural history of disease with conservative management. Progression to CP after the index ERCP was noted in 16.9% of patients overall. The probability of developing CP was similar between normal SOM and pSOD ($P = .74$). A post hoc analysis revealed that patients with pSOD have a 4-fold increased risk of developing RAP during follow-up compared with patients with normal SOM (adjusted hazard ratio, 4.3; $P<.02$). Number of AP episodes before randomization, CP in follow-up, and post-ERCP pancreatitis after index ERCP were also shown to be independent risk factors for RAP. These conclusions should be considered descriptive because the study was not powered for risk factor analysis.

As stated previously, the persistent RAP seen after intervention with DES suggests that ablation of the pancreatic sphincter is not curative in patients with pSOD. This finding argues against the theory that SOD is a direct cause of RAP, indicating instead that it may be a consequence of recurrent inflammatory episodes. PES thus cannot be recommended for treatment of SOD-associated RAP, especially because no additional benefit was seen compared with BES. In addition, a higher than expected prevalence of pSOD in the study population did not translate into a higher prevalence of CP in follow-up, indicating pSOD may not be an early marker of CP. Although SOD was found to be associated with a significantly increased risk of future AP episodes compared with normal SOM, the mechanism of progression to CP is still unclear. Because patients with both SOD and normal SOM have RAP, both groups have an increased risk of fibrosis that may potentially lead to CP. The increased risk of progression seen in pSOD may indicate this group of patients has unique genetic or environmental risk factors. Future studies should aim to build on these findings to further develop the understanding of the natural history of SOD as it relates to RAP.

A study evaluating the long-term outcomes of endoscopic therapy for patients with RAP with SOD enrolled 48 patients from 1995 to 1998 with documented mean pancreatic sphincter pressure greater than or equal to 40 mm Hg by SOM and greater than or equal to 2 episodes in the 12 months before initial evaluation.[30] Endoscopic intervention with BES, PES, or DES (at least PES since 1997) with 7-F prophylactic pancreatic stent at initial evaluation was performed at the discretion of the endoscopist. Patients were followed prospectively for 2 years, undergoing repeat ERCP and SOM in the case of RAP at the end of this period and then retrospectively 10 years after initial evaluation obtaining medical records from the patients' primary care physicians. The total follow-up period was 11.5 years ± 1.6 years, range 120 to 162 months. Eleven out of 48 patients in the study population were only followed short term for 2 years and 37 out of 48 were followed long term. After 2 years, 5 out of 37 of the long-term follow-up patients developed RAP, with 4 out of 5 going on to receive DES and 1 out of 5 receiving pancreaticojejunostomy. One patient from each treatment group remained asymptomatic for the duration of the study. Two out of 11 of the short-term follow-up patients developed recurrence and received DES. These patients remained asymptomatic throughout the 2-year follow-up period. In the long-term follow-up period, 17 out of 37 patients developed confirmed RAP, and thus recurrence in 19 out of 48 overall, including the 2 patients who developed RAP within 2 years but remained asymptomatic thereafter. Overall, time to first recurrence after initial endoscopic intervention was

3.5 years (range 3–84 months). This finding is surprising given that all study participants had frequent RAP (≥ 2 episodes in the preceding 12 months) before enrollment. In addition, the overall mean number of relapses in the long-term follow-up period was 0.65 ± 0.7 (range 0–2). This number was lower than the incidence of RAP at enrollment (2.5 ± 0.5, range 2–4), which, together with the long time to first recurrence, may indicate the efficacy of endoscopic therapy in delaying disease progression. However, these values cannot be readily compared because the former was obtained by retrospective analysis and the latter was obtained by past medical history. Furthermore, this study's small sample size limits the ability to definitively make such a conclusion. Progression to CP was confirmed in only 2 out of 37 patients, suggesting that occult CP at enrollment as a cause of RAP is unlikely. A univariate analysis of potential risk factors for RAP post-ES showed that patients who received lone BES or PES had a higher risk of recurrence compared with patients who underwent DES (12 out of 13 vs 7 out of 24, $P<.05$). This finding suggests the therapeutic superiority of DES, but a prospective randomized trial is needed to confirm this conclusion. These data also corroborate the results of previous studies, which found ES to effectively reduce the rate of RAP in the short term but to have a reduced efficacy in the long term. Here, 14% relapse was seen in the short term and 51% relapse was seen in the long term. Given this and the median 3.5 years to first recurrence, follow-up after ES for SOD-associated RAP should be at least 5 years. However, this study does not inform the efficacy of empirical ES without prior SOM.

The earlier described prospective study on IRAP conducted by Kaw and Brodmerkel[23] contains relevant findings on the efficacy of endotherapy in SOD-associated RAP.[23] Approximately half of the enrolled patients who underwent SOM were found to have SOD, all of whom were treated with BES. Seventy-eight percent of these patients had persistent pancreatic sphincter hypertension and were treated with PES. Although response rates following PES were not clearly reported, the overall response rate following ES in patients with SOD was reported at 75%. The investigators recommend PES in patients with manometrically diagnosed SOD who are unresponsive to BES.

Another interesting treatment modality for pSOD-associated RAP is endoscopic botulinum toxin injection. A prospective study conducted by Wehrmann and colleagues[31] assessed the technical feasibility, safety, and efficacy of botulinum toxin injection both in the short term and as a predictive tool for evaluating potential response to ES. In brief, 15 patients with RAP with manometrically diagnosed pSOD (8 out of 15 also with bSOD [Biliary Sphincter of Oddi dysfunction]) and greater than or equal to 2 AP episodes (median 4) in the last 6 months received a 100-mouse unit injection of botulinum toxin at the major papilla. Injection was performed successfully in all patients and only 1 developed abdominal pain not associated with enzyme level increases, which was quickly resolved. Patients were then followed prospectively with monthly clinical evaluations for 3 months. Three out of 15 (20%) patients developed RAP during this time and were termed nonresponders. The 12 out of 15 (80%) patients who remained asymptomatic and developed recurrence after 3 months post-intervention were termed botulinum toxin responders who experienced symptomatic benefit. All patients with RAP underwent repeat SOM with a blinded assessment of SOM results and pancreatic sphincterotomy with prophylactic stent placement irrespective of these results. Follow-up continued after this point, with recurrence serving as the study end point. The only 1 of the 3 nonresponders who had persistently increased pancreatic sphincter pressure was also the only nonresponder to benefit from PES. Eleven out of 12 responders followed for a median of 15 months developed RAP 6 ± 2 months postinjection, all of whom were asymptomatic after ES.

Significantly more responders experienced benefit from ES (6 PES alone and 8 DES) compared with nonresponders (11 vs 1, P<.05). Although limited by a small sample size and short follow-up period, this study suggests botulinum toxin injection is safe and may provide effective short-term symptom relief in SOD-associated RAP while also acting as a predictor of ES success in responders. Although promising, botulinum toxin injection remains an experimental treatment modality and a randomized controlled trial is needed to corroborate these results.

Overall, evidence supporting endotherapy in SOD-associated RAP remains sparse and a review of the current literature does not yield a cohesive set of recommendations regarding the use of endoscopic intervention, particularly with regard to sphincterotomy. Despite recent advances, the natural history of pSOD and the efficacy of endotherapy in treating this disorder are poorly elucidated. SOD seems to be a secondary consequence of RAP and although PES may provide marginal or no benefit when used in conjunction with BES, it may be pursued as a last resort in patients with persistent RAP who are willing to accept the risk of postprocedure pancreatitis. Studies focusing exclusively on endotherapy in pSOD-associated RAP are still few. With waning support for SOM given the risk of postprocedure pancreatitis and the requirement for both expensive equipment and special training, future studies may be hindered by the use of less accurate noninvasive diagnostic studies that may not produce valid diagnoses.

PANCREAS DIVISUM

PD is the most common congenital anomaly of the pancreas, with an overall prevalence of approximately 2.9%. It results from the failed fusion of the dorsal and ventral pancreatic ducts during weeks 6 to 8 of gestation. Pancreatic fluids drain primarily through the minor papilla, and pancreatitis secondary to PD is thought to occur because of minor papilla stenosis with a subsequent increase in intraductal pressures. Although PD has been implicated in the pathogenesis of RAP, CP, and chronic abdominal pain (CAP), most patients with PD are asymptomatic, with less than 10% developing pancreatitis.[32] As such, the role of PD as a direct cause of RAP remains controversial. Although PD is more prevalent among unexplained cases of RAP compared with control patients (8%–50% vs 3%–12%), thus indicating an association between the two conditions,[33] symptomatic PD has also been noted in greater frequency among patients with RAP with genetic abnormalities. Cases of cystic fibrosis transmembrane conductance regulator (CFTR) mutation–associated RAP in particular have significantly greater rates of PD compared with cases of idiopathic RAP and/or CP,[34] which suggests that PD itself does not lead to RAP. Instead, certain genetic and/or environmental risk factors likely predispose a subset of patients with PD to developing pancreatitis.

PD is typically diagnosed with either ERCP or secretin-enhanced MRCP. Endoscopic intervention involves minor papilla sphincterotomy, stenting, or balloon dilation in an effort to decompress the dorsal duct and decrease intraductal pressure. Because stenting necessitates reintervention for stent exchanges and introduces the risk of stent-induced dorsal duct changes with long-term use, minor papillotomy has become the preferred treatment option. Pull and free-hand needle-knife sphincterotomy techniques have been shown to be equally effective.[35] However, there is a greater risk of post-ERCP pancreatitis in minor papilla sphincterotomy compared with biliary sphincterotomy. This risk may be mitigated with the prophylactic use of small-caliber 3-F or 4-F stents and 100-mg rectal indomethacin.[33] The therapeutic benefit of endotherapy in PD-associated RAP can still be debated. Most studies on this subject are retrospective and uncontrolled, with small sample sizes, variable follow-up periods, variable types of endotherapy, and variable definitions of successful response to endotherapy. Many do not limit their definitions of symptomatic PD to only RAP and also include PD-associated CP and CAP without pancreatitis. Few describe prior evaluation for alternative causes.

Lans and colleagues[36] conducted the only randomized controlled trial evaluating endotherapy in PD-associated RAP to date. Nineteen patients were enrolled over 5 years, all of whom had complete PD diagnosed by ERCP and greater than or equal to 2 episodes of AP (abdominal pain and serum amylase greater than or equal to $2\times$ upper limit of normal). Those with identifiable alternative causes of RAP, including CP, and a history of pancreatic surgery were excluded. All patients underwent an initial ERCP to confirm PD. Failure to cannulate or introduce a guidewire into the pancreatic duct resulted in exclusion (success rate 83%). After initial evaluation, patients were randomized to receive dorsal duct stenting (10) or no intervention in the control group (9). The intervention included serial dilation with a graduated Soehendra catheter (4 to 7 F) and placement of a dorsal duct stent (5 to 7 F, 3–7 cm) with dual-sided barbs at each end. The stent and control groups were followed for a mean of 28.6 and 31.5 months, respectively. During follow-up, patients were evaluated every 4 months to obtain information about number of documented AP episodes, number of hospitalizations or emergency room visits for abdominal pain without increased pancreatic enzyme levels, and subjective feelings of health as graded by patients using a visual analog scale. After 1 year with stent exchanges every 4 months, all stents were removed and intervention group patients were simply followed. Repeat ERCP was conducted only if clinically appropriate.

The number of documented AP attacks was significantly lower in the stent group compared with the control group (1 vs 7, $P<.05$). The 1 AP episode in the stent group occurred just before the replacement of an occluded stent and was less severe than previous attacks experienced by that patient. Compared with the control group, in which there were 5 hospitalizations and 2 emergency department (ED) visits for abdominal pain alone, there were no hospitalizations for ED visits in the stent group ($P<.05$). Although 9 out of 10 patients in the stent group reported greater than or equal to 50% symptomatic improvement, only 1 of the 9 patients in the control group reported such improvement ($P<.05$). After the study period, 4 control group patients with persistent RAP and abdominal pain underwent stenting. They were followed for an additional 6 to 53 months and all remained asymptomatic during this time.

These findings support an obstructive cause for RAP in PD and further suggest that minor papilla sphincter ablation via dorsal duct stenting may be an effective short-term bridge to definitive interventions such as sphincterotomy or surgical sphincteroplasty. However, stenting requires intermittent reinterventions for stent exchanges and has risks. In addition to stent migration into or out of the pancreatic duct, long-term stenting may lead to ductal changes. Although notable for being both randomized and controlled with an assessment of outcomes in patients with PD exclusively with RAP, this study is limited by a small sample size and short-term follow-up. Moreover, subjective data collected from patients on overall wellness were likely skewed by the placebo effect because patients were not blinded.

The efficacy of MPES in reducing the frequency of RAP in patients with PD remains unclear and many think that the risk of intervention is too great given the lack of proven benefit. In order to definitively address this concern, Romagnuolo and colleagues[37] are preparing to conduct a multicenter, long-term, randomized sham-controlled trial, the pilot study for which is described here.

In 2013, Romagnuolo and colleagues[37] conducted a large prospective study, the Frequency of Recurrent Acute Pancreatitis after Minor Papilla Endoscopic Sphincterotomy (FRAMES) study, in patients with PD with IRAP. Forty patients were prospectively recruited from 6 tertiary centers. Inclusion entailed PD diagnosed on imaging and greater than or equal to 1 episode of unexplained AP ($>3\times$ normal enzyme levels) requiring hospitalization. Overall these patients had a mean of 2 (range 0–7) AP episodes in the last year. Patients with prior MPES or other significant biliary or pancreatic ductal disorder were excluded. Information on QOL and pain between AP episodes (RAPID [recurrent abdominal pain intensity and disability] score) was recorded at initial evaluation, revealing an average of 18 days of pain in the last 90 days and a median Short-Form 12 (SF-12) physical component score 0.5 standard deviation below the baseline of a normal population. All patients underwent ERCP with MPES and temporary (<4 weeks) prophylactic pancreatic stent placement. Overall minor papilla cannulation and sphincterotomy success rate was 97.5% (39 out of 40). Despite this high success rate, identification of the minor papilla was challenging, described as subtle in 42% of cases and only visible after secretin in 12%. The investigators also noted that identification could be aided by spraying methylene blue on the duodenal wall and watching as pancreatic juice washes away the dye.[33] Placed stents lacked flanges in 72% of cases and were less than 4 F in 75%. During a follow-up period of 6 months, patients were monitored for QOL, pain, and RAP. Those with pain between attacks rated greater than 5 out of 10 and occurring more than 3 d/wk were included in a separate group called FRAMES-2 (4 out of 40). At a median of 71 days (range 15–78) after intervention, 8.3% (3 out of 36) of patients had an AP episode. At 3-month follow-up, 8.3% (3 out of 36) of patients were admitted for pain, compared with 50% (2 out of 4) of patients in the FRAMES-2 group. After intervention and at end of the 6-month follow-up, there was a median 11-day decrease in the number of days with pain in the last 90 days, compared with an 80-day decrease in the FRAMES-2 group. The median RAPID score decreased from 10 at baseline to 0 at 3 and 6 months ($P = .001$). A similar decrease was seen in FRAMES-2. This study suggests that MPES with temporary stenting leads to a reduced AP recurrence rate at 6 months with reduced pain and increased QOL.

A recent systematic review examined response to endoscopic therapy in patients with RAP, CP, or CAP secondary to PD.[32] Sixteen of the 22 studies evaluated in this review included patients with PD-associated RAP. Of the 314 patients with documented outcomes, 230 were noted to be responsive. Of note, successful response to endotherapy was variably defined by study and included reduced rates of pancreatitis, hospitalization, abdominal pain, narcotic use, or eliminated need for surgical intervention. No trends were seen in response rates with respect to types of definitions for response. Type of endotherapy used also varied to include minor papilla sphincterotomy, stenting, and balloon dilation. Patients with PD-associated RAP were found to have the highest response rates, with a range of 43% to 100% (median 73%). In contrast, 21% to 80% (median 42%) of patients with CP and 11% to 55% (median 33%) of patients with CAP were responsive. Low response rates in patients with PD-associated CP may result from irreversible ductal changes that are unaffected by endoscopic intervention. Alternatively, poor response rates in patients with CP and CAP suggest that PD is not the cause of CP but instead an incidental finding, marker, or cofactor.

Focusing on some of the notable studies included in this systematic review, Chacko and colleagues[38] conducted a retrospective study examining clinical outcomes after minor papilla endotherapy (MPE) in patients with symptomatic PD. In line with the findings of the systematic review described earlier, MPE was found to be the most effective in patients with RAP with PD with or without ductal changes, resulting in a 76%

response rate. Patients with RAP experienced the same benefit whether they had ductal changes or not (75% vs 71%). In contrast, 42% of patients with CP responded to MPE, a marked but not statistically significant difference. This finding suggests that underlying ductal changes may not predict poor response to MPE. Instead, what more aptly differentiates cases of PD-associated RAP with ductal changes and PD-associated CP is the frequency of pain. Although the former has discrete pain episodes with intervening periods without symptoms, the latter involve chronic daily pain. Patients with RAP with ductal changes likely represent a subgroup of patients in transition to CP and long-term follow-up may reveal a decrease in response rates. Additional studies are needed to assess this. These findings further suggest that changes in pain perception as a result of differing pain patterns likely contribute more significantly to differences in response rates than was previously expected.

In 2014, Mariani[39] published the largest prospective controlled study to date assessing outcomes of endotherapy compared with conservative management in PD-associated RAP. Over 5 years, 36 patients were enrolled, all with ss-MRCP–diagnosed PD and RAP ($\geq$2 episodes of abdominal pain with serum amylase and/or lipase levels $\geq$2$\times$ the normal limit) with no evidence of CP on EUS. Patients underwent evaluation to rule out alternative causes for RAP, including a thorough history, genetic screening for CFTR mutations, serum IgG4, and fecal elastase assays. Those with suspected alternative causes and previous pancreatic surgery or pancreatic sphincterotomy were excluded. Patients were divided into 2 groups: a recent RAP group (22 out of 36) in which patients had greater than or equal to 1 episode of RAP in the past year, and a previous RAP group (14 out of 36) in which patients did not have RAP in the past year. The former received MPES and the latter received conservative management. MPES included the prophylactic dorsal duct placement of a 5-F, 2-cm to 3-cm single-flange plastic pancreatic stent with a duodenal pigtail or a 5-F unflanged stent to prevent post-ERCP pancreatitis. All patients received pharmacologic prophylaxis. Only those with successful dorsal duct drainage on intervention were included in subsequent analyses. Successful response to endotherapy was defined as lack of recurrence. Unsuccessful response to endotherapy was defined as RAP in follow-up. Endotherapy failure was defined as inability to drain the dorsal duct or cannulate the minor papilla. Three of the 36 recruited patients were excluded from analyses, including 1 who refused follow-up after a failed second ERCP and 2 who had a failed index MPES. Dilated main pancreatic ducts defined as being greater than or equal to 3 mm in caliber were noted on initial evaluation in both the recent (12 out of 22) and previous RAP (6 out of 14) groups.

Patients were followed for a mean of 4.5 years (range 2–6.7 y) with clinical and biochemical evaluation as well as EUS after each year of follow-up. Patients who developed RAP received ERCP and EUS with each episode of recurrence. Recurrence in the previous RAP group was treated with MPES. Recurrence in the recent RAP group after the index MPES was treated with a second MPES with extension of the papillary orifice in the case of inadequate sphincterotomy along with short-term stenting to prevent post-ERCP orifice narrowing. Alternatively, in the case of adequate sphincterotomy, patients were treated with long-term stenting. Short-term stenting was defined as placement of a 7-F, 3-cm to 4-cm plastic pancreatic stent for less than or equal to 1 month and long-term stenting was defined as placement of a 7-F, 3-cm to 7-cm plastic pancreatic stent for 3 months with exchanges every 3 months for 1 year.

Of the 22 patients who underwent MPES in the recent RAP group, cannulation and sphincterotomy was achieved in 20 at the index procedure and in 19 out of 20 at reintervention. RAP was seen in 57.9% (11 out of 19) after the index ERCP, 31.6% (6 out of 19) after the second ERCP, and 26.3% (5 out of 19) after the third ERCP. Thus, after 2 or 3 interventions, 14 out of 19 patients remained free of recurrence for an overall success rate of 73.7% (14 out of 19). Five patients had persistent RAP despite multiple interventions. No recurrence was observed in the previous RAP group, with 64.3% (9 out of 14) of patients progressing to CP. Although greater rates of RAP were seen in patients without main pancreatic duct dilatation (37.5%) compared with those with dilatation (18.2%) at baseline, this difference was not significant. Ten out of 19 patients in the recent RAP group were treated with long-term stenting, half of whom developed recurrence. The other 9 patients in this group received either no stenting or only short-term stenting. Overall, 20 out of 33 (60.6%) patients progressed to CP as diagnosed by EUS (≥ 4 Wiersema criteria), including 11 out of 19 (57.9%) in the recent RAP group and 9 out of 14 (64.3%) in the previous RAP group, a nonsignificant difference. Following intervention with multiple ERCPs, EUS signs suggestive of CP were noted in 42.8% (6 out of 14) of patients without and 100% (5 out of 5) of patients with RAP in follow-up ($P = .04$). For patients receiving stent therapy, CP developed in 80% (8 out of 10) of those treated with long-term stenting and 33.3% (3 out of 9) of those treated with no or only short-term stenting. The mean time to CP after a patient's first AP episode, which did not differ significantly between the recent and previous RAP groups, was 6.1 ± 1.4 years. The most frequent abnormal findings on EUS suggestive of CP were side branch dilatation, hyperechoic main pancreatic duct margins, and hyperechoic strands and foci.

As described earlier, previous studies strongly suggest that the subset of patients with PD who develop RAP are the most likely to respond to endotherapy. This study sought to determine the extent to which endoscopic intervention improves outcomes and prevents progression to CP in these patients, something that has been poorly studied thus far. The investigators found that neither dorsal duct dilatation nor time from last episode of pancreatitis could predict progression to CP, indicating that some additional disorder aside from that affecting the pancreatic ducts must result in RAP and subsequently CP. However, successful endotherapy did result in a significant reduction in frequency of CP compared with unsuccessful ERCP, suggesting at least some degree of an obstructive pathogenic component. Moreover, lower rates of CP were observed in patients who received intervention compared with those who received conservative management (42.8% vs 64.3%). These findings suggest the presence of 2 potential subgroups within patients with PD-associated RAP, one with persistent inflammation in which intervention slows progression to CP and one with inactive disease in which endotherapy yields a lower response rate. Note that long-term stenting itself may have resulted in findings suggestive of CP, potentially resulting in the greater rates of CP compared with MPES with or without the short-term stenting seen here (80% vs 33.3%). However, rates of CP in long-term stenting compared with observation are similar (60% vs 64%). Although limited by a small samples size and short follow-up period, this study provides compelling evidence that endotherapy is most effective in patients with PD-associated RAP with recent AP episodes with or without ductal dilatation. Although about 60% of patients with PD with either recent or previous RAP developed CP over a 6-year period, successful MPES in patients with PD and recent RAP reduced rates of recurrence as well as risk of progression to CP. Additional studies are needed to confirm these findings.

A recent meta-analysis conducted by Michailidis[40] that included 23 studies assessing the efficacy of endoscopic therapy for PD reported a pooled success rate of 67.5% with a pooled post-ERCP pancreatitis rate of 10.1%. By subgroup, pooled success rates following endoscopic intervention were 76% for RAP, 52.4% for CP, and 48% for pancreatic-type pain. These findings suggest that the subset

Table 2
Summary of included studies and results

IRAP/SOD	Author, Date	Randomized	Sample Size (n = Total)	Endoscopic Intervention	Follow-up (y)	Response (%)
Retrospective	Das et al,[17] 2016	N	50	BES and/or PES	7	42
	Wehrmann,[30] 2011	N	37	BES, PES, DES	11.5	60
Prospective	Coté et al,[16] 2012	Y	89	BES, DES	6.5	51.50
	Jacob et al,[22] 2001	Y	34	PSt	2.75	89.00
	Wehrmann,[30] 2011	N	48	BES, PES, DES	2	85
	Testoni et al,[24] 2000	N	40	BES, PES, MPES, PSt	2.25–6	78.60
	Kaw & Brodmerkel,[23] 2002	N	126	BES, PES, MPES	2.47	67–100
	Wehrmann,[31] 2000	N	15	Major papilla Botulinum toxin >PES/DES	1.25	80

PD + RAP	Author, Date	Randomized	Sample Size (n = Total)	Endoscopic Intervention	Follow-up (y)	Response (%)
Prospective	Lans et al,[36] 1992	Y	19	MPSt	2.4	90
	Mariani,[39] 2014	N	36	MPES ± long-term/short-term stent	4.5	73.70
	Romagnuolo et al,[37] 2013	N	40	MPES	0.5	91.70
	Kaw & Brodmerkel,[23] 2002	N	9 (PD)	MPES	2.47	89
	Testoni et al,[24] 2000	N	3 (PD)	BES + MPSt, MPES	2.25–6	Unavailable

Response: for initial therapy or after multiple interventions, definition varies by study to include lack of recurrence and reduced rates of pancreatitis, hospitalization, abdominal pain, or narcotic use, or eliminated need for surgical intervention.
Abbreviations: BES, biliary ES; DES, dual ES; MPSt, minor papilla stenting; N, no; PES, pancreatic ES; Y, yes.

of patients with PD with RAP is the most likely to benefit from endotherapy, a conclusion that is well supported by previous studies. A meta-regression analysis revealed that therapy with dorsal duct stenting alone and a longer follow-up period were the only factors predictive of response to endotherapy. Although dorsal duct stenting may reduce the risk of post-ERCP pancreatitis, this does not fully explain the benefit observed here. Note that only 2 of the 17 studies included in the regression analysis assessed therapy with dorsal duct stenting alone[36,41]; these were early studies conducted in 1990 and 1992 with small sample sizes. The benefit seen with extended follow-up may be explained by additional endoscopic interventions or more frequent assessment by providers. Funnel plot analysis also revealed the likely presence of publication bias in the literature, with most studies reporting a positive effect. This meta-analysis was limited by the significant heterogeneity seen among the included studies. Moreover, most studies were case series prone to selection and reporting bias.

SUMMARY REGARDING ENDOSCOPIC APPROACH TO RECURRENT ACUTE PANCREATITIS

The answer to the central question regarding the true utility of endoscopic intervention in treating RAP continues to be elusive. Recent studies reviewed here suggest that, with regard to IRAP, treatment with ES is at best questionably beneficial and at worst unlikely to alter the natural history of disease. Although prior prospective studies indicate that treatment with ES results in remission or a reduced frequency of attacks, many of these studies lack control groups and are limited by small sample sizes and short follow-up periods. Furthermore, in SOD-related RAP, DES seems to have no added benefit compared with BES alone, although, as with IRAP, prior studies suggest otherwise. Despite the poorly defined efficacy of sphincterotomy, stenting seems to be a highly effective means of preventing recurrence, albeit with likely continued pancreatic-type pain. Larger studies are required to corroborate these findings. In PD-related RAP, preliminary studies provide some evidence supporting the efficacy of MPES, but a definitive long-term prospective randomized controlled trial has yet to be completed. Minor papilla stenting seems to provide short-term benefits and may be a viable bridge to MPES. In addition, a few generalities have also become apparent. For instance, certain patient characteristics, such as greater numbers of attacks before therapy, are likely predictive of persistent RAP postintervention. In addition, patients should be followed for at least 5 years postintervention to evaluate for RAP, particularly in the case of SOD-related RAP. RAP is a challenging entity to study, with multiple possible causes, unpredictable disease patterns, and still uncertain treatment modalities, but there has been significant progress. Continued efforts are sure to yield further advances in understanding, which will guide clinical practice (**Table 2**).

REFERENCES

1. Singer MV, Gyr K, Sarles H. Revised classification of pancreatitis. Report of the second international symposium on the classification of pancreatitis in Marseille, France, March 28-30, 1984. Gastroenterology 1985;89:683–5.
2. Whitcomb DC. Mechanisms of disease: advances in understanding the mechanisms leading to chronic pancreatitis. Nat Clin Pract Gastroenterol Hepatol 2004;1:46–52.
3. Machicado JD, Yadav D. Epidemiology of recurrent acute and chronic pancreatitis: similarities and differences. Dig Dis Sci 2017;62:1683–91.

4. Yadav D, Lowenfels AB. The epidemiology of pancreatitis and pancreatic cancer. Gastroenterology 2013;144:1252–61.

5. Sankaran SJ, Xiao AY, Wu LM, et al. Frequency of progression from acute to chronic pancreatitis and risk factors: a meta-analysis. Gastroenterology 2015; 149:1490–500.e1.

6. Etemad B, Whitcomb DC. Chronic pancreatitis: diagnosis, classification, and new genetic developments. Gastroenterology 2001;120:682–707.

7. Guda NM, Romagnuolo J, Freeman ML. Recurrent and relapsing pancreatitis. Curr Gastroenterol Rep 2011;13:140–9.

8. da Costa DW, Bouwense SA, Schepers NJ, et al. Same-admission versus interval cholecystectomy for mild gallstone pancreatitis (PONCHO): a multicentre randomised controlled trial. Lancet 2015;386:1261–8.

9. van Geenen EJM, van der Peet DL, Mulder CJJ, et al. Recurrent acute biliary pancreatitis: the protective role of cholecystectomy and endoscopic sphincterotomy. Surg Endosc 2009;23:950–6.

10. Takeyama Y. Long-term prognosis of acute pancreatitis in Japan. Clin Gastroenterol Hepatol 2009;7:S15–7.

11. Nordback I, Pelli H, Lappalainen-Lehto R, et al. The recurrence of acute alcohol-associated pancreatitis can be reduced: a randomized controlled trial. Gastroenterology 2009;136:848–55.

12. Yadav D, Hawes RH, Brand RE, et al. Alcohol consumption, cigarette smoking, and the risk of recurrent acute and chronic pancreatitis. Arch Intern Med 2009; 169:1035–45.

13. Rebours V, Boutron-Ruault MC, Schnee M, et al. The natural history of hereditary pancreatitis: a national series. Gut 2009;58:97–103.

14. Christian JB, Arondekar B, Buysman EK, et al. Determining triglyceride reductions needed for clinical effect/affect in severe hypertriglyceridemia. Am J Med 2014;127:36–44.e1.

15. Vipperla K, Somerville C, Furlan A, et al. Clinical profile and natural course in a large cohort of patients with hypertriglyceridemia and pancreatitis. J Clin Gastroenterol 2017;51:77–85.

16. Coté GA, Imperiale TF, Schmidt SE, et al. Similar efficacies of biliary, with or without pancreatic, sphincterotomy in treatment of idiopathic recurrent acute pancreatitis. Gastroenterology 2012;143:1502–9.e1.

17. Das R, Clarke B, Tang G, et al. Endoscopic sphincterotomy (ES) may not alter the natural history of idiopathic recurrent acute pancreatitis (IRAP). Pancreatology 2016;16(5):770–7.

18. Garg PK, Tandon RK, Madan K. Is biliary microlithiasis a significant cause of idiopathic recurrent acute pancreatitis? A long-term follow-up study. Clin Gastroenterol Hepatol 2007;5:75–9.

19. Nøjgaard C, Becker U, Matzen P, et al. Progression from acute to chronic pancreatitis: prognostic factors, mortality, and natural course. Pancreas 2011;40: 1195–200.

20. Amann ST, Yadav D, Barmada MM, et al. Physical and mental quality of life in chronic pancreatitis: a case-control study from the North American Pancreatitis Study 2 cohort. Pancreas 2013;42:293–300.

21. Gardner TB, Kennedy AT, Gelrud A, et al. Chronic pancreatitis and its effect on employment and health care experience: results of a prospective American multicenter study. Pancreas 2010;39:498–501.

22. Jacob L, Geenen JE, Catalano MF, et al. Prevention of pancreatitis in patients with idiopathic recurrent pancreatitis: a prospective nonblinded randomized study using endoscopic stents. Endoscopy 2001;33:559–62.
23. Kaw M, Brodmerkel GJ. ERCP, biliary crystal analysis, and sphincter of Oddi manometry in idiopathic recurrent pancreatitis. Gastrointest Endosc 2002;55: 157–62.
24. Testoni PA, Caporuscio S, Bagnolo F, et al. Idiopathic recurrent pancreatitis: long-term results after ERCP, endoscopic sphincterotomy, or ursodeoxycholic acid treatment. Am J Gastroenterol 2000;95:1702–7.
25. Heetun ZS, Zeb F, Cullen G, et al. Biliary sphincter of Oddi dysfunction: response rates after ERCP and sphincterotomy in a 5-year ERCP series and proposal for new practical guidelines. Eur J Gastroenterol Hepatol 2011;23:327–33.
26. Yaghoobi M, Romagnuolo J. Sphincter of Oddi dysfunction: updates from the recent literature. Curr Gastroenterol Rep 2015;17:31.
27. Hall TC, Dennison AR, Garcea G. The diagnosis and management of sphincter of Oddi dysfunction: a systematic review. Langenbecks Arch Surg 2012;397: 889–98.
28. Gong J-Q. Management of patients with sphincter of Oddi dysfunction based on a new classification. World J Gastroenterol 2011;17:385.
29. Park S-H, Watkins JL, Fogel EL, et al. Long-term outcome of endoscopic dual pancreatobiliary sphincterotomy in patients with manometry-documented sphincter of Oddi dysfunction and normal pancreatogram. Gastrointest Endosc 2003;57:483–91.
30. Wehrmann T. Long-term results (≥ 10 years) of endoscopic therapy for sphincter of Oddi dysfunction in patients with acute recurrent pancreatitis. Endoscopy 2011;43:202–7.
31. Wehrmann T, Schmitt TH, Arndt A, et al. Endoscopic injection of botulinum toxin in patients with recurrent acute pancreatitis caused by/because of pancreatic sphincter of Oddi dysfunction. Aliment Pharmacol Ther 2000;14:1469–77.
32. Kanth R, Samji NS, Inaganti A, et al. Endotherapy in symptomatic pancreas divisum: a systematic review. Pancreatology 2014;14(4):244–50.
33. Roberts JR, Romagnuolo J. Endoscopic therapy for acute recurrent pancreatitis. Gastrointest Endosc Clin North Am 2013;23:803–19.
34. Bertin C, Pelletier AL, Vullierme MP, et al. Pancreas divisum is not a cause of pancreatitis by itself but acts as a partner of genetic mutations. Am J Gastroenterol 2012;107:311–7.
35. Attwell A, Borak G, Hawes R, et al. Endoscopic pancreatic sphincterotomy for pancreas divisum by using a needle-knife or standard pull-type technique: safety and reintervention rates. Gastrointest Endosc 2006;64:705–11.
36. Lans JI, Geenen JE, Johanson JF, et al. Endoscopic therapy in patients with pancreas divisum and acute pancreatitis: a prospective, randomized, controlled clinical trial. Gastrointest Endosc 1992;38:430–4.
37. Romagnuolo J, Durkalski V, Fogel EI, et al. Mo1427 outcomes after minor papilla endoscopic sphincterotomy (MPES) for unexplained acute pancreatitis and pancreas divisum: final results of the multicenter prospective FRAMES (frequency of recurrent acute pancreatitis after minor papilla endoscopic sphincterotomy) study. Gastrointest Endosc 2013;77:AB379.
38. Chacko LN, Chen YK, Shah RJ. Clinical outcomes and nonendoscopic interventions after minor papilla endotherapy in patients with symptomatic pancreas divisum. Gastrointest Endosc 2008;68:667–73.

39. Mariani A. Outcome of endotherapy for pancreas divisum in patients with acute recurrent pancreatitis. World J Gastroenterol 2014;20:17468.
40. Michailidis L. The efficacy of endoscopic therapy for pancreas divisum: a meta-analysis. Ann Gastroenterol 2017. https://doi.org/10.20524/aog.2017.0159.
41. Siegel JH, Ben-Zvi JS, Pullano W, et al. Effectiveness of endoscopic drainage for pancreas divisum: endoscopic and surgical results in 31 patients. Endoscopy 1990;22:129–33.

Systematic Review of Endoscopic Cyst Gastrostomy

Steven Shamah, MD[a], Patrick I. Okolo III, MD, MPH[b],*

KEYWORDS

- Pancreatic fluid collection • WOPN • LAMs • Cyst gastrostomy • Necrosis
- Necrosectomy • Pseudocyst

KEY POINTS

- Accurate typification of fluid collection is paramount, as it allows accurate prediction of endoscopic outcome and clinical course.
- Endoscopic ultrasound has become the main therapeutic option for cyst gastrostomy/duodenostomy formation with lower morbidity and higher resolution rates than surgical interventions.
- Pseudocysts without solid debris can be safely and effectively drained using plastic stent placement over the current trend of metal stent insertion.
- Transpapillary drainage may be indicated only if cross-sectional imaging suggests pancreatic duct disruption.
- With the advent of lumen-apposing metal stents, repeated necrosectomy can be carried out, thereby increasing resolution rates of walled-off necrosis.

INTRODUCTION

Since the original description of pancreatic fluid collection (PFC) in 1761 by Morgagni,[1] the diagnosis, description, and management have continued to evolve. The mainstay of therapy for symptomatic PFCs has been the creation of a communication between a PFC and the stomach (duodenum, jejunum), to enable drainage. Surgical creation of these drainage conduits (cyst gastrostomy, duodenostomy, or jejunostomy) had been the gold standard of therapy; however, there has been a paradigm shift in recent years with an increasing role of endoscopic drainage. The techniques of endoscopic

Neither of the above authors have any conflicts of interest or financial incentives to declare.
a University of Chicago Medical Center, CERT Division, 5700 South Maryland Avenue, MC 8043, Chicago, IL 60637, USA; b Division of Gastroenterology, Lenox Hill Hospital, 100 East 77th Street, 2nd Floor, New York, NY 10075, USA
* Corresponding author.
E-mail address: pokolo@northwell.edu

Gastrointest Endoscopy Clin N Am 28 (2018) 477–492
https://doi.org/10.1016/j.giec.2018.06.002
1052-5157/18/© 2018 Elsevier Inc. All rights reserved.

giendo.theclinics.com

drainage have evolved from blind fluid aspiration to include endoscopic necrosectomy and the placement of lumen-apposing metal stents (LAMS).

REVISED ATLANTA CLASSIFICATION

The Atlanta Classification, originally published in 1992, attempted to offer a global consensus on the classification of acute pancreatitis and PFCs. Understanding that treatment success may differ based on the type of fluid collection, changes to the classification were made in 2012.[2]

The distinction between the 2 forms of acute pancreatitis, interstitial and necrotizing, discerned by cross-sectional imaging, remained. Additional discriminators in the revised classification were the categorizations of PFC in relation to time of onset of symptoms as well as the presence or absence of necrosis within the collection. In a patient who may be classified as having interstitial edematous pancreatitis, a collection that develops less than 4 weeks after symptom onset would be considered an acute PFC and more than 4 weeks a pseudocyst. In a patient with necrosis present, early collections less than 4 weeks are acute necrotic collections (ANC) and more than 4 weeks can be considered walled-off necrosis (WON or WOPN).[2]

The distinction about timing of development also helps delineate the timing of drainage, if indicated. If drainage of a PFC is required, it should be undertaken after at least 4 weeks to allow for encapsulation potentially reducing the risk of adverse events. A study of 242 patients found that mortality was reduced as the time from hospital admission to intervention of the PFC was increased (0–14 days: 56% to >29 days: 15%; $P<.001$).[3]

Approximately 10% to 20% of patients with acute pancreatitis will develop pancreatic necrosis. A third of these patients will become infected.[2,3] There is no clear correlation among the extent of necrosis, the risk of infection, and duration of symptoms.[4] Although it may be difficult to differentiate between ANC and acute PFC at initial presentation, sequential imaging may be useful to characterize the evolution or stability of these acute collections. ANCs may appear loculated, with variable amounts of debris within the fluid. Although acute PFCs appear more homogeneous, WON, which appears more than 4 weeks after the initial pancreatitis, typically will have a mature enhancing wall formed from reactive tissue. These distinctions allow for proper classification of PFCs.[2]

Accurate typification of fluid collection is paramount, as it allows accurate prediction of endoscopic outcome and clinical course. A study of 211 patients who underwent endoscopic drainage of PFCs noted that pseudocysts have a higher drainage success rate and a lower adverse event rate than those patients with WON (93.5% vs 63.2%, $P<.0001$, and 15.8% vs 5.2%, $P = .02$, respectively).[5]

INDICATIONS FOR CYST GASTROSTOMY

Most acute PFCs will remain sterile and resolve spontaneously without intervention. As such, PFCs of recent onset that lack a mature encapsulation should not be drained. These collections are considered high risk for peritoneal spillage if drainage is attempted, thus should be managed expectantly. ANCs carry similar risk of adverse event if drainage is carried out before the development of a mature enhancing wall. Overall, the risk associated with the drainage of PFCs decreases with increasing remoteness from the onset of the initial pancreatic injury.[3]

Before considering drainage of a PFC, a thorough radiologic and/or endosonographic examination should be performed. A multimodality approach will help confirm that the PFC does not represent a cystic neoplasm. Cyst neoplasms should not be generally drained and can carry significant morbidity if drained into the gastrointestinal tract.[6] Drainage of PFCs (WON and pseudocysts) causing symptoms such as abdominal pain, biliary or gastrointestinal obstruction, and anorexia warrant drainage. Size alone is no longer an indication for drainage.[7]

Infection in the context of a WON, on the other hand, may be a secondary indication for drainage.[8] In severe acute pancreatitis, disturbed gastrointestinal motility may lead to bacterial overgrowth and failure of the structural mucosal barrier, which leads to bacterial translocation.[9] This is thought to be the mechanism by which WON becomes infected. Clinical symptoms of infected necrosis usually become apparent 2 to 4 weeks after onset of pancreatitis. Signs of infected necrosis include new-onset or persistent sepsis, clinical deterioration despite adequate support and no alternative source of infection, or gas bubbles within the PFC on radiologic imaging.[8] With mortality of patients who develop infected WON approaching 40%, it is imperative that these patients undergo endoscopic or surgical debridement. The optimal approach to these collections is discussed in the next section.

What Is the Optimal Approach to Cyst Gastrostomy Creation?

Surgical approach to cyst gastrostomy

Since the early 1980s, surgery was the gold standard in the management of PFCs.[10] In a cumulative review of 1032 patients, mortality was recorded at 5.8%, with a recurrence rate approaching 5% and a complication rate of 24%.[11] Three main laparoscopic surgical approaches exist: transgastric (anterior) cyst gastrostomy, lesser sac (posterior) cyst gastrostomy, and cyst jejunostomy. Despite improvements in tools and technique, 10% of laparoscopic approaches need to be converted to open procedures.[12]

An anterior gastrostomy is made over the area of maximal bulge by the PFC, usually along the greater curvature of the stomach. An 18-gauge to 22-gauge needle is used to access the pseudocyst and entered into the posterior wall of the stomach. Biopsy of the wall of the cyst is performed to exclude concurrent malignancy. The posterior wall of the stomach is sutured to the pseudocyst and the anterior gastrostomy is sutured closed.[12] A similar approach has been described using intraluminal guidance using an endoscope.[13] Enthusiasm for this approach has been largely tempered by the development of a premature anastomotic stenosis that can be seen following this approach, thus favoring a lesser sac approach.[12]

The lesser sac or posterior approach to laparoscopic cyst gastrostomy has been described as an alternative technique to PFC drainage. Anterior approach necessitates a wide contact surface between the pseudocyst and the posterior gastric wall, lesser sac approach only requires pseudocyst to be in contact with the posterior gastric wall.[12] Several investigators believe that this approach allows for better visibility, less bleeding, larger anastomosis creation, and less premature anastomotic closure.[14]

Cyst jejunostomy is generally reserved for cases in which the pseudocyst is not in close proximity to the stomach. The creation of an enteric-enteric anastomosis and a flexible Roux limb allows juxtaposition of the jejunum to the pseudocyst with minimal tension on the anastomosis.[15] Despite the absence of prospective trials, laparoscopic technique, in comparison with open, offers certain benefits, such as improved pain, decreased length of stay, and decreased wound infections.[12]

Advances in therapeutic endoscopy has pushed surgery to second line, with endoscopy taking center stage, reserving surgery for those patients who fail endoscopic therapy. Although endoscopy and moreover endoscopic ultrasonography (EUS), is just as effective as laparoscopic cystgastrostomy, it has a lower length of stay, cost, complication rate, and recurrence, as noted in a recent prospective comparison between both techniques.[16] Recent advances in EUS resolution and stent design have started to expand the efficacy gap between these techniques, formulating an easier choice of technique.

There does remain one instance in which surgical management may be the initial therapeutic option, which is when a necrotic collection does not abut the gastric/duodenal wall with retroperitoneal extension into the pelvis. Video-assisted retroperitoneal debridement is indicated and preferred in this particular circumstance. Deep necrotic debridement is conducted under direct visualization, while leaving a drain behind for frequent irrigation.[17] This remains the only preferable instance when surgery is indicated over endoscopic management.

Endoscopic approach to cyst gastrostomy
Pre-procedure Anticoagulant and antiplatelet medications (other than aspirin) should ideally be discontinued before endoscopy because endoscopic drainage and necrosectomy have been associated with acute and delayed bleeding. A team of interventional radiologists and surgeons should be available if severe bleeding or uncontrolled perforation should ensue.[18]

Endoscopic drainage techniques
Transmural "blind" approach Transmural drainage of a pseudocyst using a gastroscope involves "blind" puncture technique. The puncture is made beyond the wall at the site of maximum bulge, or cystic compression of the gastrointestinal (GI) tract. The technique does not permit full visual evaluation for presence of vasculature along the trajectory of the puncture needle. In a randomized trial, the use of EUS altered the planned trajectory of the needle in 33% of cases.[19] In another study, EUS was noted to have a higher technical success rate in comparison with the transmural esophago-gastro-duodenoscopy (EGD) approach.[20] Given these results and their generalizability, EUS is preferred and when available should be first-line approach for pseudocyst drainage.

Is endoscopic retrograde cholangiopancreatography needed before the endoscopic ultrasonography approach? Historically, endoscopic retrograde cholangiopancreatography (ERCP) has been an essential part of the algorithm to direct the proper endoscopic approach for drainage, whether transmural versus transpapillary. ERCP enables the identification of the pancreatic duct, a ductal communication or obstruction, which provides a clear correlation with the failure and successes of pseudocyst drainage.[21] As the prevalence of post-ERCP pancreatitis rises to 8% and increases in those patients who may be difficult to cannulate, less ductal manipulation is paramount.[22] With refined imaging techniques and the ready availability of MRCP, noninvasive assessment of ductal anatomy is preferred.[23]

Transpapillary drainage: when is it indicated? Transpapillary stenting of the pancreatic duct (PD) with or without a sphincterotomy had been routinely attempted, as it was initially thought to assist in pseudocyst drainage. The placement of the stent across the papilla offers a path of least resistance to pancreatic secretions and leads them out of the PD, instead of flowing into the pseudocyst through the ductal disruption, if present. Early studies suggested that transpapillary drainage (TPD) combined with transmural drainage offered best chance at successful resolution of PFC, especially if main PD disruption was noted.[24,25] A study in 2010 echoed these results when they assessed 110 patients who underwent pseudocyst drainage, 40 of whom underwent TPD with stent placement. At 8 weeks, those who underwent PD stent placement had better resolution (97% vs 80%) than those who had not undergone TPD.[26]

In a recent retrospective study looking at 375 patients who underwent transmural drainage (TMD) versus combined drainage (CD), which consisted of TMD and TPD, TMD alone was performed in 95 (55%) and CD in 79 (45%) pseudocysts. TMD alone was successful in 92 (97%) versus CD in 35 (44%) and there had been no difference in overall symptomatic resolution (69% vs 62%). Therefore, the investigators concluded based on this recent data set that there was no added benefit of TPD to EUS-guided TMD drainage.[27] As Shrode and colleagues[28] noted in 2013, those and only those patients with radiologic or endosonographic evidence of PD disruption should undergo TPD combined with TMD.

Endoscopic ultrasound–guided cyst gastrostomy or duodenostomy The EUS-guided approach enables direct visualization and approximation of the pseudocyst or WON with access obtained through the gastric or duodenal wall, depending on location of collection. The tract is then dilated and followed by stent placement. Detailed description of the current technique is defined as follows.

A therapeutic linear echoendoscope (with a 3.7-mm working channel) with color Doppler is preferred for the initial assessment and approximation of the pseudocyst.[29] However, puncturing the gastric wall at a sharp angle may impede the technical success of the procedure. The sharp angle coupled with the force exerted on the needle on insertion may push the gastric wall away from the endoscope. The forward-viewing echoendoscope may be used to overcome these physical factors and has been evaluated in several retrospective studies.[30]

Initial assessment of the pancreatic fluid collections The location of the pseudocyst usually can be discerned by endoscopic examination of the gastric cavity and identification of luminal bulge. Using the echoendoscope, the PFC is then examined to confirm the diagnosis, as a homogeneous anechoic structure without septations. This step will also allow for identification of solid debris, which will help decide on the type and number of stents (plastic vs metal) that will be placed and if nasocystic drainage will be needed.

Identification of the ideal puncture site Ideal position is with the gastric wall juxtaposed to the pseudocyst or WON wall no more than 6.0 mm apart without vascular structures in the puncture site, using Doppler flow. If that cannot be obtained, other stations should be assessed to see if a more ideal puncture site may exist in the duodenum.

Puncture with a 19-gauge needle Once the initial assessment confirms that there is no vasculature at the puncture site, a 19-gauge needle is inserted through the instrument channel and under endosonographic visualization, with a quick jab, the needle is introduced through the gastric (or duodenal) wall into the cystic cavity. Once access is obtained, aspiration of fluid should be obtained to confirm diagnosis of pseudocyst and ruling out malignancy with cytology and carcinoembryonic antigen level.[31] If suspicion of cystic neoplasm exists, no further drainage should be carried out. Assessment for infection or hemorrhage by examination of cystic fluid appearance is also helpful.

Passage of guidewire into the cystic cavity Passage of a 0.035-inch guidewire into the cyst, confirmation can be confirmed using fluoroscopy or endosonography. Once confirmed, enough of the guidewire should be passed into the cyst to allow for coiling. The needle is withdrawn, leaving the guidewire in place, bridging the lumen and the cystic structure. If in step 1, multiple stents are deemed necessary for successful drainage, a biliary brush catheter with the brush removed can be used to facilitate multiple guidewire insertion through one puncture site.[32]

Dilation of the tract Balloons of 8 to 10 mm are used to dilate the fistula tract to allow for passage of one or multiple plastic stents (PSs).[33] If larger stents are indicated or being used, larger dilation may be needed. After the initial dilation, one may observe a spurt of cystic fluid into the gastrointestinal lumen. Several variations to balloon dilation exist, namely cystotome,[34] needle knife,[35] modified needle wire,[36] fistulotome,[37] or graded dilators.[38]

Insertion of double-pigtail plastic stent(s) After the tract has been dilated, a double-pigtail stent is passed over the guidewire. One pigtail is then deployed in the cystic cavity with the proximal pigtail in the GI tract lumen, thereby keep the stent anchored in place. Stent size between 7 and 10 French are used to facilitate proper cyst drainage. Although most endoscopists will place more than one stent, there appears to be no relationship between the technical success rate and the number or characteristic of stents used in patients undergoing endoscopic transmural drainage of uncomplicated pancreatic pseudocysts.[39] If a nasocystic drainage catheter is being deployed to irrigate the cavity to remove necrotic debris, then 100 mL of normal saline is flushed until the aspirate is clear.[40]

Repeat cross-sectional imaging Repeat imaging 4 to 6 weeks after stent placement to confirm resolution of PFC. Once resolution of PFC is confirmed on radiologic imaging, EGD may be scheduled for removal of the stents placed. During EGD, Rat Tooth forceps or cold snare can be used to remove each stent that had been placed. No repeat imaging is needed unless clinical deterioration is noted.

Evolution of stent technology: does it matter?
Transluminal drainage is effective only if the fistula tract is kept patent by placement of stents through the tract under EUS, fluoroscopic, and endoscopic guidance. Traditionally, double-pigtail PSs have been used for this purpose, but fully covered self-expanding metal stents (FcSEMS) have been increasingly used instead, and recently LAMS that are specifically designed for PFC drainage have been introduced. With the overall efficacy of transmural stenting with a PS more than 90%,[16] are other stents needed to ensure proper PFC drainage?

Biliary FcSEMS have been added to the armamentarium for the treatment of PFC, both pseudocysts and WON. With their larger diameter (10 mm), FcSEMS offer a larger tract for drainage while needing only 1 stent instead of multiple PSs. Use of FcSEMS also reduces the overall steps of the procedure.[41] Stent migration is still a major complication of the use of FcSEMS. To overcome this risk, stents with anti-migratory fins have been developed.[42] The placement of a double-pigtail stent across a FcSEMS has also been described to prevent stent migration (**Fig. 1**).[43] Despite all these innovations, a recent randomized study failed to demonstrate superiority of FcSEMS over PS for pseudocyst drainage (91% vs 87%, respectively, $P = .97$).[44] A meta-analysis further confirmed these results, looking at 881 patients, noting a similar treatment success rate between PS and metal stents (85% vs 83%, respectively).[45] Without significant increase of treatment success with the use of FcSEMS, the cost and risk of migration, which approaches 15%,[43] does not seem to represent an improvement over current PS technology, and therefore for simple pseudocysts should not be used. On the other hand, FcSEMS do have a role in the treatment success of WON and will be discussed later.

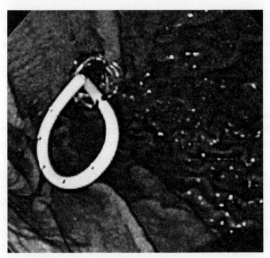

Fig. 1. Cyst gastrostomy with FcSEMS with double-pigtail stent anchor. (*From* Lee BU, Song TJ, Lee SS, et al. Newly designed fully covered metal stents for endoscopic ultrasound (EUS)-guided transmural drainage of peripancreatic fluid collections: a prospective randomized study. Endoscopy 2012;46:1078–84; with permission.)

To address some of the concerns raised by the FcSEMS, LAMS with a unique dumbbell shape, recruits the walls of the collection and the lumen to stabilize the position of the stent. In animal studies before the approval of the stents by the Food and Drug Administration, Binmoeller and Shah[46] demonstrated in animal models that the stent withstood various vector forces without migration. The stent was also noted to be easily removed without tissue damage. The stent is currently approved for the 10-mm and 15-mm diameters, with the 15-mm diameter better for those pseudocysts with necrotic debris (**Fig. 2**).[47]

In 2012, the initial retrospective study that noted clinical success of PFC resolution in all 15 patients who underwent LAMS (AXIOS) placement.[48] Follow-up larger studies noted similar clinical success rates of pseudocyst drainage in 93% of patients attempted, with a complication rate up to 10% to 15%.[47] A similar study was conducted using a NAGI stent in a European cohort noted 93% successful drainage of PFC

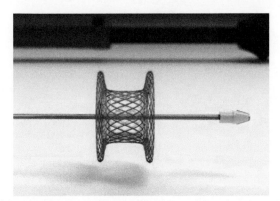

Fig. 2. AXIOS lumen-apposing metal stent. (*Courtesy of* Boston Scientific, Marlborough, MA; with permission.)

(**Fig. 3**).[49] The AXIOS stent is a LAMS approved in the United States, whereas the NAGI stent is approved in Europe, Asia, and the Middle East. Despite impressive clinical success rates and diminished procedure times, should LAMS replace PS in the drainage of homogeneous pseudocysts?[50] Due to cost, complication rate, and equal success rate to PSs, PSs are still favored for homogeneous pseudocysts without evidence of necrotic debris, where repeated endoscopies are not warranted.

Walled-off necrosis

Necrotic fluid collections necessitate both the creation of a cyst gastrostomy (or duodenostomy) and maintenance of the tract for repeat endoscopic debridement procedures. This requirement has become the most actively researched aspect of PFCs. As noted previously, with current stents there exists a disparity between clinical success between pseudocyst and WON drainage (93.5% vs 63.2%, respectively).[5] The advancement in stent technology has helped increase the clinical success rate for WON to 87%.[51]

The steps needed to establish access to WON is similar to those described previously in cyst gastrostomy for pseudocyst drainage. Where the steps differ is with the type of stent inserted to keep the fistula tract open to allow for future endoscopic debridement sessions. Recent data suggest that the use of PSs is insufficient for this requirement.[52] Once the guide wire is in place and the tract is dilated, either an FcSEMS is placed creating the cyst gastrostomy or an LAMS is deployed bringing the 2 lumens together. With FcSEMS reporting high migration rates that seem to be reduced with LAMS, LAMS seem to be a preferred choice for fistula creation in patients who require repeat endoscopic intervention.[52] Following successful placement of an LAMS and observed egress of necrotic fluid (**Fig. 4**), most endoscopists will dilate the stent to its maximum diameter (at either 10 or 15 mm). Current recommendation is to dilate the tract and allow time for the stent to mold to the tissue before performing endoscopic intervention, decreasing risk of inadvertent dislodgement.[53]

Multiple recent studies have demonstrated improved outcomes for the treatment of WON with LAMS, fewer endoscopic necrosectomy sessions required to achieve resolution, reduced surgical interventions, and fewer adverse events. The largest retrospective trial looking at utilization of LAMS for WON was conducted including 17 hospitals between 2014 and 2015. A total of 107 (87.6%) of the 124 patients enrolled in the study obtained clinical success with WON resolution at the end of a 4-month

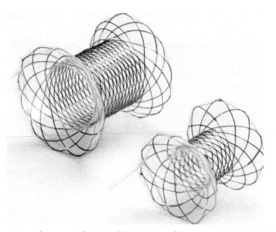

Fig. 3. NAGI lumen-apposing metal stent. (*Courtesy of* Taewoong Medical Co, Gyeonggi-do, South Korea; with permission.)

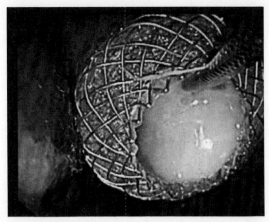

Fig. 4. EUS-guided cyst gastrostomy with drainage of infected collection with purulent debris.

period. Higher resolution rate was noted with the use of 15-mm LAMS then a 10 mm. The adverse event rate was 11.3% for fewer than 30 days after placement and 7.2% for more than 30 days post placement, and this consisted of mostly stent occlusion. Stent migration recorded at 5.6%.[51] Similar data had been published in a mixed cohort of patients, but a subset analysis noted clinical success in 85.7% with WON with use of LAMS.[53] An interim audit in one randomized study has raised some serious concerns; adverse event rate after enrolling 12 patients in the LAMS group was 50%. This consisted of 3 patients with significant upper GI bleeding, 2 patients with buried stent syndrome, and 1 with obstructive jaundice due to CBD compression by stent.[54] Although these are preliminary results, one will have to wait to full enrollment before judging overall efficacy and safety of LAMS in treatment of WON. Based on published clinical data, the use of LAMS for cyst gastrostomy in WON is the most efficacious stent in clinical practice.

Another technique described that may offer a higher clinical success rate is multiple transluminal gateway technique (MTGT), which involves creating multiple transmural tracts, with one reserved for nasocystic lavage (**Fig. 5**). Multiple stents are placed into the other tracts to allow for proper drainage of necrotic debris. A study of 60 patients with WON found that MTGT demonstrated a higher rate of clinical success compared with single orifice stenting, which also included nasocystic lavage (91.7% vs 52.1% $P = .01$).[55] Follow-up study attempted to replicate the results; however, they used the MTGT technique with multiple LAMS. One stent was placed transmurally in the stomach and the second tract established in the duodenum. Reported clinical success rate was 87.1% compared with 91.7% in the single LAMS group.[56] Larger studies will be needed to comment on whether increasing the number of transmural tracts will increase rates of clinical success; however, at this time, this approach incurs a higher cost without offering a higher clinical success to standard techniques.

Necrosectomy

Creation of the cyst gastrostomy is simply an initial step when treating WON. The preponderance of necrotic material within a WON is adherent and not freely mobile, and as such will not drain spontaneously. This is in contrast to the smaller fraction of freely mobile debris that will drain spontaneously via the fistula. Historically, surgical debridement carried up to a 39% mortality, through recent advancements the

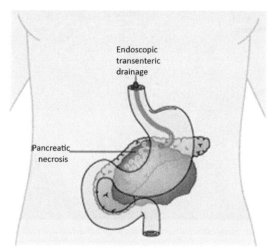

Fig. 5. MTGT. (*From* Varadarajulu S, Phadnis MA, Christein JD, et al. Multiple transluminal gateway technique for EUS-guided drainage of symptomatic walled off pancreatic necrosis. Gastrointest Endosc 2011;74:74–80; with permission.)

mortality has decreased but still remains high at 10%.[12] In 1996, Baron and colleagues[40] described the first series of successful endoscopic drainage of necrotic PFCs. The cavity is entered through the created fistula, preferably with a forward-viewing endoscope, and the necrotic pancreatic tissue is removed from the cavity (**Figs. 6** and **7**). Careful removal of necrotic debris needs to be performed, as the splenic vein and artery course closely to the body and tail of the pancreas, and damage to such structures can cause massive hemhorrage.[57]

Sharaiha and colleagues[51] and Siddiqui and colleagues[53] conducted 2 large multi-center studies that evaluated the utility of EUS-inserted LAMS (AXIOS) to create a cyst gastrostomy. The aim of each study was to evaluate LAMS for necrosectomy in the treatment of WON. A technical success rate of 100% and 85.7%, respectively, was

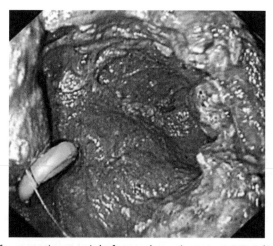

Fig. 6. Walled-off pancreatic necrosis before endoscopic necrosectomy. (*From* Voermans RP, Besselink MG, Fockens P. Endoscopic management of walled-off necrosis. J Hepatobiliary Pancreat Sci 2015;22:20–6; with permission.)

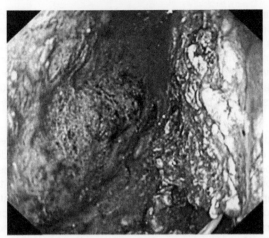

Fig. 7. Walled-off pancreatic necrosis cavity after endoscopic necrosectomy. (*From* Voermans RP, Besselink MG, Fockens P. Endoscopic management of walled-off pancreatic necrosis. J Hepatobiliary Pancreat Sci 2015;22:20–6; with permission.)

noted with a clinical resolution rate of 86.7% and 100%, respectively. The studies prove that the use of LAMS in the setting of WON is both cost-effective and highly efficacious, findings not reproduced with the treatment of pseudocysts.[52,53]

The necessity of debridement has been a longstanding debate. In 2009, Gardner and colleagues[58] conducted a study to examine the difference in WON resolution between active debridement using forceps, snares, and tripods versus just creating the cyst gastrostomy and allowing debris to drain passively. Clinical resolution was accomplished in 88% of the active group compared with 45% of the passive group; concluding that direct endoscopic necrosectomy achieves higher rates of resolution, without a concomitant change in the number of endoscopic procedures, complication rate, or time to resolution.

Another technique to increase clinical success rate in placement of a nasocystic irrigation catheter, this will provide constant irrigation to the cystic cavity. Normal or sterile saline will be flushed through the catheter 100 mL at a time until the effluent returns clear. This may be particularly helpful if the necrosis is infected. A retrospective study examining the difference between nasocystic drainage plus PS and PS alone, noted a higher resolution rate with nasocystic catheter placement (85% vs 63%, respectively), with a lower rate of stent occlusion (13% vs 33%).[59] It is unclear if this will offer any advantage to drainage with use of a large-diameter LAMS. LAMS alone increases resolution by approximately 10% to 15% as compared with PS (95% vs 80%).[60] Two small case series noted that endoscopic irrigation of the necrotic debris with a solution of hydrogen peroxide has demonstrated a reduction in the need for mechanical debridement by breaking up necrotic and devascularized tissue.[61,62]

A small case series described a novel technique to assist with WON cavity closure that has since fallen by the wayside for pancreatic necrosis, but has gained traction in the treatment of postsurgical leaks: an endoscopic-deployed vacuum-assisted closure system using a surgical sponge attached to Salem sump attached to suction.[63] This apparatus is deployed to the cavity after necrosectomy; suction allows for collapse of the cavity and formation of granulation tissue. Downsizing of the sponge every 2 to 3 days allows for stepwise closure of the cavity (see: https://www.bbraun.com/en/products/b0/endo-sponge.html).[64]

Upper GI bleeding is a not infrequent adverse event during endoscopic cyst gastrostomy and necrosectomy for WON, occurring in up to 20% of the procedures. Careful Doppler survey at initial assessment for regional vasculature minimizes bleeding risk. Most of the bleeding events occur during the fistula creation and dilation of the tract and can be controlled with injection of epinephrine, APC, or hemoclip placement. The rate of bleeding has decreased substantially with the introduction of the Hot AXIOS delivery system, which delivers the initial puncture of the AXIOS system with a cutting current.[65]

Outcomes

Pseudocyst Outcomes after attempted drainage of pseudocysts are greatly dependent on the type of collection drained and the expertise of the endoscopist. In the hands of an experienced endoscopist, treatment success ranges from 82% to 100%, with complication rates of 15% and recurrence rates up to 10%.[40,66] A randomized trial comparing 20 patients undergoing surgical cyst gastrostomy and 20 patients undergoing endoscopic cyst gastrostomy found no recurrence in the endoscopic group and 1 recurrence in the surgical group. The endoscopic group had a lower length of stay and a much lower cost ($7000 vs $15,000).[16] Although the new innovative stents marginally increase the clinical success of pseudocyst gastrostomy formation, PS insertion should be favored (90% vs 93%).[16,47]

Walled-off necrosis WON is the more difficult PFC to treat, as the frequent need for repeat procedures for necrosectomy. Historically, what had been a poor clinical success rate of 63.2%, now, with recent innovations in stent structure, has increased the clinical success rate to 87.6%.[5,51] A randomized controlled trial of 22 patients with infected necrotizing pancreatitis found that patients treated with endoscopic necrosectomy had a much-reduced inflammatory response, a significantly reduced incidence of new-onset multiple-organ failure, and a significant reduction in the number of pancreatic fistulas compared with the surgically treated group.[67] The role of LAMS within the meshwork of a multimodality approach may prove to yield the highest clinical success rate and has yet to be defined.

SUMMARY

EUS-guided formation of cyst gastrostomy or duodenostomy has become the mainstay of treatment for symptomatic PFCs or WON. Recent advances in stent design (FcSEMS and LAMS) has allowed for quicker, more effective resolution of WON. These stents also allow for repeat access to gastrostomy cavity for prudent necrotic debridement. Simple PFCs can effectively be drained with the use of double-pigtail PSs. Surgery is reserved for those necrotic collections that do not abut the gastrointestinal tract and may be found in the retroperitoneal space. More randomized studies with larger numbers of patients need to be conducted to further evaluate the role of combined approaches.

REFERENCES

1. Morgagni JB. De sedibuset causis morborum per anatomen indagatis, vol. 4. Paris: 1821. p. 86–123.
2. Banks PA, Bollen TL, Dervenis C, et al. Classification of acute pancreatitis-2012. Revision of the Atlanta classification and definition by international concensus. Gut 2013;62:102–11.
3. Van Santvoort HC, Bakker OJ, Bollen TL, et al. A conservative and minimally invasive approach to necrotizing pancreatitis improves outcome. Gastroenterology 2011;141:1254–63.

4. Besselink MG, van Santvoort HC, Boermeester MA, et al. Timing and impact of infections in acute pancreatitis. Br J Surg 2009;96:267–73.
5. Varadarajulu S, Bang JY, Phadnis MA, et al. Endoscopic transmural drainage of peripancreatic fluid collections: outcomes and predictors of treatment success in 211 consecutive patients. J Gastrointest Surg 2011;15:2080–8.
6. Scott J, Martin I, Redhead D, et al. Mucinous cystic neoplasms of the pancreas: imaging features and diagnostic difficulties. Clin Radiol 2000; 55(3):187–92.
7. Working Group IAPAPAAPG. IAP/APA evidence-based guidelines for the management of acute pancreatitis. Pancreatology 2013;13:e1–15.
8. Van Brunschot S, Bakker OJ, Besselink MG, et al. Treatment of necrotizing pancreatitis. Clin Gastroenterol Hepatol 2012;10:1190–201.
9. Dervenis C, Smailis D, Hatzitheoklitos E. Bacterial translocation and its prevention in acute pancreatitis. J Hepatobiliary Pancreat Surg 2003;10:415–8.
10. Vtas GJ, Sarr MG. Selected management of pancreatic pseudocysts; operative versus expectant management. Surgery 1992;111(2):123–30.
11. Gumaste VV, Pitchumoni CS. Pancreatic pseudocyst. Gastroenterologist 1996; 4(1):33–43.
12. Bergman S, Melvin S. Operative and non-operative management of pancreatic pseudocysts. Surg Clin North Am 2007;87:1447–60.
13. Park AE, Heniford BT. Therapeutic laparoscopy of the pancreas. Ann Surg 2002; 236(2):149–58.
14. Barragan B, Love L, Wachel M, et al. A comparison of anterior and posterior approaches for the surgical management of pseudocysts of the pancreas using laparoscopic cystgastrostomy. Surg Laparosc Endosc Percutan Tech 2002; 12(6):433–6.
15. Texeira J, Gibbs KE, Vaimakis S, et al. Laparoscopic Rou en Y pancreatic cyst-jejunostomy. Surg Endosc 2003;17(12):1910–3.
16. Varadarajulu S, Bang JY, Sutton BS, et al. Equal efficacy of endoscopic and surgical cystgastrostomy for pancreatic pseudocyst: a randomized control trial. Gastroenterology 2013;145:583–90.
17. Logue JA, Carter CR. Minimally invasive necrosectomy techniques in severe acute pancreatitis: role of percutaneous necrosectomy and video assisted retroperitoneal debridement. Gastroenterol Res Pract 2015;2015:693040.
18. Acosta RD, Abraham NS, Chandrasekhara V, et al, ASGE Standards of Practice Committee. Management of antithrombotic agents for endoscopic procedures. Gastrointest Endosc 2016;83:3–16.
19. Khahelah M, Shami VM, Conaway MR, et al. Endoscopic ultrasound drainage of pancreatic pseudocyst: a prospective comparison with conventional endoscopic drainage. Endoscopy 2006;38:355–9.
20. Vadarajulu S, Christein JD, Tamhane A, et al. Prospective randomized trial comparing EUS and EGD for transmural drainage of pancreatic pseuodcysts (with videos). Gastrointest Endosc 2008;68:1102–11.
21. Nealon WH, Walser E. Main PD anatomy can direct choice of modality for drainage of pancreatic pseudocysts (surgery versus percutaneous). Ann Surg 2002;235:751–8.
22. Wang P, Li ZS, Ren X, et al. Risk factors for ERCP-related complications: a prospective multi-center study. Am J Gastroenterol 2009;104:31–40.
23. Zerem E, Hauser G, Loga-zec S, et al. Minimally invasive management of pancreatic pseudocyst. World J Gastroenterol 2015;21(22):6850–60.

24. Catalano MF, Greenen JE, Schmalz JM, et al. Treatment of pancreatic psedocysts with ductal communication by transpapillary pancreatic duct endoprosthesis. Gastrointest Endosc 1995;42:214–8.
25. Binmoeller K, Seifert H. Transpapillary and transmural drainage of pancreatic pseudocysts. Gastrointest Endosc 1995;42:219–24.
26. Trevino M, Tamhane A, Varadarjulu S, et al. Successful stenting in ductal disruption favorably impacts treatment outcomes in patients undergoing drainage of peripancreatic fluid collections. J Gastroenterol Hepatol 2010; 25:526–31.
27. Yang D, Amin S, Gonazalez S, et al. Transpapillary drainage has no added benefit on treatment outcomes in patients undergoing EUS drainage of pseudo-cyst. Gastrointest Endosc 2016;83:720–9.
28. Shrode CW, Macdonough P, Gaidhane M, et al. Multi-modality endoscopic treat-ment of pancreatic duct disruption with stenting and pseudocyst drainage: how efficacious is it? Dig Liver Dis 2013;45:129–33.
29. Antillon MR, Shah RJ, Stiegmann G, et al. Single step EUS guided transmural drainage of simple and complicated pancreatic pseudocysts. Gastrointest En-dosc 2006;63:797–883.
30. Fusaroli P, Ceroni L, Caletti G. Forward-view endoscopic ultrasound; a systematic review of diagnostic and therapeutic applications. J Gastrointestin Liver Dis 2011; 20:216–7.
31. Hun Oh S, Lee JK, Lee KT, et al. The combination of cyst fluid carcinoembryonic antigen, cytology and viscosity increase the diagnostic accuracy of mucinous cystic neoplasm. Gut Liver 2017;11(2):283–9.
32. Khasab MA, Lennon AM, Singh VK, et al. Endoscopic ultrasound (EUS) guided pseudocyst drainage as a one-step procedure using novel multiple wire insertion technique (with video). Surg Endosc 2012;26:3320–3.
33. Seewald S, Groth S, Omar S, et al. Aggressive endoscopic therapy of pancreatic necrosis and pancreatic abscess: a new and safe treatment and effective algo-rithm (videos). Gastrointest Endosc 2005;62:92–100.
34. Ahlawat SK, Charabaty-Pishvanian A, Jackson PG, et al. Single-step EUS-guided pancreatic pseudocyst drainage using a large channel linear echoendoscope and cystotome: results in 11 patients. JOP 2006;7:616–24.
35. Azar RR, Oh YS, Janec EM, et al. Wire-guided pancreatic pseudocyst drainage by using a modified needle knife and therapeutic echoendoscope. Gastrointest Endosc 2006;63:688–92.
36. Kruger M, Schneider AS, Manns MP, et al. Endoscopic management of pancre-atic pseudocyst or abscesses after an EUS-guided 1-step procedure for initial access. Gastrointest Endosc 2006;63:409–16.
37. Lopes CV, Pesenti C, Bories E, et al. Endoscopic-ultrasound-guided endoscopic transmural drainage of pancreatic pseudocyst or abscesses. Scand J Gastroen-terol 2007;42:524–9.
38. Ang TL, Teo EK, Fock FM. EUS-guided drainage of infected pancreatic pseudocyst: use of a 10 F soehendra dilator to facilitate double wire tech-nique for initial gastric access (with videos). Gastrointest Endosc 2008;68: 192–4.
39. Bang JY, Wilcox CM, Trevino JM, et al. Relationship between stent characteristics and treatment outcomes in endoscopic transmural drainage of uncomplicated pseudocysts. Surg Endosc 2014;28:2877–83.
40. Baron TH, Thaggard WG, Morgan DE, et al. Endoscopic therapy for organized pancreatic necrosis. Gastroenterology 1996;111:755–64.

41. Talreja JP, Shami VM, Ku J, et al. Transenteric drainage of pancreatic fluid collections with fully covered self-expanding stents (with video). Gastrointest Endosc 2008;68:1199–203.
42. Raijman I, Tarnasky PR, Patel S, et al. Endoscopic drainage of pancreatic fluid collections using a fully covered expandable metal stent with antimigratory fins. Endosc Ultrasound 2015;4:213–8.
43. Penn DE, Draganov PV, Wagh MS, et al. Prospective evaluation of the use of fully covered self-expanding metal stents for EUS-guided transmural drainage of pancreatic pseudocysts. Gastrointest Endosc 2012;76:679–84.
44. Lee BU, Song TJ, Lee SS, et al. Newly designed fully covered metal stents for endoscopic ultrasound (EUS)-guided transmural drainage of peripancreatic fluid collections: a prospective randomized study. Endoscopy 2012;46:1078–84.
45. Bang JY, Hawes R, Bartoluci A, et al. Efficacy of metal and plastic stents for transmural drainage of pancreatic fluid collections: a systematic review. Dig Endosc 2015;27:486–98.
46. Binmoeller K, Shah J. A novel lumen apposing stent for transluminal drainage of non-adherent extra-luminal fluid collections. Endoscopy 2011;43:337–42.
47. Shah RJ, Shah JN, Waxman I, et al. Safety and efficacy of EUS guided drainage of pancreatic fluid collections. Clin Gastroenterol Hepatol 2015;13:747–52.
48. Itoi T, Binmoeller KF, Shah RJ, et al. Clinical evaluation of a novel lumen apposing metal stent for endosonography guided pancreatic pseudocyst and gall bladder drainage (with videos). Gastrointest Endosc 2012;75:870–6.
49. Walter D, Will U, Sanchez-Yague A, et al. Novel lumen apposing metal stent for EUS guided drainage of pancreatic fluid collections. Endoscopy 2015;47:63–7.
50. Gornals JB, De la Serna-Higuera C, Sanchez-Yague A, et al. Endosonography guided drainage of pancreatic fluid collections with an novel lumen apposing stent. Surg Endosc 2013;27:1428–34.
51. Sharaiha R, Tyberg A, Khashab M, et al. Endoscopic therapy with LAM is safe and effective with pancreatic walled off necrosis. Clin Gastroenterol Hepatol 2017;14:1797–803.
52. Voermans RP, Besselink MG, Fockens P. Endoscopic management of walled-off pancreatic necrosis. J Hepatobiliary Pancreat Sci 2015;22:20–6.
53. Siddiqui AA, Adler D, Nieto J, et al. EUS guided drainage of peripancreatic fluid collections and necrosis using a novel lumen apposing metal stent; a large retrospective multi-center US experience. Gastrointest Endosc 2016;4:699–707.
54. Bang J, Hasan M, Navaneethan L, et al. Lumen-apposing metal stents (LAMS) for pancreatic fluid collection drainage. GUT 2016.
55. Varadarajulu S, Phadnis MA, Christein JD, et al. Multiple transluminal gateway technique for EUS-guided drainage of symptomatic walled off pancreatic necrosis. Gastrointest Endosc 2011;74:74–80.
56. Kerdsirichairat T, Amateau S, Mallery S, et al. Outcomes of multiple gateway versus single gateway transluminal endoscopic drainage and necrosectomy in patients with necrotizing pancreatitis and walled off necrosis (WON) using lumen apposing metal stents: results from an endoscopic step up approach cohort. Gastro Endosc 2017;85:AB98.
57. Gardner TB, Coelho-Prabhu N, Grodon SR, et al. Direct endoscopic necrosectomy for the treatment of walled off pancreatic necrosis: results from a multicenter US case series. Gastrointest Endosc 2011;73:718–26.
58. Gardner TB, Chahal P, Papachristou GI, et al. A comparison of direct endoscopic necrosectomy with transmural endoscopic drainage for the treatment of walled off pancreatic necrosis. Gastrointest Endosc 2009;69:1085–94.

59. Siddiqui AA, Dewitt JM, Strongin A, et al. Outcomes of EUS-guided drainage of debris-containing pancreatic pseudocysts by using combined endoprosthesis and a nasocystic drain. Gastrointest Endosc 2013;75:589–95.

60. Siddiqui AA, Kowalski TE, Loren DE, et al. Fully covered self-expanding metal stents versus lumen apposing fully covered self-expanding metal stent versus plastic stents for endoscopic drainage of pancreatic walled off necrosis: clinical outcomes and success. Gastrointest Endosc 2017;85:758–65.

61. Siddiqui AA, Easler J, Strongin A, et al. Hydrogen peroxide-assisted endoscopic necrosectomy for walled-off pancreatic necrosis: a dual center pilot experience. Dig Dis Sci 2014;59:687–90.

62. Abdelhafez M, Elnegouly M, Hasab Allah MS, et al. Transluminal retroperitoneal endoscopic necrosectomy with the use of hydrogen peroxide and without external irrigation: a novel approach for the treatment of walled-off pancreatic necrosis. Surg Endosc 2013;27:3911–20.

63. Kuehn F, Loske G, Schiffman L, et al. Endoscopic vacuum therapy of various defects of the upper gastrointestinal tract. Surg Endosc 2017;31(9):3449–58.

64. Wedemeyer J, Kubicka S, Lankisch TO, et al. Transgastrically placed endoscopic vacuum-assisted closure system as an addition to transgastric necrosectomy in necrotizing pancreatitis. Gastrointest Endosc 2012;76(6):123841.

65. Ryan BM, Vekatachalapathy SV, Huggett MT, et al. Safety of lumen-apposing metal stents (LAMS) for pancreatic fluid collection drainage. Gut 2017. https://doi.org/10.1136/gutjnl-2016-313388.

66. Beckingham IJ, Krige JE, Bornman PC, et al. Long term outcome of endoscopic drainage of pancreatic pseudocysts. Am J Gastroenterol 1999;94:71–4.

67. Bakker OJ, van Santvoort HC, van Brunschot S, et al. Endoscopic transgastric vs surgical necrosectomy for infected necrotizing pancreatitis: a randomized trial. JAMA 2012;307:1053–61.

Management of Autoimmune Pancreatitis

Kamraan Madhani, MD[a,b], James J. Farrell, MD[c],*

KEYWORDS

- Autoimmune pancreatitis • Lymphoplasmacytic sclerosing pancreatitis
- Idiopathic duct centric pancreatitis • IgG-4 • Corticosteroids • Immunomodulator
- Azathioprine • Rituximab

KEY POINTS

- Autoimmune pancreatitis (AIP) can affect the pancreas primarily; however, it can also present as part of a systemic disease related to IgG-4.
- AIP is primarily a histologic diagnosis; however, currently AIP is diagnosed using clinical characteristics.
- The mainstay of therapy for AIP is corticosteroids.
- Relapse rates following corticosteroid therapy are high.
- Treatment of steroid-refractory AIP includes immunomodulators in conjunction with steroids, or rituximab.

INTRODUCTION

Autoimmune pancreatitis (AIP) is a disease with characteristic clinical (eg, obstructive jaundice, acute pancreatitis, and abdominal pain), radiological (eg, diffusely enlarged pancreas or pancreatic mass), and serologic features (elevated serum immunoglobulin-4 [IgG-4]) affecting primarily the pancreas with the ability to involve other organs. Given these clinical presentations, the exclusion of pancreatic cancer is necessary before considering the diagnosis of AIP.

The international consensus diagnostic criteria (ICDC) classified AIP as type 1, type 2, and AIP not otherwise specified (NOS).[1] In type 1 AIP, the pancreas is affected as part of a systemic IgG-4–positive disease, also known as lymphoplasmacytic sclerosing pancreatitis (LPSP). Type 2 AIP is characterized by histologically confirmed

Disclosure Statement: The authors have nothing to disclose.
a Department of Medicine, Yale School of Medicine, 333 Cedar Street, New Haven, CT 06510, USA; b Department of Medicine, Waterbury Internal Medicine Residency Program, Waterbury Hospital, Yale New Haven Hospital, Main 3, 64 Robbins Street, Waterbury, CT 06708, USA; c Section of Digestive Diseases, Yale University School of Medicine, Yale Center for Pancreatic Disease, Yale University, LMP 1080, 15 York Street, New Haven, CT 06510, USA
* Corresponding author.
E-mail address: james.j.farrell@yale.edu

Gastrointest Endoscopy Clin N Am 28 (2018) 493–519
https://doi.org/10.1016/j.giec.2018.05.002
giendo.theclinics.com

idiopathic duct centric pancreatitis (IDCP) often with granulocytic epithelial lesions (GELs) with or without granulocytic acinar inflammation along with absent (0–10 cells/high-power field [HPF]) IgG-4–positive cells, and without systemic involvement. There is a strong association between AIP and other immune-mediated diseases, including IgG-4–associated cholangitis (IAC), salivary gland disorders, mediastinal fibrosis, retroperitoneal fibrosis, tubulointerstitial disease, and inflammatory bowel disease (IBD).

Multiple pathophysiological mechanisms for AIP have been proposed, including it being an autoimmune disorder demonstrated by the predominance of immune cells, including B-lymphocyte antigen CD 20, into various tissues, including the pancreas, and the characteristic response to corticosteroids.[2] Other associated disease mechanisms associated with AIP include disease susceptibility–related factors, such as human leukocyte antigen serotypes, molecular mimicry, and specific regulatory immune pathways involving regulatory T cells.[3] Recently a drug-induced immune-based pancreatitis has been reported in association with other systemic immune adverse effects, including colitis, in patients being treated with immune check-point inhibitors (ICI), such as cytotoxic T-lymphocyte–associated protein 4 (CTLA-4) and programmed death-ligand 1 (PD-L1) inhibitors.[4,5] Initial experience suggests that discontinuation of the ICI medication with or without steroid therapy may be effective.

Accurate assessments of incidence and prevalence of AIP remain largely unknown, although one study in Japan estimates that the incidence of AIP was approximately 1 per 100,000.[6] The rate of undiagnosed AIP in large cohorts of patients undergoing pancreatic surgical resection of presumed pancreatic cancer is approximately 2%.[7,8] Although most cohorts have described adult patients, there is a growing, although limited, recognition of children who present with AIP, the largest of which reported the average age at diagnosis of 13 years, with presentations similar to type 2 AIP.[9]

Most patients with either type of AIP can be successfully managed with corticosteroid therapy rather than immune modulation or surgical intervention.[10] However, in patients who do not tolerate or whose disease is refractory to steroid therapy, there is an evolving understanding for the role of immune modulation, rituximab, and more invasive interventions.

Although this review article includes discussion of the clinical, radiologic, serologic, and pathologic features useful in making the diagnosis of AIP, this has been discussed in greater detail in another recent review.[11] We will therefore aim to emphasize management strategies for this complex disease.

CLINICAL CHARACTERISTICS
Clinical Presentation

Patients with either type of AIP commonly present with obstructive jaundice, abdominal pain, and/or biochemical evidence of pancreatitis, although those with type I AIP typically present at an older age (on average 16 years older).[12] The study of a large cohort of 731 patients found that obstructive jaundice was the presenting symptom in 75% of patients with type 1 AIP compared with abdominal pain being the most common presentation in 68% of patients with type 2 AIP.[12] The obstructive jaundice may be related to pancreatic swelling and compression of the biliary tree, or due to proximal extrahepatic and intrahepatic duct stricture, which can be part of an associated IAC.[13] The abdominal pain is typically mild and may or may not be associated with documented attacks of acute pancreatitis. AIP is not a common cause for idiopathic recurrent pancreatitis.

Pancreatic Imaging

Pancreatic imaging abnormalities are found in up to 85% of all patients with AIP.[14] Imaging findings range from either diffuse (typical) or focal (atypical) pancreatic involvement, often with evidence of other organ involvement (OOI), including hilar lymphadenopathy, extrapancreatic biliary duct involvement, or renal masses.

Traditional modes for radiographic evaluation have included computed tomography (CT) and MRI; however, ductal imaging with endoscopic retrograde cholangiopancreatography (ERCP) and magnetic resonance cholangiopancreatography (MRCP), transabdominal ultrasound, and endoscopic ultrasound (EUS) have relevant roles in the evaluation of AIP.

Typical features suggestive of AIP on CT or MRI are diffuse parenchymal enlargement (sausage shape) with delayed enhancement sometimes associated with rimlike enhancement (low attenuation halo) (**Fig. 1**).[15] Indeterminate or atypical imaging of the pancreas includes segmental or focal enlargement with delayed enhancement, which should prompt investigation for alternative diagnosis, such as pancreatic cancer.[1] Rarely, peripancreatic vascular involvement is described, which can be confused with features of locally advanced pancreatic malignancy.[14,16]

It may be difficult to distinguish AIP from pancreatic cancer on imaging alone. A recent prospective study with 3 radiologists independently comparing 32 patients with AIP with a control population of patients with pancreatic adenocarcinoma based on CT imaging features, found that the most common findings seen on CT in patients with AIP were common bile duct stricture (63%), bile duct wall hyperenhancement (47%), and diffuse parenchymal enlargement (41%). Conversely, in the control population of patients with pancreatic ductal adenocarcinoma, the most common features were focal mass (78%) and pancreatic ductal dilatation (69%). In the 10 patients with pathologically confirmed AIP, a misdiagnosis of pancreatic adenocarcinoma was made based on the presence of a focal mass, which was seen in 9 patients (90%).[17]

Ductal imaging with either ERCP and MRCP can provide limited collateral evidence in diagnosing AIP in cases in which parenchymal imaging is noncontributory. Typical features on ERCP are long or multiple strictures of the pancreatic duct without marked upstream dilatation[1,18] (**Fig. 2**). Similarly, a focal stricture of the proximal or distal common bile duct (CBD) or irregular narrowing of the intrahepatic ducts can be found due

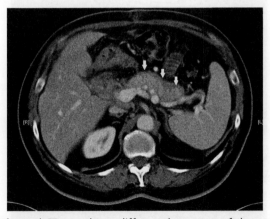

Fig. 1. Contrast-enhanced CT scan shows diffuse enlargement of the pancreas with sharp borders and minimal peripancreatic stranding (*arrows*). The hypoenhancing rim "the halo" is strongly suggestive of autoimmune pancreatitis.

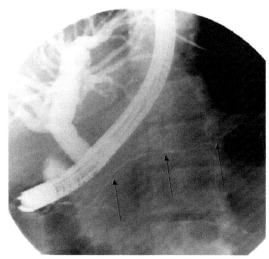

Fig. 2. ERCP shows focal stricture in distal CBD with diffuse narrowing of PD without upstream dilatation (*arrows*).

to the association with IAC. Stenosis that extends beyond the lower bile duct in to extrahepatic and even intrahepatic biliary tree may require further consideration of serology (eg, IgG-4), age of onset, and liver biopsy, to differentiate from primary sclerosing cholangitis (PSC) or cholangiocarcinoma.[19]

Ultrasound has also been used to evaluate the parenchyma of the pancreas in patients presenting with pancreatic mass (**Fig. 3**).[16,20] Abdominal ultrasound, with contrast enhancement where available, is often a useful and inexpensive initial diagnostic study for patients presenting with a pancreatic mass.[21] In a study comparing characterization using contrast-enhanced ultrasound on focal pancreatic mass

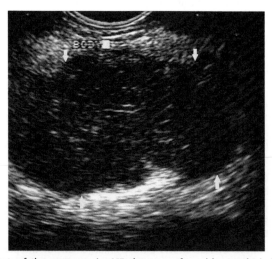

Fig. 3. EUS imaging of the pancreas in AIP shows profound hypoechoic infiltration of the pancreas body. Normal-sized PD shown (*arrows*).

lesions in patients with histologically confirmed AIP, as well as in patients with pancreatic ductal adenocarcinoma, lesions in AIP were consistently iso-enhancing in arterial phase and hyperenhancing or iso-enhancing during late phase compared with those in pancreatic ductal adenocarcinoma, which were hypoenhancing throughout.[22]

On EUS, imaging features include diffuse hypoechoic pancreatic enlargement in 57% of cases and a focal, irregular hypoechoic mass in the remaining 43%.[16] EUS can also be used to evaluate the pancreatic parenchyma as well as bile and pancreatic ducts. One study suggests that EUS imaging can be used to differentiate between AIP and malignancy by considering the length of dilatation of the main pancreatic duct (PD) (>3 mm), paired with level of carbohydrate antigen (CA) 19–9, and the presence of a capsule-like rim sign.[23,24] Details about the role of EUS guided biopsy in the diagnosis of AIP will be discussed in the section on histology.

Serology

IgG-4 typically accounts for less than 5% of the total serum IgG in healthy individuals and is typically less than 140 mg/dL. Elevations in IgG-4 or serum antinuclear antibody (ANA) levels can be expected in patients with AIP, with some cohorts demonstrating IgG-4 levels ≥10 times the upper limit of normal.[1,25]

By evaluating patients with AIP and comparing them with age-matched and sex-matched patients who were healthy, the median IgG-4 level in patients with AIP was 663 mg/dL compared with 51 mg/dL in healthy patients.[25] In a separate cohort, 45 patients with AIP had a mean serum IgG-4 of 550 mg/dL compared with 69.5 mg/dL among 135 patients with pancreatic cancer.[26] Furthermore, serum IgG-4 levels were found to be elevated in 13 (10%) of 135 of the patients with pancreatic cancer but only 1% of this group had IgG-4 level >280 mg/dL compared with 53% of the AIP subset. An IgG-4 level greater than 280 mg/dL (level 1 evidence per ICDC guidelines) corresponds with a sensitivity and specificity of 53% and 99%, respectively, whereas IgG-4 level >140 mg/dL (level 2 evidence per ICDC guidelines) has sensitivity and specificity of 76% and 93%, respectively. It is agreed that although significant IgG-4 elevation can be seen rarely in conditions such as pancreatic cancer, chronic pancreatitis, primary biliary cirrhosis, PSC, and Sjogren syndrome, the levels of elevation seen compared with AIP are striking (**Fig. 4**).[25] In contrast to type 1 AIP, IgG-4 levels are not well correlated with type 2 AIP and are traditionally not elevated in this condition. Other antibodies measured in patients with AIP, including anti-plasminogen-binding protein, carbonic anhydrase II antigen, and lactoferrin, do not have the sufficient sensitivity and specificity to separate out patients with AIP from pancreatic malignancy.[27–29]

Other Organ Involvement

Given the growing body of evidence supporting type 1 AIP as a manifestation of IgG-4–related disease (IgG4-RD), a significant portion of patients with AIP have some degree of extrapancreatic involvement.[30] More common extrapancreatic manifestations include involvement of the lacrimal and salivary glands and retroperitoneal fibrosis, with involvement of biliary tree, kidneys, pituitary, and prostate also described (**Table 1**).[30,31] This is in contrast to type 2 AIP, which carries a characteristically strong association with IBD, although not exclusively.[32] On histologic evaluation, extrapancreatic organs have marked lymphoplasmacytic infiltration with fibrosis and without granulocytic infiltration, with storiform fibrosis, obliterative phlebitis, or abundant (>10 cells/HPF) IgG-4–positive cells.[1]

Initially, AIP was thought to be associated with PSC; however, the intrahepatic and extrahepatic biliary tract abnormalities with stricture seen in AIP are most often related

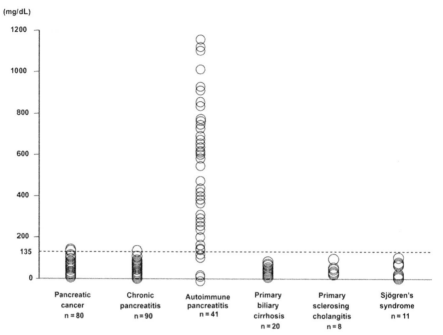

Fig. 4. Scattergram of serum IgG-4 values in various conditions, including AIP. (*From* Hamano H, Kawa S, Horiuchi A, et al. High serum IgG4 concentrations in patients with sclerosing pancreatitis. N Engl J Med 2001;344(10):735; with permission.)

to an IAC, often with associated elevations of serum IgG-4. PSC biliary strictures are typically bandlike with a beaded or pruned appearance, whereas those seen in IAC are typically segmental, long strictures with a prestenotic dilatation, and more commonly seen in the distal CBD. In addition, AIP-related biliary strictures are more likely to

Table 1
Prevalence of extrapancreatic lesions complicating AIP

Organ	No. of Cases	Frequency, %
Total extrapancreatic lesions	83/90	92.2
Lacrimal or salivary gland	38/80	47.5
Hilar lymph node (CT)	54/69	78.3
Hilar lymph node (Ga-67 scintigraphy)	60/80	75.0
Lung	25/46	54.3
Bile duct	63/81	77.8
Peripancreatic or para-aortic lymph node	51/90	57.0
Kidney	13/90	14.4
Retroperitoneum	17/86	19.8
Ligamentum teres	2/90	2.2
Prostate	8/80	10.0

From Fujinaga Y, Kadoya M, Kawa S, et al. Characteristic findings in images of extra-pancreatic lesions associated with autoimmune pancreatitis. Eur J Radiol 2010;76(2):229; with permission.

respond to steroids.[33,34] This distinction from PSC has been confirmed by a pathology study of gallbladders from patients with AIP, PSC, and pancreatic carcinoma. Dense extramural infiltrates were detected in 41% of gallbladders of AIP cases, compared with only 4% of patients with pancreatic carcinoma and 0% in patients with PSC. Additionally, specimens from patients with AIP showed a higher IgG-4/IgG ratio compared with PSC and pancreatic carcinoma counterparts.[35]

IBD is primarily associated with type 2 AIP; however, there are reports of patients with type 1 AIP concurrently diagnosed with IBD. According to a multicenter international study that compared 204 patients with type 1 AIP and 64 patients with type 2 AIP, patients with type 2 AIP were more likely to have concurrent IBD, specifically ulcerative colitis (UC), 16% versus 1%, respectively.[12,36,37] This was confirmed by another multicenter study showing that although most patients with AIP and IBD had type 2 AIP, two-thirds of patients have UC, often with proctitis and one-third of patients have Crohn disease, often with inflammatory features. Patients with IBD and AIP in this study had higher rates of colectomy than patients with IBD alone.[38]

Histology

The characteristic histologic feature of type 1 AIP is an LPSP, whereas type 2 AIP, also known as IDCP, is more classically associated with GELs with or without granulocytic acinar inflammation along with absent (0–10 cells/HPF) IgG-4–positive cells (**Fig. 5**). However, GELs are not entirely specific for type 2 AIP, and may be found in up to 27% of type 1 AIP cases.[39] Additional histologic features of AIP include obliterative phlebitis, storiform fibrosis, and abundant (>10 cells/HPF) IgG-4–positive cells.[1] Level 1 and level 2 evidence (per ICDC guidelines) necessary for making a diagnosis of type 1 AIP includes, respectively, 3 and 2 of the following histologic features: periductal lymphoplasmacytic infiltrate without granulocytic infiltration, obliterative phlebitis, storiform fibrosis, and abundant (>10 cell/HPF) IgG4-positive cells. To confirm a

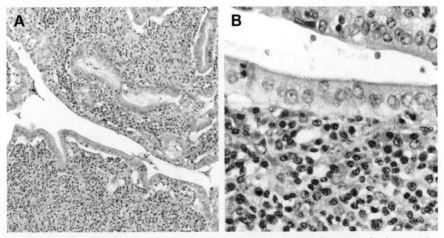

Fig. 5. (*A*) Surgical resection. Photomicrograph showing typical pancreatic findings with a heavy periductal lymphocytic and plasmacytic infiltration around the PDs. There is a lesser degree of neutrophilic inflammation in duct lumens (hematoxylin-eosin [H&E], original magnification ×40). (*B*) Higher-power photomicrograph showing periductal infiltration (H&E, original magnification ×100).

diagnosis of type 2 AIP histologically, both granulocytic infiltration of duct wall (with GEL) with or without granulocytic acinar inflammation, and absent or scant (0–10 cell/HPF) IgG4-positive cells need to be present (level 1 evidence, per ICDC guidelines).

The method of acquiring tissue for histologic evaluation is focused on using minimally invasive methods, such as EUS with core biopsy. There is growing evidence of the ability of EUS with fine-needle core biopsy to obtain at least level 2, and occasionally level 1 histologic evidence to make a diagnosis of AIP (**Fig. 6**).[16,40–42] The finding of lymphoplasmacytic infiltrates with immunostaining for IgG-4 in extrapancreatic tissue also may support the diagnosis of AIP.[43]

Diagnostic Trial of Corticosteroids

Only after pancreatic malignancy has been ruled out should a diagnostic steroid trial be conducted.[1] For a diagnostic corticosteroid trial to be considered positive, a rapid (within 2 weeks) improvement in radiologic pancreatic/extrapancreatic manifestations should be demonstrated in response to a dose of 0.6 to 1.0 mg/kg per day of oral prednisolone administered for 2 to 4 weeks followed by a gradual taper.[44]

The spontaneous resolution of symptoms or radiologic features in patients with AIP in the absence of steroid treatment, which can occasionally be seen, is not considered a diagnostic criterion. Spontaneous relapsing and remitting symptoms or imaging features without steroid administration has been described in the literature, most recently in a cohort of 51 patients with clinically diagnosed AIP, in which a single patient who presented with classic parenchymal imaging for AIP, OOI, and histology ruling against pancreatic adenocarcinoma, had a spontaneous improvement in symptoms without steroid administration.[45]

DIAGNOSIS

Numerous guidelines have evolved to reasonably differentiate AIP from pancreatic cancer preoperatively including Japanese Pancreas Society (JPS-2006,[46] JPS-2011[47]), Korean Criteria,[48] Asian Criteria,[49] HISORt[50] and most recently the ICDC.[1]

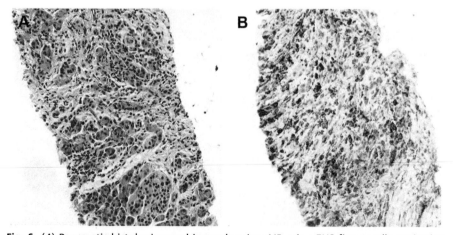

Fig. 6. (A) Pancreatic histologic core biopsy showing AIP using EUS fine-needle aspiration (FNA) biopsy (H&E, original magnification ×40). (B) Pancreatic histologic core biopsy showing IgG-4 immunostaining of plasma cells in AIP using EUS FNA biopsy (original magnification ×40).

Using varying combinations of histology, parenchymal and ductal imaging, serology, OOI, and response to corticosteroids, the diagnosis of definite or probable AIP can be confirmed using criteria stated above.[46-50]

Unlike older criteria, ICDC does not require typical pancreatic imaging to make the diagnosis, instead providing multiple avenues, which can be taken depending on available data, in order to make definite or probable diagnosis (**Table 2**). For example, unlike type 1, the lack of association between type 2 AIP and elevated levels of IgG-4 and OOI requires tissue to confirm the diagnosis of type 2 AIP and to avoid a misdiagnosis of pancreatic malignancy.[1]

The ICDC[1] uses the 5 cardinal features of AIP:

1. Pancreatic imaging of either parenchyma (P) or ducts (D)
2. Serology (S)
3. OOI
4. Histology of the pancreas (H)
5. Response to corticosteroid therapy (Rt)

Validation of clinical diagnostic guidelines including the ICDC is difficult owing to the need for histology to confirm the disease, "the gold standard." However recent validation studies comparing the diagnostic sensitivity and specificity of the major criteria using a cohort of patients with AIP and control groups with pancreatic cancer, showed that the ICDC guidelines[1] have the greatest sensitivity (74.5% to 95.1%) compared with Korean[48] (90.2%), JPS-2011[47] (86.9%), Asian[49] (83.6%), and HISORt[50] (83.6%), as well as the greatest specificity, up to 97%.[39,45,47]

MANAGEMENT
Who Should Be Treated for Autoimmune Pancreatitis?

Even after a definite or probable diagnosis of AIP has been made, constant review of the diagnosis and the possibility of underlying malignancy are important both during and after treatment have been completed. AIP is still a very uncommon disease, relative to more common mimickers, such as pancreatic cancer. Currently there are no subgroups of patients in whom treatment is not recommended; however, treating for isolated elevations in IgG-4, amylase, and lipase levels in the absence of additional information to support a diagnosis of AIP is not advocated.

Several treatment indications and recommendations exist for induction and maintenance of remission, and the treatment of relapse. However, there is a paucity of high-quality data on which to base these recommendations. A therapeutic algorithm has been proposed by the International Consensus for the Treatment of AIP, including the exclusion of malignancy, consideration of corticosteroid use, and immune-modulating agents, as well as relapse instructions (**Fig. 7**).[44]

In addition to helping confirm a diagnosis of AIP in patients who may be asymptomatic and management of symptoms in others, there is growing evidence supporting proactive management of patients with both symptomatic and asymptomatic AIP to decrease risk of relapse and prevent long-term complications, such as impaired glucose tolerance, associated with AIP.[51]

Although a minority of patients with AIP are asymptomatic, consensus guidelines from the international consensus on the treatment of IgG4-RD as well as the International Association of Pancreatology treatment guidelines for AIP published in 2017 recommend that certain asymptomatic patients (eg, persistent pancreatic mass on imaging or persistent abnormalities on liver function testing indicating IAC, asymptomatic lymphadenopathy, or mild submandibular gland enlargement) be initiated with

Table 2
Diagnosis of definitive and probable type 1 autoimmune pancreatitis using international consensus diagnostic criteria

Criterion	Level 1	Level 2
P: Parenchymal imaging	Typical: Diffuse enlargement with delayed enhancement (sometimes associated with rimlike enhancement)	Indeterminate (including atypical[a]): Segmental/focal enlargement with delayed enhancement
D: Ductal imaging (ERP)	Long (>1/3 length of the main pancreatic duct) or multiple strictures without marked upstream dilatation	Segmental/focal narrowing without marked upstream dilatation (duct size, <5 mm)
S: Serology	IgG-4 >2 × upper limit of normal value a or b	IgG-4, 1–2 × upper limit of normal value a or b
OOI: Other organ involvement	a. Histology of extrapancreatic organs Any 3 of the following: 1. Marked lymphoplasmacytic infiltration with fibrosis and without granulocytic infiltration 2. Storiform fibrosis 3. Obliterative phlebitis 4. Abundant (>10 cells HPF) IgG-4-positive cells b. Typical radiological evidence At least 1 of the following: 1. Segmental/multiple proximal (hilar/intrahepatic) or proximal and distal bile duct stricture 2. Retroperitoneal fibrosis	a. Histology of extrapancreatic organs including endoscopic biopsies of bile duct[b]: Both of the following: 1. Marked lymphoplasmacytic infiltration without granulocytic infiltration 2. Abundant (>10 cells HPF) IgG-4-positive cells b. Physical or radiological evidence At least 1 of the following: 1. Symmetrically enlarged salivary/lachrymal glands 2. Radiological evidence of renal involvement described in association with AIP

H: Histology of the pancreas	LPSP (core biopsy resection)	LPSP (core biopsy)
	At least 3 of the following:	Any 2 of the following:
	1. Periductal lymphoplasmacytic infiltrate without granulocytic infiltration	1. Periductal lymphoplasmacytic infiltrate without granulocytic infiltration
	2. Obliterative phlebitis	2. Obliterative phlebitis
	3. Storiform fibrosis	3. Storiform fibrosis
	4. Abundant (>10 cells/HPF) IgG-4–positive cells	4. Abundant (>10 cells/HPF) IgG-4–positive cells
Response to steroid (Rt)[c]	Diagnostic steroid trial	
	Rapid (≤2 wk) radiologically demonstrable resolution or marked improvement in pancreatic/extrapancreatic manifestations	

Abbreviations: AIP, autoimmune pancreatitis; ERP, endoscopic retrograde pancreatography; HPF, high-power field; Ig, immunoglobulin; LPSP, lymphoplasmacytic sclerosing pancreatitis; Rt, response to corticosteroid therapy.

[a] Atypical: Some AIP cases may show low-density mass, pancreatic ductal dilatation, or distal atrophy. Such atypical imaging findings in patients with obstructive jaundice and/or pancreatic mass are highly suggestive of pancreatic cancer. Such patients should be managed as pancreatic cancer unless there is strong collateral evidence for AIP, and a thorough workup for cancer is negative (see algorithm).

[b] Endoscopic biopsy of duodenal papilla is a useful adjunctive method because ampulla often is involved pathologically in AIP.

[c] Diagnostic steroid trial should be conducted carefully by pancreatologists with caveats (see text) only after negative workup for cancer including endoscopic ultrasound-guided line needle aspiration.

From Shimosegawa T, Chari ST, Frulloni L, et al. International consensus diagnostic criteria for autoimmune pancreatitis: guidelines of the International Association of Pancreatology. Pancreas 2011;40(3):354; with permission.

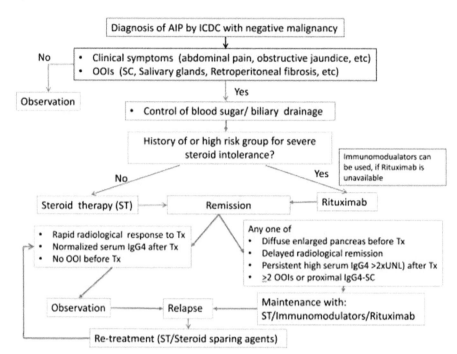

Fig. 7. Therapeutic algorithm for AIP. SC, sclerosing cholangitis; Tx, treatment. (*From* Okazaki K, Chari ST, Frulloni L, et al. International consensus for the treatment of autoimmune pancreatitis. Pancreatology 2017;17(1):5; with permission.)

therapy.[44,52] This is based on the rationale of preventing the progression of pancreatic involvement to a progressive fibrotic stage with possible irreversible pancreatic exocrine or endocrine-associated gland dysfunction, or proximal biliary strictures resulting in infectious cholangitis or irreversible hepatic fibrosis and cirrhosis.[52] Interestingly, the international consensus treatment for IgG4-RD also recommend steroid treatment for subclinical lesions, as these may lead to severe, irreversible manifestations in the kidney, aorta, mediastinum, retroperitoneum, mesentery, and other organs.[52] The other rationale for treatment in asymptomatic individuals is the likely benefit of decreasing the risk of future relapse.[10,53] Although it has been demonstrated that 10% to 25% of asymptomatic patients will experience spontaneous remission without therapy, due to the concerns outlined, it may be reasonable to consider a treatment trial in all asymptomatic patients with either a definite or probable diagnosis of AIP with a view to decrease the risk of persistent or progressive disease, as well as preemptively managing patients who do not resolve spontaneously.[52] If there are concerns about toxicity associated with short-term or long-term use of steroids, often this may need to be balanced with potential benefits in patients with AIP who are asymptomatic.

Patients with AIP exhibiting systemic manifestations indicating pancreatic involvement (eg, obstructive jaundice, abdominal pain, back pain) or OOI (eg, jaundice from IAC, salivary gland enlargement, retroperitoneal fibrosis) should receive treatment for AIP.[10] Studies suggest that those with significant symptomatic disease who are not treated are more likely to develop unfavorable long-term events (eg, obstructive jaundice, pancreatic pseudocyst, sclerogenic changes of extrapancreatic bile ducts, hydronephrosis, or interstitial nephritis).[54]

Even though there are growing data to support treating both asymptomatic and symptomatic patients with AIP, there have been efforts to identify patients in whom spontaneous remission may be seen without the administration of steroids. In a cohort of more than 600 patients with AIP, 97 were assigned to a wait-and-see approach. More than half (55.7%) of this group experienced transient remission. Furthermore, the wait-and-see subgroup was composed of patients who were older and had lower disease activity (eg, lower incidence of jaundice, diffuse pancreas swelling, sclerosing cholangitis [SC], and stent placement).[55] Although no recommendation or consensus advocating withholding steroids exists, some patients with type 1 AIP may experience transient remission without steroid administration, and efforts to reliably identify patients in whom spontaneous remission may be clinically useful.

Caution should also be practiced when considering treatment of AIP in patients concurrently infected with hepatitis B virus (HBV). Administration of immune-modulating agents, corticosteroids, or rituximab can lead to reactivation of HBV. Thus, patients at risk for HBV reactivation should be monitored with HBV DNA during immunosuppression medication use.[56]

How Should Steroids Be Used to Induce Remission?

Often patients with an initial diagnosis of AIP undergo treatment as part of a "diagnostic trial of steroids," which also constitutes their initial treatment if the diagnosis is correct. Incidentally, this also skews the known response rates to steroids in presumed AIP, as a response to steroids is often required to confirm the diagnosis.

For a diagnostic corticosteroid trial to be considered positive, a rapid (within 2 weeks) improvement in radiologic pancreatic and/or extrapancreatic manifestations should be demonstrated in response to a dose of 0.6 to 1.0 mg/kg per day of oral prednisolone administered for 2 to 4 weeks followed by a gradual taper.[1,44,57] The role of a 2-week steroid trial is also valuable in cases in which the diagnosis of AIP is uncertain. In a study of 22 patients with atypical parenchymal imaging for AIP not yet differentiated from pancreatic cancer, the 15 patients who improved after steroids were found to have a diagnosis of AIP, whereas the remaining 7 who did not improve all had pancreatic cancer, supporting the concept that a 2-week steroid trial may be helpful in confirming a diagnosis of AIP, especially in cases that resulted in improvement in narrowing of the main PD and reduction in the size of the pancreatic mass.[58]

Most recommendations advocating for standard dose, 0.6 to 1.0 mg/kg/day of corticosteroids, are based on trials demonstrating exceptional induction rates. This dose has been validated, including by a multicenter national study in Japan, which retrospectively studied a cohort of 459 patients who were treated with 0.6 mg/kg of prednisolone. They recorded a remission rate of 98% among this treatment group compared with a remission rate of 74% of patients who were not treated with corticosteroids.[53] In the international multicenter study, similar high rates of remission were reported (99.6% in type 1 [n = 684] and 92.3% in type 2 [n = 52]). Furthermore, patients with pancreatic and bile duct lesions in the setting of AIP treated medically with corticosteroid therapy compared with surgical intervention have been shown to have effective improvements in these lesions, although up 19% will have recurrences.[59]

Alternative dosing strategies, including lower and higher steroid dosing, and the utilization of pulse-dose steroids have been suggested. However, low-dose prednisone (20 mg/d), high-dose prednisone (60 mg/d), or early utilization of pulse-dose steroids (2 courses of 500 mg/d for 3 days with a 4-day interval) has not demonstrated equal or greater efficacy than standard dosing (30–40 mg/d) at inducing remission or improving pancreatic lesion size.[51,53,54,57,60–63] In these studies, however, it was noted that in patients who received pulse-dose prednisone, there was a significant improvement in lower biliary duct strictures after 2 weeks of treatment.[63] Nonetheless, pulse-dose prednisone is not a standard therapeutic regimen that is commonly used by practitioners worldwide.

How Should Steroids Be Tapered?

The International Consensus treatment recommendation is to administer standard dose steroid therapy for 2 to 4 weeks, then initiate a taper by 5 mg every 1 to 2 weeks while monitoring clinical response (eg, symptoms, IgG-4 levels) and imaging data (eg, ultrasound, CT, MRCP, ERCP).[52] An alternative method for tapering steroids is to taper by 5 to 10 mg/d every 1 to 2 weeks, then to slowly taper down from 20 mg/d by decreasing daily dosing by 5 mg/d every 2 weeks.[52,57] Another acceptable regimen is to administer 40 mg/d for 4 weeks, then taper by 5 mg/wk. Using any of the proposed regimens results in total steroid administration of approximately 12 weeks (**Table 3**).[64] In cases in which rapid and substantial clinical evidence of disease remission is evident, quicker tapering strategies may be used in an effort to minimize the adverse effects of prolonged steroid therapy. Occasionally during a steroid taper, the patient will develop a recurrence of symptoms or progression of imaging findings. One option is to increase the dose of steroids for a period of time and then repeat the steroid taper or to use a pulse-dose strategy.

How Can Treatment Response Be Assessed?

Markers for treatment response include serum IgG-4 levels as well as surveillance imaging monitoring for improvement in pancreatic swelling. Support for the surveillance of serum IgG-4 comes from a study of 12 patients with sclerosing pancreatitis (AIP), in which average serum IgG-4 values was 742 mg/dL before corticosteroid therapy compared with 223 mg/dL after 4 weeks of therapy, suggesting its role in monitoring treatment response.[25,65]

Table 3
Management strategy of autoimmune pancreatitis: comparison of Japanese and Asian countries with American and European countries

Time	0–12 wk	12 wk–6 mo	6 mo-3 y
Japan and Asian Countries			
Objective	Induction of remission		Maintenance therapy
Drug	Prednisolone		Prednisolone
Dose	0.6 mg/kg per day for 2–4 wk, tapered by 5 mg every 1–2 wk to maintenance dose		2.5–5 mg/d
American and European Countries			
Objective	Induction of remission	Maintenance therapy	Observation
Drug	Prednisolone	Prednisolone	Immunomodulator/ rituximab (when relapsing)
Dose	30–40 mg/d for 2–4 wk, tapered by 5 mg every 1–2 wk to a maintenance dose	5.0–7.5 mg/d	Undetermined

From Cai O, Tan S. From pathogenesis, clinical manifestation, and diagnosis to treatment: an overview on autoimmune pancreatitis. Gastroenterol Res Pract 2017;2017:3246459; with permission.

Surveillance imaging can also be used to assess for the likelihood of response to treatment.[57] Radiologic features predictive of a favorable response include diffuse swelling with a halo (ie, a hypo-attenuating rim surrounding the pancreas) on CT, whereas factors predicting a suboptimal response include focal pancreatic ductal stricture and a persistent focal mass swelling after resolution of diffuse changes. Pathologically, it is hypothesized that an early inflammatory phase is associated with a favorable response to corticosteroid treatment, and that a suboptimal response may be associated with progressive irreversible tissue fibrosis.[66]

As mentioned before, a lack of objective treatment response or improvement in symptoms should prompt additional clinical reevaluation, especially to rule out malignancy of the pancreas or biliary tree. This may include repeat pancreatic biopsy to either rule out malignancy or to try to specifically rule in a histologic diagnosis of either type of AIP.[23]

When Should Other First-Line Agents for Induction Therapy Be Considered?

For a small number of patients, steroid treatment will not be a reasonable first-line treatment option due to side-effect profile. Rituximab can be used without coadministration of corticosteroid therapy, and other than corticosteroids is the only other single drug that can be used for induction of remission. The effectiveness and mechanism of action of rituximab support that B-lymphocytes and CD 20 antigen play a central role in the pathogenesis of AIP and has been successfully used to treat patients with IgG4-RD.[67] Although rituximab can be given independently of steroids, in cases with obstructive jaundice, patients may benefit from overlapping steroid therapy, given the delayed onset of action of rituximab.[68] In a study of 12 patients with relapsing disease intolerant of immune-modulating therapy or corticosteroid therapy who were treated with rituximab, 83% achieved complete remission with no relapses while on maintenance therapy with rituximab.[68] However, 25% of patients reported side effects, including a mild infusion reaction and late-onset neutropenia.[68] Proposed dosing includes 2 separate infusions of 1000 mg, 15 days apart, or alternatively, 375 mg/m^2 once per week for 4 weeks.[69,70] This administration has resulted in 77%[70] to 90% of cases demonstrating significant improvement measured using the IgG4-RD Responder Index.[71,72]

Steroid-sparing therapy with immune-modulating agents represent a group of modalities for which no consensus or large trial has demonstrated superiority in maintaining remission compared with continued or repeat corticosteroid administration alone.[68,73] To date, comparative studies among azathioprine, 6-mercaptopurine (6-MP), and mycophenolate mofetil (MMF) are ill defined, with recommendations regarding dosing and duration lacking.[44]

Is Long-Term Maintenance Therapy Beneficial?

To prevent disease relapse in patients considered at increased risk, it may be reasonable to consider proactive treatment with maintenance therapy following a successful course of induction therapy. Patients with otherwise low level of disease activity, defined by lesions isolated to the pancreas without OOI or rapid resolution of symptoms and/or pancreatic mass and/or elevations in serum IgG-4, are more likely to remain in remission without continuation of maintenance steroids compared with patients with type 1 AIP demonstrating diffuse pancreatic enlargement, delayed resolution in radiographic or serologic markers of AIP (eg, IgG-4 level greater than twice the upper limit of normal following steroid therapy), more than 2 OOI, or associated IgG-4 SC before treatment.[44]

Maintenance steroids (2.5–7.5 mg/d) after successful induction of remission appear to decrease the risk of relapse. In one cohort study of 377 patients with AIP following successful induction therapy, maintenance steroids resulted in statistically significant lower subsequent relapses in 23%, compared with a relapse rate in 34% among patients whose steroid therapy had been discontinued.[53,59] However, another study from South Korea reported a higher relapse rate of 33% (13/40 patients) among patients who had previously achieved remission with maintenance steroids.[74] So whereas relapse while on maintenance steroid therapy has been demonstrated to occur less frequently (18%) compared with relapse following steroid discontinuation (67%) or during steroid taper (15%), it does occur and it may occur late.[53] Even in patients treated for at least 3 years without relapse, significant risk for relapse exists following steroid discontinuation as demonstrated among a cohort of 21 patients followed for a median of 43 months, of whom 10 (47.6%) relapsed.[75]

The decision to use long-term steroid maintenance therapy must consider both short-term and long-term side effects. To address these issues, a prospective randomized controlled trial randomized patients with AIP who had achieved remission to either continued maintenance steroid therapy with 5.0 to 7.5 mg/d of oral prednisolone for 3 years or no additional treatment beyond 26 weeks (**Fig. 8**A). Relapse rates in patients assigned to the cessation arm occurred in 57.9% (11 of 19 patients) within 3 years compared with 23.3% (7 of 30 patients) in the maintenance arm (**Fig. 8**B). Patients treated with maintenance therapy relapsed at a significantly lower rate over 3 years and had longer relapse-free survival, without any short-term adverse events from steroid use.[76] Overall, this study suggests that maintenance corticosteroid therapy may decrease relapses in patients with AIP compared with those not treated with maintenance therapy. However, the results of this study have not become widely accepted due to geographic differences in practices and concerns about the study design, including lack of statistical power, heterogeneous treatment options, insufficient numbers to properly identify subsets at increased risk of relapse, and the lack of data relating to the long-term side effects of steroids.[77,78]

Can We Predict Who Will Relapse?

The vast majority of relapses occur within 3 years of starting steroid therapy, as reported by a multicenter Japanese study that followed 99 cases of relapse (56% within 1 year, 76% within 2 years, and 92% within 3 years).[53] A large international multicenter study examined relapse rates among type 1 and type 2 AIP and reported nearly 31% (302 of 978 patients) of patients with type 1 and 9% (8 of 89 patients) of patients with type 2 experienced at least 1 relapse episode, with the timing of relapse being closely related to the discontinuation of steroids, as opposed to relapses occurring during steroid tapering or while on maintenance steroids, which were reported to be 15% and 18%, respectively.[10] Furthermore, overall relapse rates approach a plateau of 70.2% after 8 years (**Fig. 9**).[79] There does not appear to be a dose-related relationship influencing relapse rate, as a study comparing patients treated with 40 mg/d versus 30 mg/d of steroid showed no statistically significant difference in relapse rates between the higher-dose arm (19%) compared with lower-dose arm (23%).[53]

Other parameters that have been implicated in predicting relapsing disease include high level of disease activity, defined by elevated IgG-4 values greater than 4 times the upper limit of normal or persistent elevations despite steroid therapy, extensive extrapancreatic disease including proximal biliary strictures, lack of maintenance steroid therapy, focal pancreatic enlargement, and prior history of relapse (**Table 4**).[44,79]

Persistent elevation in serum IgG-4 values despite corticosteroid therapy has been suggested as a predictor of relapsing AIP by several studies, including a cohort study

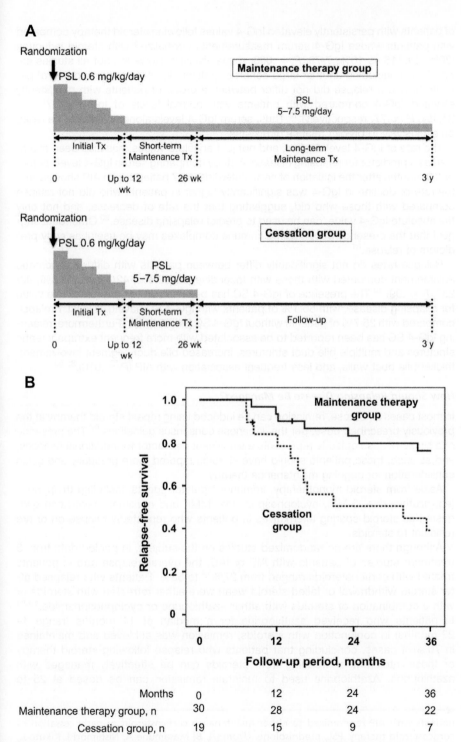

Fig. 8. (A) Trial design of randomized clinical trial comparing maintenance dosing versus early cessation of corticosteroids in induction therapy for AIP. (B) Relapse-free survival in

of patients with persistently elevated IgG-4 values following steroid therapy compared with patients whose IgG-4 serum measurements normalized with steroid induction (30%, 34/115 vs 10%, 7/79, $P = .003$, respectively).[53] However, not all studies are conclusive, including another large cohort of patients in which the proportion of patients having a relapse did not differ between a group of patients with persistently elevated IgG-4 compared with patients with normal levels of IgG-4 (32.7% vs 31.4%, $P = .77$, respectively).[10] Thus, serum IgG-4 levels alone should not be relied on exclusively to predict relapse of disease.

The rate of IgG-4 level decline, and not just absolute values, has also been examined as a predictor for relapsing disease. A study comparing serum IgG-4 levels before and 2 months after the initiation of corticosteroids in 47 patients with AIP showed that the rate of decline in IgG-4 was significantly higher in patients who did not relapse compared with those who did, suggesting that the rate of decrease, and not only the absolute IgG-4 value, can be used to predict relapsing disease.[80] Other data suggest that the presence of circulating immune complexes may be useful as early predictors of relapse.[81]

Relapse rates do not significantly differ between patients with diffuse pancreatic enlargement compared with those with focal disease (32.3%, 42/440 vs 32.3%, 92/285, $P = .99$).[10] The presence of IgG-4 SC has been shown to carry predictive value for relapsing disease, with 56.1% of patients with IgG-4 SC having at least 1 relapse compared with 25.7% of patients without IgG-4 SC ($P<.001$).[10,82] Furthermore, relapsing IgG-4 SC has been reported to be associated with more frequent extrapancreatic strictures and multiple bile duct strictures, increased bile duct segment involvement, thicker bile duct walls, and less-frequent association with AIP ($P = .016$).[82,83]

How Should Relapsing Disease Be Managed?

In most cases of relapse, remission can be induced using repeat steroid therapy at the previously prescribed dose, per the Japanese consensus guidelines.[57] The presence of a single relapse episode represents a significant risk factor for additional relapses, and as such, these patients should have steroids tapered more gradually and given consideration for ongoing maintenance therapy.

Aside from steroid monotherapy, immunomodulator agents, including thiopurines (eg, azathioprine, 5-MP), cyclophosphamide, MMF and rituximab have been suggested as steroid-sparing alternatives in patients who repeatedly relapse on or are resistant to steroids.

Although there are no randomized studies on the subject, in pooled data from 3 treatment studies of patients with AIP or IAC, the overall relapse rate in patients treated with corticosteroids ranged from 27%[14] to 53%. Patients who relapsed after steroid withdrawal or failed steroid wean were either retreated with steroids or with a combination of steroids with either azathioprine or cyclophosphamide.[13,84] In patients who received azathioprine for a median of 14 months (range 1–27 months) in conjunction with steroids, remission was achieved and maintained in 70% of cases, concluding that patients who relapse following steroid therapy or those intolerant of weaning from steroids can be effectively managed with azathioprine. Azathioprine used to maintain remission can be dosed at 25 to

patients with AIP randomized to either maintenance corticosteroid or early cessation of corticosteroid therapy. PSL, prednisolone. (*From [A, B]* Masamune A, Nishimori I, Kikuta K, et al. Randomised controlled trial of long-term maintenance corticosteroid therapy in patients with autoimmune pancreatitis. Gut 2017;66(3):489–92; with permission.)

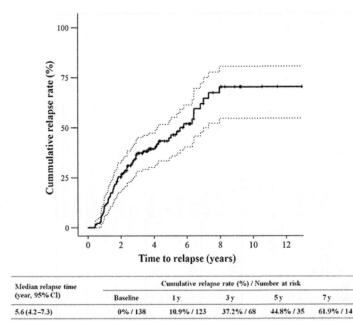

Median relapse time	Cumulative relapse rate (%) / Number at risk				
(year, 95% CI)	Baseline	1 y	3 y	5 y	7 y
5.6 (4.2–7.3)	0% / 138	10.9% / 123	37.2% / 68	44.8% / 35	61.9% / 14

Fig. 9. Timing of relapse in type 1 AIP. (*From* Lee HW, Moon SH, Kim MH, et al. Relapse rate and predictors of relapse in a large single center cohort of type 1 autoimmune pancreatitis: long-term follow-up results after steroid therapy with short-duration maintenance treatment. J Gastroenterol 2018. [Epub ahead of print]; with permission.)

50 mg/d with increases of 25 mg every 3 to 7 days to achieve a target dose of 2.0 to 2.5 mg/kg per day.[85] Contradictory to these studies, a separate analysis of disease-free survival among 116 patients with type 1 AIP demonstrated that disease-free survival was not significantly different between patients treated with combination steroids plus immune-modulating therapy and steroid monotherapy alone ($P = .23$).[68] In addition, azathioprine carries a significant side-effect profile, including pancreatitis, thereby making therapy with azathioprine for AIP confusing, especially in patients who relapse while on this medication. So overall, it has not been demonstrated conclusively that the use of steroids in conjunction with immunosuppressant medications prolongs disease-free survival compared with treating relapses of AIP with steroids alone.[68]

Rheumatologists, in the setting of organ transplantation, IBD, and rheumatoid arthritis, have frequently used MMF given inhibition of T-cell and B-cell proliferation. However, the theoretic role of MMF in the treatment of steroid-refractory AIP has yet to be extensively studied, and sufficient data beyond case reports on safety and efficacy are lacking.[86] Case reports have described patients with AIP who benefit from MMF due to azathioprine-induced pancreatitis, steroid intolerance due to concurrent diabetes mellitus, or consistently relapsing disease with steroid taper. Additional prospective trials are needed before MMF can become a mainstay of therapy for AIP. There are also experimental data (but currently no clinical data) suggesting that cyclosporine A and rapamycin may be more effective than azathioprine as steroid alterantives.[87]

Although there is growing evidence for the role of rituximab in the induction of remission of AIP, there is limited information about its role in the treatment of relapse. In

Table 4
Relapse rates and predictors of relapse in type 1 AIP

Study First Author, Year	Setting	No. of Patients with AIP	Subtyping	Relapse Rate, %	Follow-up Duration, mo, Median	Significant Predictors of Relapse
Kamisawa et al,[53] 2009	Japan, multicenter	563	N-A	24% with steroids 42% without steroids	N-A	No steroid therapy Stopped maintenance steroids Persistent elevation of sIgG4 after steroids
Frulloni et al,[27] 2009	Italy, single center	87	N-A	25	89 (mean)	Focal pancreatic enlargement Smoker Elevated sIgG4
Sah et al,[93] 2010	US, single center	78	Type 1	47	42	Proximal bile duct involvement Diffuse pancreatic enlargement No pancreaticoduodenectomy
Maire et al,[66] 2011	France, single center	44	Type 1 (28) Type 2 (16)	27	41	Elevated sIgG4 (>ULN) No acute pancreatitis Other organ involvement
Hart, 2013	International, multicenter	978	Type 1	31	N-A	IgG-4-related sclerosing cholangitis
Buijs et al,[89] 2015	Netherlands, multicenter	96	Type 1	55	75	N-A
Culver et al,[94] 2016	UK, single center	58[a]	Type 1	58	31	Elevated sIgG4 (>2 × ULN)
Kubota et al,[95] 2017	Japan, multicenter	510	Type 1	31	61 (mean)	No maintenance steroids Diffuse pancreatic enlargement
Lee et al,[79] 2018[b]	Korea, single center	138	Type 1	48	60	Other organ involvement Proximal bile duct involvement

Some cohorts with AIP are mixed with type 2 autoimmune pancreatitis.
Abbreviations: Ig, immunoglobulin; N-A, not available; sIgG4, serum IgG-4; ULN, upper limit of normal.
[a] Patients with IgG-4-related disease (not confined to type 1 AIP).
[b] Data from Lee and colleagues excluding surgically treated patients.

From Lee HW, Moon SH, Kim MH, et al. Relapse rate and predictors of relapse in a large single center cohort of type 1 autoimmune pancreatitis: long-term follow-up results after steroid therapy with short-duration maintenance treatment. J Gastroenterol 2018. https://doi.org/10.1007/s00535-018-1434-6; with permission.

patients with IgG4-RD that remains refractory despite the standard therapy with either corticosteroids or rituximab, there is currently a clinical trial, the TIGR2 trial, investigating the role of combination rituximab with lenalidomide, an immune-modulating agent that may inhibit the secretion of proinflammatory cytokines in AIP, on sustaining disease remission. Data collection and analysis are currently ongoing.

Management of Endocrine and Exocrine Dysfunction in Autoimmune Pancreatitis

As the duration of AIP lengthens, permanent parenchymal fibrosis of the pancreas becomes possible, which can lead to impaired exocrine gland function manifesting with weight loss, fat malabsorption, and fat-soluble vitamin deficiencies. Fecal elastase 1 levels (FE-1) are a proposed marker for developing pancreas exocrine dysfunction as described among a cohort of 21 patients with AIP. With treatment, all patients (100%) demonstrated increased FE-1 levels, although 7 patients (33%) continued to demonstrate manifestations of pancreatic insufficiency (ie, weight loss).[88] In this same cohort, markedly low FE-1 levels (1–19 μg/g in stool) correlated with the presence of diabetes mellitus. Following steroid therapy, only 4 of these patients continued to require insulin therapy for hyperglycemia.[88]

Interestingly, with steroid administration, it may be possible to reverse exocrine and endocrine dysfunction. There has been demonstration of a paradoxic effect of steroid therapy leading to improvement in glycemic control. This was demonstrated in a cohort of 47 patients with AIP and impaired glucose tolerance treated with steroid therapy. Glucose tolerance was improved or unchanged in 81%, concluding that early administration of steroid therapy is preferable given the increased likelihood of recovering insulin secretion abilities of the pancreas.[51]

Management of Cancer Risk

The correlation between AIP and the development of a variety of malignancies, including gastric, prostate, and pancreatic, is not clear. Although some cohorts have reported cases of pancreatic cancer developing in patients with AIP after 1 year, others have not demonstrated any evidence of pancreatic cancer among patients who had been followed for several years for AIP.[89,90] However, it is important to emphasize that both conditions can coexist, and that the exclusion of pancreatic cancer before the consideration for AIP, especially in those who do not respond to corticosteroid therapy, is vital.[10]

When Should Endoscopic Intervention Be Considered?

The management of biliary obstruction represents a unique treatment challenge, seen in up to 63% of patients initially presenting with AIP. In cases with otherwise low disease activity, performing biliary stenting endoscopically has been reported to induce remission in 71% of cases of type 1 AIP without the concurrent use of corticosteroids.[10] This likely reflects the spontaneous resolution of the biliary obstruction during the period of biliary stenting done for management of obstructive jaundice. ERCP performed at the time of biliary stenting also has the benefit of allowing for biliary stricture brushing and biopsy to rule out malignancy.

Alternatively, biliary obstruction associated with type 1 AIP also can be safely managed with corticosteroids without biliary stenting. In a Japanese study involving patients with obstructive jaundice, it was demonstrated that outcomes did not drastically differ between those treated with steroids alone (0.6 ± 0.12 mg/kg per day) compared with those treated with steroids (0.6 ± 0.17 mg/kg per day) in combination with biliary drainage.[53] In one particular North American series, 15 patients with jaundice related to type 1 AIP were all successfully managed with steroids, without the use of biliary stenting. Complete resolution of jaundice biochemically was noted between 15 and 54 days, and there were no cases of cholangitis or other infectious complications during steroid treatment.[91]

When Should Surgical Treatment Be Considered?

Surgical intervention should be considered in the setting of suspicion for pancreatic or biliary malignancy based on masslike lesions or ambiguous imaging.[7,8] However, significant data are lacking, advocating early or routine surgical management of known AIP, instead supporting early prioritization of medical management strategies. Indications for surgical intervention include patients in whom extrapancreatic fibrosis is extensive, and surgical debulking is desired.[57] Additionally, in patients who have repeat relapses despite maximum medical therapy or failed biliary stenting; palliative pancreatectomy can be considered.[44,92]

SUMMARY

Several international groups have evaluated AIP in an effort to produce diagnostic guidelines that can be universally applied by specialists and nonspecialists alike. The ICDC, similar to the preceding guidelines, cite the 5 cardinal features of AIP and draw on evidence from each of those features in the diagnosis of AIP. Other than histologic confirmation, the use of evidence from a single cardinal feature should not be used in isolation and instead should be paired with other evidence, as outlined by ICDC in the diagnosis of AIP.

Although steroids remain the mainstay of treatment for patients diagnosed with AIP, immune-modulating agents in conjunction with rituximab or rituximab monotherapy have been shown to induce remission in those intolerant of steroid maintenance or weaning. Relapsing disease is common, and retreatment with steroids often is sufficient to reinduce remission. In patients not responding to induction therapy, reapplication of diagnostic guidelines and reconsideration of diagnosis is paramount to ensure malignancy is not overlooked.

REFERENCES

1. Shimosegawa T, Chari ST, Frulloni L, et al. International consensus diagnostic criteria for autoimmune pancreatitis: guidelines of the International Association of Pancreatology. Pancreas 2011;40(3):352–8.
2. Pezzilli R, Pagano N. Pathophysiology of autoimmune pancreatitis. World J Gastrointest Pathophysiol 2014;5(1):11–7.
3. Stone JH, Zen Y, Deshpande V. IgG4-related disease. N Engl J Med 2012;366(6): 539–51.
4. Michot JM, Ragou P, Carbonnel F, et al. Significance of immune-related lipase increase induced by antiprogrammed death-1 or death ligand-1 antibodies: a brief communication. J Immunother 2018;41(2):84–5.
5. Ikeuchi K, Okuma Y, Tabata T. Immune-related pancreatitis secondary to nivolumab in a patient with recurrent lung adenocarcinoma: a case report. Lung Cancer 2016;99:148–50.
6. Uchida K, Masamune A, Shimosegawa T, et al. Prevalence of IgG4-related disease in Japan Based on Nationwide Survey in 2009. Int J Rheumatol 2012; 2012:358371.
7. Weber SM, Cubukcu-Dimopulo O, Palesty JA, et al. Lymphoplasmacytic sclerosing pancreatitis: inflammatory mimic of pancreatic carcinoma. J Gastrointest Surg 2003;7(1):129–37 [discussion: 129–37].

8. Hardacre JM, Iacobuzio-Donahue CA, Sohn TA, et al. Results of pancreaticoduodenectomy for lymphoplasmacytic sclerosing pancreatitis. Ann Surg 2003; 237(6):853–8 [discussion: 858–9].

9. Scheers I, Palermo JJ, Freedman S, et al. Autoimmune pancreatitis in children: characteristic features, diagnosis, and management. Am J Gastroenterol 2017; 112(10):1604–11.

10. Hart PA, Kamisawa T, Brugge WR, et al. Long-term outcomes of autoimmune pancreatitis: a multicentre, international analysis. Gut 2013;62(12):1771–6.

11. Madhani K, Farrell JJ. Autoimmune pancreatitis: an update on diagnosis and management. Gastroenterol Clin North Am 2016;45(1):29–43.

12. Kamisawa T, Chari ST, Giday SA, et al. Clinical profile of autoimmune pancreatitis and its histological subtypes: an international multicenter survey. Pancreas 2011; 40(6):809–14.

13. Ghazale A, Chari ST, Zhang L, et al. Immunoglobulin G4-associated cholangitis: clinical profile and response to therapy. Gastroenterology 2008;134(3):706–15.

14. Raina A, Yadav D, Krasinskas AM, et al. Evaluation and management of autoimmune pancreatitis: experience at a large US center. Am J Gastroenterol 2009; 104(9):2295–306.

15. Lee-Felker SA, Felker ER, Kadell B, et al. Use of MDCT to differentiate autoimmune pancreatitis from ductal adenocarcinoma and interstitial pancreatitis. AJR Am J Roentgenol 2015;205(1):2–9.

16. Farrell JJ, Garber J, Sahani D, et al. EUS findings in patients with autoimmune pancreatitis. Gastrointest Endosc 2004;60(6):927–36.

17. Zaheer A, Singh VK, Akshintala VS, et al. Differentiating autoimmune pancreatitis from pancreatic adenocarcinoma using dual-phase computed tomography. J Comput Assist Tomogr 2014;38(1):146–52.

18. Sugumar A, Levy MJ, Kamisawa T, et al. Endoscopic retrograde pancreatography criteria to diagnose autoimmune pancreatitis: an international multicentre study. Gut 2011;60(5):666–70.

19. Nishino T, Oyama H, Hashimoto E, et al. Clinicopathological differentiation between sclerosing cholangitis with autoimmune pancreatitis and primary sclerosing cholangitis. J Gastroenterol 2007;42(7):550–9.

20. Numata K, Ozawa Y, Kobayashi N, et al. Contrast-enhanced sonography of autoimmune pancreatitis: comparison with pathologic findings. J Ultrasound Med 2004;23(2):199–206.

21. De Robertis R, D'Onofrio M, Crosara S, et al. Contrast-enhanced ultrasound of pancreatic tumours. Australas J Ultrasound Med 2014;17(3):96–109.

22. Dong Y, D'Onofrio M, Hocke M, et al. Autoimmune pancreatitis: imaging features. Endosc Ultrasound 2017;7(3):196–203.

23. Sugimoto M, Takagi T, Suzuki R, et al. Endoscopic ultrasonography-guided fine needle aspiration can be used to rule out malignancy in autoimmune pancreatitis patients. J Ultrasound Med 2017;36(11):2237–44.

24. Irie H, Honda H, Baba S, et al. Autoimmune pancreatitis: CT and MR characteristics. AJR Am J Roentgenol 1998;170(5):1323–7.

25. Hamano H, Kawa S, Horiuchi A, et al. High serum IgG4 concentrations in patients with sclerosing pancreatitis. N Engl J Med 2001;344(10):732–8.

26. Ghazale A, Chari ST, Smyrk TC, et al. Value of serum IgG4 in the diagnosis of autoimmune pancreatitis and in distinguishing it from pancreatic cancer. Am J Gastroenterol 2007;102(8):1646–53.

27. Frulloni L, Lunardi C, Simone R, et al. Identification of a novel antibody associated with autoimmune pancreatitis. N Engl J Med 2009;361(22):2135–42.

28. Kim KP, Kim MH, Song MH, et al. Autoimmune chronic pancreatitis. Am J Gastro-enterol 2004;99(8):1605–16.
29. Kino-Ohsaki J, Nishimori I, Morita M, et al. Serum antibodies to carbonic anhydrase I and II in patients with idiopathic chronic pancreatitis and Sjogren's syndrome. Gastroenterology 1996;110(5):1579–86.
30. Fujinaga Y, Kadoya M, Kawa S, et al. Characteristic findings in images of extrapancreatic lesions associated with autoimmune pancreatitis. Eur J Radiol 2010; 76(2):228–38.
31. Ralli S, Lin J, Farrell J. Autoimmune pancreatitis. N Engl J Med 2007;356(15): 1586 [author reply: 1587].
32. Maconi G, Dominici R, Molteni M, et al. Prevalence of pancreatic insufficiency in inflammatory bowel diseases. Assessment by fecal elastase-1. Dig Dis Sci 2008; 53(1):262–70.
33. Nakazawa T, Ohara H, Sano H, et al. Cholangiography can discriminate sclerosing cholangitis with autoimmune pancreatitis from primary sclerosing cholangitis. Gastrointest Endosc 2004;60(6):937–44.
34. Nakazawa T, Ohara H, Sano H, et al. Clinical differences between primary sclerosing cholangitis and sclerosing cholangitis with autoimmune pancreatitis. Pancreas 2005;30(1):20–5.
35. Wang WL, Farris AB, Lauwers GY, et al. Autoimmune pancreatitis-related cholecystitis: a morphologically and immunologically distinctive form of lymphoplasmacytic sclerosing cholecystitis. Histopathology 2009;54(7):829–36.
36. Hamano H, Arakura N, Muraki T, et al. Prevalence and distribution of extrapancreatic lesions complicating autoimmune pancreatitis. J Gastroenterol 2006;41(12): 1197–205.
37. Nishino T, Toki F, Oyama H, et al. Biliary tract involvement in autoimmune pancreatitis. Pancreas 2005;30(1):76–82.
38. Lorenzo D, Maire F, Stefanescu C, et al. Features of autoimmune pancreatitis associated with inflammatory bowel diseases. Clin Gastroenterol Hepatol 2018; 16(1):59–67.
39. Sumimoto K, Uchida K, Mitsuyama T, et al. A proposal of a diagnostic algorithm with validation of International Consensus Diagnostic Criteria for autoimmune pancreatitis in a Japanese cohort. Pancreatology 2013;13(3):230–7.
40. Levy MJ, Reddy RP, Wiersema MJ, et al. EUS-guided trucut biopsy in establishing autoimmune pancreatitis as the cause of obstructive jaundice. Gastrointest Endosc 2005;61(3):467–72.
41. Iwashita T, Yasuda I, Doi S, et al. Use of samples from endoscopic ultrasound-guided 19-gauge fine-needle aspiration in diagnosis of autoimmune pancreatitis. Clin Gastroenterol Hepatol 2012;10(3):316–22.
42. Kanno A, Ishida K, Hamada S, et al. Diagnosis of autoimmune pancreatitis by EUS-FNA by using a 22-gauge needle based on the International Consensus Diagnostic Criteria. Gastrointest Endosc 2012;76(3):594–602.
43. Deheragoda MG, Church NI, Rodriguez-Justo M, et al. The use of immunoglobulin g4 immunostaining in diagnosing pancreatic and extrapancreatic involvement in autoimmune pancreatitis. Clin Gastroenterol Hepatol 2007;5(10): 1229–34.
44. Okazaki K, Chari ST, Frulloni L, et al. International consensus for the treatment of autoimmune pancreatitis. Pancreatology 2017;17(1):1–6.
45. Madhani K, Felker S, Felker ER, et al. Evaluation of international consensus diagnostic criteria in the diagnosis of autoimmune pancreatitis: a single center North American Cohort Study. JOP 2017;18(4):327–34.

46. Okazaki K, Kawa S, Kamisawa T, et al. Clinical diagnostic criteria of autoimmune pancreatitis: revised proposal. J Gastroenterol 2006;41(7):626–31.

47. Maruyama M, Watanabe T, Kanai K, et al. International consensus diagnostic criteria for autoimmune pancreatitis and its Japanese Amendment have improved diagnostic ability over existing criteria. Gastroenterol Res Pract 2013;2013: 456965.

48. Kim KP, Kim MH, Kim JC, et al. Diagnostic criteria for autoimmune chronic pancreatitis revisited. World J Gastroenterol 2006;12(16):2487–96.

49. Otsuki M, Chung JB, Okazaki K, et al. Asian diagnostic criteria for autoimmune pancreatitis: consensus of the Japan-Korea Symposium on Autoimmune Pancreatitis. J Gastroenterol 2008;43(6):403–8.

50. Chari ST, Smyrk TC, Levy MJ, et al. Diagnosis of autoimmune pancreatitis: the Mayo Clinic experience. Clin Gastroenterol Hepatol 2006;4(8):110–1016.

51. Hirano K, Isogawa A, Tada M, et al. Long-term prognosis of autoimmune pancreatitis in terms of glucose tolerance. Pancreas 2012;41(5):691–5.

52. Khosroshahi A, Wallace ZS, Crowe JL, et al. International consensus guidance statement on the management and treatment of IgG4-related disease. Arthritis Rheumatol 2015;67(7):1688–99.

53. Kamisawa T, Shimosegawa T, Okazaki K, et al. Standard steroid treatment for autoimmune pancreatitis. Gut 2009;58(11):1504–7.

54. Hirano K, Tada M, Isayama H, et al. Long-term prognosis of autoimmune pancreatitis with and without corticosteroid treatment. Gut 2007;56(12):1719–24.

55. Kubota K, Kamisawa T, Hirano K, et al. Clinical course of type 1 autoimmune pancreatitis patients without steroid treatment: a Japanese multicenter study of 97 patients. J Hepatobiliary Pancreat Sci 2018;25(4):223–30.

56. Shouval D, Shibolet O. Immunosuppression and HBV reactivation. Semin Liver Dis 2013;33(2):167–77.

57. Kamisawa T, Okazaki K, Kawa S, et al. Amendment of the Japanese consensus guidelines for autoimmune pancreatitis, 2013 III. Treatment and prognosis of autoimmune pancreatitis. J Gastroenterol 2014;49(6):961–70.

58. Moon SH, Kim MH, Park DH, et al. Is a 2-week steroid trial after initial negative investigation for malignancy useful in differentiating autoimmune pancreatitis from pancreatic cancer? A prospective outcome study. Gut 2008;57(12): 1704–12.

59. Wakabayashi T, Kawaura Y, Satomura Y, et al. Long-term prognosis of duct-narrowing chronic pancreatitis: strategy for steroid treatment. Pancreas 2005; 30(1):31–9.

60. Buijs J, van Heerde MJ, Rauws EA, et al. Comparable efficacy of low- versus high-dose induction corticosteroid treatment in autoimmune pancreatitis. Pancreas 2014;43(2):261–7.

61. Matsushita M, Yamashina M, Ikeura T, et al. Effective steroid pulse therapy for the biliary stenosis caused by autoimmune pancreatitis. Am J Gastroenterol 2007; 102(1):220–1.

62. Sugimoto M, Takagi T, Suzuki R, et al. Efficacy of steroid pulse therapy for autoimmune pancreatitis type 1: a retrospective study. PLoS One 2015;10(9): e0138604.

63. Tomiyama T, Uchida K, Matsushita M, et al. Comparison of steroid pulse therapy and conventional oral steroid therapy as initial treatment for autoimmune pancreatitis. J Gastroenterol 2011;46(5):696–704.

64. Cai O, Tan S. From pathogenesis, clinical manifestation, and diagnosis to treatment: an overview on autoimmune pancreatitis. Gastroenterol Res Pract 2017; 2017:3246459.

65. Kawa S, Hamano H. Clinical features of autoimmune pancreatitis. J Gastroenterol 2007;42(Suppl 18):9–14.

66. Maire F, Le Baleur Y, Rebours V, et al. Outcome of patients with type 1 or 2 autoimmune pancreatitis. Am J Gastroenterol 2011;106(1):151–6.

67. Topazian M, Witzig TE, Smyrk TC, et al. Rituximab therapy for refractory biliary strictures in immunoglobulin G4-associated cholangitis. Clin Gastroenterol Hepatol 2008;6(3):364–6.

68. Hart PA, Topazian MD, Witzig TE, et al. Treatment of relapsing autoimmune pancreatitis with immunomodulators and rituximab: the Mayo Clinic experience. Gut 2013;62(11):1607–15.

69. Majumder S, Takahashi N, Chari ST. Autoimmune pancreatitis. Dig Dis Sci 2017; 62(7):1762–9.

70. Carruthers MN, Topazian MD, Khosroshahi A, et al. Rituximab for IgG4-related disease: a prospective, open-label trial. Ann Rheum Dis 2015;74(6):1171–7.

71. Khosroshahi A, Carruthers MN, Deshpande V, et al. Rituximab for the treatment of IgG4-related disease: lessons from 10 consecutive patients. Medicine (Baltimore) 2012;91(1):57–66.

72. Carruthers MN, Stone JH, Deshpande V, et al. Development of an IgG4-RD responder index. Int J Rheumatol 2012;2012:259408.

73. Ghazale A, Chari ST. Optimising corticosteroid treatment for autoimmune pancreatitis. Gut 2007;56(12):1650–2.

74. Park DH, Kim MH, Oh HB, et al. Substitution of aspartic acid at position 57 of the DQbeta1 affects relapse of autoimmune pancreatitis. Gastroenterology 2008; 134(2):440–6.

75. Hirano K, Tada M, Isayama H, et al. Outcome of long-term maintenance steroid therapy cessation in patients with autoimmune pancreatitis: a prospective study. J Clin Gastroenterol 2016;50(4):331–7.

76. Masamune A, Nishimori I, Kikuta K, et al. Randomised controlled trial of long-term maintenance corticosteroid therapy in patients with autoimmune pancreatitis. Gut 2017;66(3):487–94.

77. Hart PA, Chari ST. Preventing disease relapses in autoimmune pancreatitis with maintenance steroids: are we there yet? Gut 2017;66(3):394–6.

78. Frulloni L, de Pretis N, Amodio A. Maintenance therapy in autoimmune pancreatitis: a weak light into the darkness. Ann Transl Med 2017;5(17):367.

79. Lee HW, Moon SH, Kim MH, et al. Relapse rate and predictors of relapse in a large single center cohort of type 1 autoimmune pancreatitis: long-term follow-up results after steroid therapy with short-duration maintenance treatment. J Gastroenterol 2018;53:1–11.

80. Shimizu K, Tahara J, Takayama Y, et al. Assessment of the rate of decrease in serum IgG4 level of autoimmune pancreatitis patients in response to initial steroid therapy as a predictor of subsequent relapse. Pancreas 2016;45(9):1341–6.

81. Kawa S, Hamano H, Ozaki Y, et al. Long-term follow-up of autoimmune pancreatitis: characteristics of chronic disease and recurrence. Clin Gastroenterol Hepatol 2009;7(11 Suppl):S18–22.

82. You MW, Kim JH, Byun JH, et al. Relapse of IgG4-related sclerosing cholangitis after steroid therapy: image findings and risk factors. Eur Radiol 2014;24(5): 1039–48.

83. Ito T, Nishimori I, Inoue N, et al. Treatment for autoimmune pancreatitis: consensus on the treatment for patients with autoimmune pancreatitis in Japan. J Gastroenterol 2007;42(Suppl 18):50–8.

84. Sandanayake NS, Church NI, Chapman MH, et al. Presentation and management of post-treatment relapse in autoimmune pancreatitis/immunoglobulin G4-associated cholangitis. Clin Gastroenterol Hepatol 2009;7(10):1089–96.

85. de Pretis N, Amodio A, Bernardoni L, et al. Azathioprine maintenance therapy to prevent relapses in autoimmune pancreatitis. Clin Transl Gastroenterol 2017;8(4): e90.

86. Sodikoff JB, Keilin SA, Cai Q, et al. Mycophenolate mofetil for maintenance of remission in steroid-dependent autoimmune pancreatitis. World J Gastroenterol 2012;18(18):2287–90.

87. Schwaiger T, van den Brandt C, Fitzner B, et al. Autoimmune pancreatitis in MRL/ Mp mice is a T cell-mediated disease responsive to cyclosporine A and rapamycin treatment. Gut 2014;63(3):494–505.

88. Frulloni L, Scattolini C, Katsotourchi AM, et al. Exocrine and endocrine pancreatic function in 21 patients suffering from autoimmune pancreatitis before and after steroid treatment. Pancreatology 2010;10(2–3):129–33.

89. Buijs J, Cahen DL, van Heerde MJ, et al. The long-term impact of autoimmune pancreatitis on pancreatic function, quality of life, and life expectancy. Pancreas 2015;44(7):1065–71.

90. Shiokawa M, Kodama Y, Yoshimura K, et al. Risk of cancer in patients with autoimmune pancreatitis. Am J Gastroenterol 2013;108(4):610–7.

91. Bi Y, Hart PA, Law R, et al. Obstructive jaundice in autoimmune pancreatitis can be safely treated with corticosteroids alone without biliary stenting. Pancreatology 2016;16(3):391–6.

92. Clark CJ, Morales-Oyarvide V, Zaydfudim V, et al. Short-term and long-term outcomes for patients with autoimmune pancreatitis after pancreatectomy: a multi-institutional study. J Gastrointest Surg 2013;17(5):899–906.

93. Sah RP, Chari ST, Pannala R, et al. Differences in clinical profile and relapse rate of type 1 versus type 2 autoimmune pancreatitis. Gastroenterology 2010;139: 140–8.

94. Culver EL, Sadler R, Simpson D, et al. Elevated serum IgG4 levels in diagnosis, treatment response, organ involvement, and relapse in a prospective IgG4-related disease UK cohort. Am J Gastroenterol 2016;111:733–43.

95. Kubota K, Kamisawa T, Okazaki K, et al. Low-dose maintenance steroid treatment could reduce the relapse rate in patients with type 1 autoimmune pancreatitis: a long-term Japanese multicenter analysis of 510 patients. J Gastroenterol 2017; 52:955–64.

Pancreatic Insufficiency
What Is the Gold Standard?

Maisam Abu-El-Haija, MD[a,b,*], Darwin L. Conwell, MD, MS[c]

KEYWORDS

- Pancreatic insufficiency • Endoscopic function testing • Pancreatic function testing
- Chronic pancreatitis

KEY POINTS

- Endoscopic pancreatic function testing is a valuable tool to assess for exocrine insufficiency and chronic pancreatitis.
- Pancreatic fluid is assessed for volume, electrolytes, or enzyme components to evaluate for pancreatic insufficiency.
- Different pancreatic function protocols are available in the literature, with limited studies on validation or comparisons of those protocols.
- Indirect pancreatic function tests have limited sensitivity and specificity in early disease stages.
- Newer techniques using MRI to measure pancreas function show promise for evaluating pancreatic diseases.

INTRODUCTION

Exocrine pancreatic insufficiency (EPI) is the inability of the pancreas to generate the secretory capacity of secreting enzymes, bicarbonate, and enough fluid volumes to assist in food digestion, resulting in steatorrhea or diarrhea and weight loss.[1–3] EPI

Disclosures: In-kind support for investigator-initiated grant from ChiRhoClin, Inc was received for the MR study (M. Abu-El-Haija). The National Pancreas Foundation funded parts of the Pancreatic Function Studies using MRI (M. Abu-El-Haija). This study was supported by the National Cancer Institute and National Institute of Diabetes and Digestive and Kidney Diseases under award number U01DK108327 (D.L. Conwell). The content is solely the responsibility of the authors and does not necessarily represent the official views of the National Institutes of Health.

[a] Department of Pediatrics, University of Cincinnati College of Medicine, Cincinnati, OH, USA; [b] Division of Gastroenterology, Hepatology and Nutrition, Cincinnati Children's Hospital Medical Center, 3333 Burnet Avenue, Cincinnati, OH, USA; [c] Department of Internal Medicine, Division of Gastroenterology, Hepatology and Nutrition, Ohio State University Wexner Medical Center, Columbus, OH, USA
* Corresponding author. Cincinnati Children's Hospital Medical Center, 3333 Burnet Avenue, Cincinnati, OH.
E-mail address: Maisam.Haija@cchmc.org

Gastrointest Endoscopy Clin N Am 28 (2018) 521–528
https://doi.org/10.1016/j.giec.2018.05.004
1052-5157/18/© 2018 Elsevier Inc. All rights reserved.

can result from multiple congenital or acquired pathologic conditions, and has negative implications for the health and overall wellbeing of the individuals with this condition.[4,5] There is limited knowledge on the incidence and prevalence of EPI and it is generally thought to be underrecognized.[6] Etiologic factors for EPI include congenital and acquired syndromes that manifest as the patient ages from childhood to adulthood. Cystic fibrosis is the most common etiologic factor of congenital EPI in both children and adults.[7] Other conditions that cause EPI in children include but are not limited to Shwachman-Diamond syndrome,[8] Pearson Marrow syndrome, and Jeune syndrome.[9] **Box 1** highlights congenital diseases that are associated with EPI. Acute recurrent pancreatitis and chronic pancreatitis (CP) with a combined incidence of 1 to 5 out of 100,000 population are increasingly important causes of EPI.[10,11] EPI is the gold standard for diagnosing CP.[12] EPI diagnosis by direct function testing is a sensitive method to test for early CP, when mild changes are not easily detectable on imaging.[13]

CP is a morbid condition with poor quality of life; significant pain; and a negative impact on growth, health, and overall wellbeing.[4,5,14,15] Late stages of the disease, manifested by parenchymal fibrosis and loss of exocrine function, are easier to diagnose than mild and early stages (minimal change disease). If CP is recognized early, therapies to treat mild disease and halt the progression to EPI could be applied.[16–19] As such, studies geared toward early detection are needed to identify early-stage disease and allow therapeutic interventions to be applied.

Diagnosing EPI accurately in early-stage disease, remains a challenge in clinical practice. It is of particular importance to recognize the differences in pancreatic function testing (PFT) available in terms of performance, methodology, and interpretation, with the endpoint of facilitating patient management. In general, PFT is thought of in 2 major entities: indirect tests that measure the consequences of EPI and direct PFT that measures the pancreatic function directly.[20] This article summarizes the evolution of PFT over the years and highlights areas for future research.

INDIRECT PANCREATIC FUNCTION TESTING

Indirect PFT is used in clinical practice to screen for a pancreatic disease but seldom confirms the presence of the disease in the pancreas. In general, indirect testing is noninvasive but not as sensitive and specific to pancreatic disease. Indirect testing has a low sensitivity in mild pancreatic disease and has a better sensitivity in more advanced disease.[21,22] Some of the indirect methods that can be used in assessing pancreatic function include fecal fat, fecal elastase, fecal chymotrypsin, and serum markers, including trypsinogen, each of which has its limitations. Studies have shown

---

Box 1
Congenital syndromes leading to exocrine pancreatic insufficiency

- Cystic fibrosis
- Shwachman-Diamond syndrome
- Johanson-Blizzard syndrome
- Pearson bone marrow syndrome
- Jeune syndrome
- Fetal or congenital infections
- Agenesis of the pancreas

poor correlation of fecal testing with direct PFT, with a low sensitivity, specificity, and a limited positive predictive value.[23–25]

Fecal fat is used to diagnose steatorrhea when a 72-hour collection of stool has greater than 7 g of fat in an adult patient who consumes 100 g of fat per day. Different cutoffs are used for the pediatric population, and these depend on age and fat intake. In general, in patients over 6 months of age, excretion of fecal fat of more than 7% of the intake is considered abnormal.[26]

Serum markers, including the cationic trypsinogen, have been studied for EPI and are more sensitive and specific in diagnosing advanced or late stages of the disease. A test of less than 20 ng/mL was specific for pancreatic steatorrhea, compared with levels higher than 20 ng/mL.[27]

Fecal elastase is a commonly used test in practice, with a sensitivity close to 41%, specificity of 49%, and a positive predictive value of 14% in 1 pediatric study when compared with endoscopic PFT (ePFT). It also had a poor correlation of ($r = 0.19$) in that cohort.[24] Other studies in adults showed comparable numbers of fecal elastase for detecting EPI, with 26.3% sensitivity and 88.7% specificity. The positive predictive value of the fecal elastase was 45.5% with a significant discordance between ePFT and fecal elastase results.[23] Despite these known limitations, fecal elastase remains among the most commonly performed indirect pancreas function tests in the clinical practice. **Box 2**, highlights available indirect PFT.

DIRECT PANCREATIC FUNCTION TESTING

Direct PFT involves stimulation of the pancreas with a secretagogue, such as secretin or cholecystokinin (CCK), and the subsequent collection and analysis of pancreatic fluid to quantify pancreatic secretory content (eg, pancreatic fluid for volume, electrolyte components, and/or enzyme concentrations or activities, or combinations of these elements.) Direct PFT is the reference standard for diagnosis of EPI. This is a challenge because direct tests require either placement of duodenal and gastric tubes, according to the method developed by Dreiling,[28,29] or endoscopic suctioning of duodenal fluid (with ePFT).[16,30] Secretagogues used in direct PFT mainly include hormonal compounds of secretin, CCK, or both.[31–33]

Box 2
Indirect pancreatic function testing

Serum tests

- Lipase

- Amylase

- Cationic trypsinogen

Breath test

- Hydrogen and 13 carbon

Stool tests

- 72-hour fecal fat collection

- Qualitative stool fat

- Fecal elastase

- Fecal chymotrypsin

THE TUBE COLLECTION METHOD

In the late 1940s, Dreiling[28,29] described the first method of direct PFT. The test involves a double-lumen system, with a gastric portion connected to suction and a duodenal portion that collects the fluid every 15 minutes over 60 to 80 minutes. A peak bicarbonate secretion of less than 80 mEq/L is considered in the EPI range, and values less than 50 mEq/L are considered severe EPI. This method is not available at most centers, requires radiologic confirmation for tube placement, and is unpleasant for the patient. The lumen collecting method has been mostly replaced by ePFT due to these limitations.

ENDOSCOPIC PANCREATIC FUNCTION TESTING

The Dreiling method for direct PFT is not widely used,[28,34] and ePFT is gaining greater attention over the last 2 decades because it does not require radiation and can be performed under sedation.[35]

Studies comparing the Dreiling tube method with ePFT in healthy adults and patients with CP showed that ePFT was safe, shorter in duration, and had a lower cost of $1890 compared with the Dreiling method for collection (more than $2000 per patient cost).[16] Since the mid-1990s, these data showing the benefits of ePFT have affected the practice of evaluating patients with pancreatic disease. This work was supported by studies that compared ePFT with the lumen tube collection methods and showed that results are similar for the 2 methods.[36,37]

After stimulation with CCK as an infusion of 40 ng/kg/h, lipase concentrations between 2 collection methods, Dreiling and ePFT, in healthy subjects (1,612,500 vs 1,670,324 IU/L, respectively) and subjects with CP (369,594 vs 478,956 IU/L, respectively) were not different.[16] Other studies have evaluated bicarbonate secretion by ePFT[36] or enzyme activites.[23]

Different secretagogue dosages with secretin, CCK, or combinations have been used to stimulate the pancreatic secretions with varying results. Studies have shown that for enzyme measurements using CCK versus secretin versus a both, similar enzyme concentrations were produced.[38,39] The administration of CCK or secretin has also varied in different studies because some investigators used an infusion and others used a bolus.[23] The administration of the secretagogue affects the length of the test, the duration varied from 15 minutes in length to 80 minutes in length using ePFT. A recently published pediatric study of 508 children showed that enzyme activities for amylase, lipase, chymotrypsin, and trypsin, peaked at 5 minutes, and the levels at 10 and 15 minutes were not different.[23] The pH and protein content affects the enzyme activities. A pH of greater than 7 is required for optimal enzyme acitivities.[40]

Pancreas function testing is not needed in advanced stages of pancreatitis, in which calcification and ductal irregularities are seen on imaging. It is, however, of extreme utility in the work up of early-stage CP. The most sensitive test for early CP, ePFT, is considered the gold standard for diagnosing CP.[12] Other markers for early CP are needed to help advance pancreatitis management in the future.

MAGNETIC RESONANCE TESTING

Magnetic resonance cholangiopancreatography (MRCP) has been shown to be a useful tool in the assessment of the pancreatic parenchyma, pancreatic ductal anatomy, and the surrounding tissues. The use of secretin stimulation MRCP (sMRCP) has been described as a means to both improve pancreatic duct visualization and to qualitatively assess exocrine pancreatic function.[41,42] Among adult patients, there are also data to support the use of sMRCP as a noninvasive means to quantify pancreatic exocrine function; this is known as magnetic resonance PFT (MR PFT).[43–47] Different doses of secretin were used with no major difference in the total excreted volume after stimulation on MRCP.[48] Different grading systems have been used in adult studies for MR PFT. Matos and colleagues[49] presented data on pancreatic fluid volume that increased linearly with time with a mean pancreatic fluid output of 6.8 mL/min (SD 1.4 mL/min) and a mean total excreted volume of 97 mL (SD 22 mL).[50] The grading by Mensel and colleagues[43] (mean secretion of 111.8 ± 49.8 mL in response to secretin) has also been adequately described. There is also a growing experience in using MRCP for studying pancreatic function in the pediatric population.[51] Trout and colleagues[51] were able to measure fluid volume to assess the pancreatic function in 97% of the pediatric age population that needed this study, with a great correlation between readers.

MR PFT holds promise for allowing the study of the pancreatic function in a noninvasive method, which is free of radiation and does not require anesthesia in most cases. MR PFT studies need to be validated on a larger sample size of subjects because it can be of value in the follow-up of acute pancreatitis and CP. The direction of MR PFT would benefit from study of the ideal protocol, the best location, and the ideal secretin dose for measuring the pancreatic fluid volumes required to assess for function.

FUTURE RESEARCH

PFT is needed to assess the presence and extent pancreatic diseases in cases of EPI. The indications of PFT vary between adults and children but are needed in both populations. There is a gap in knowledge of the best protocol for PFT by ePFT. There is a lack of consensus on the secretagogues used, the dosage and administration of the CCK or secretin, collection methods, and (finally) the duration of the testing. There is also a lack of agreement on the best measure of EPI: is it pancreatic fluid volume as measured by the tube collection or by MR PFT? Is it the bicarbonate concentration, or the enzyme concentration or activities, as shown in different studies? There is an increasing role for noninvasive testing using sMRCP in studying the exocrine secretory capacity in children and adults. These tests can serve EPI management by stratifying disease severity (early or late stage), which will potentially facilitate biomarker discovery. Accurate diagnosis of CP will open the opportunity for targeted therapies directed at retarding or slowing CP progression.

REFERENCES

1. Hart PA, Conwell DL. Diagnosis of exocrine pancreatic insufficiency. Curr Treat Options Gastroenterol 2015;13(3):347–53.
2. Kolodziejczyk E, Wejnarska K, Dadalski M, et al. The nutritional status and factors contributing to malnutrition in children with chronic pancreatitis. Pancreatology 2014;14(4):275–9.
3. Rana M, Wong-See D, Katz T, et al. Fat-soluble vitamin deficiency in children and adolescents with cystic fibrosis. J Clin Pathol 2014;67(7):605–8.
4. Somaraju UR, Solis-Moya A. Pancreatic enzyme replacement therapy for people with cystic fibrosis. Cochrane Database Syst Rev 2014;(10):CD008227.
5. Arya VB, Senniappan S, Demirbilek H, et al. Pancreatic endocrine and exocrine function in children following near-total pancreatectomy for diffuse congenital hyperinsulinism. PLoS One 2014;9(5):e98054.

6. Levy P, Dominguez-Munoz E, Imrie C, et al. Epidemiology of chronic pancreatitis: burden of the disease and consequences. United European Gastroenterol J 2014;2(5):345–54.

7. Haupt ME, Kwasny MJ, Schechter MS, et al. Pancreatic enzyme replacement therapy dosing and nutritional outcomes in children with cystic fibrosis. J Pediatr 2014;164(5):1110–5.e1.

8. Kathuria R, Poddar U, Yachha SK. Shwachman-Diamond syndrome: are we missing many? Indian Pediatr 2012;49(9):748–9.

9. Cormier V, Rotig A, Quartino AR, et al. Widespread multi-tissue deletions of the mitochondrial genome in the Pearson marrow-pancreas syndrome. J Pediatr 1990;117(4):599–602.

10. Morinville VD, Husain SZ, Bai H, et al. Definitions of pediatric pancreatitis and survey of present clinical practices. J Pediatr Gastroenterol Nutr 2012;55(3):261–5.

11. Bai HX, Lowe ME, Husain SZ. What have we learned about acute pancreatitis in children? J Pediatr Gastroenterol Nutr 2011;52(3):262–70.

12. Wu B, Conwell DL. The endoscopic pancreatic function test. Am J Gastroenterol 2009;104(10):2381–3.

13. Stevens T, Dumot JA, Zuccaro G Jr, et al. Evaluation of duct-cell and acinar-cell function and endosonographic abnormalities in patients with suspected chronic pancreatitis. Clin Gastroenterol Hepatol 2009;7(1):114–9.

14. Amann ST, Yadav D, Barmada MM, et al. Physical and mental quality of life in chronic pancreatitis: a case-control study from the North American Pancreatitis Study 2 cohort. Pancreas 2013;42(2):293–300.

15. Schwarzenberg SJ, Bellin M, Husain SZ, et al. Pediatric chronic pancreatitis is associated with genetic risk factors and substantial disease burden. J Pediatr 2015;166(4):890–6.e1.

16. Conwell DL, Zuccaro G Jr, Vargo JJ, et al. An endoscopic pancreatic function test with cholecystokinin-octapeptide for the diagnosis of chronic pancreatitis. Clin Gastroenterol Hepatol 2003;1(3):189–94.

17. Abu Dayyeh BK, Conwell D, Buttar NS, et al. Pancreatic juice prostaglandin e2 concentrations are elevated in chronic pancreatitis and improve detection of early disease. Clin Transl Gastroenterol 2015;6:e72.

18. Pelley JR, Gordon SR, Gardner TB. Abnormal duodenal [HCO3-] following secretin stimulation develops sooner than endocrine insufficiency in minimal change chronic pancreatitis. Pancreas 2012;41(3):481–4.

19. Sendler M, Beyer G, Mahajan UM, et al. Complement component 5 mediates development of fibrosis, via activation of stellate cells, in 2 mouse models of chronic pancreatitis. Gastroenterology 2015;149(3):765–76.e10.

20. Walkowiak J, Nousia-Arvanitakis S, Henker J, et al. Indirect pancreatic function tests in children. J Pediatr Gastroenterol Nutr 2005;40(2):107–14.

21. Chowdhury RS, Forsmark CE. Review article: pancreatic function testing. Aliment Pharmacol Ther 2003;17(6):733–50.

22. Taylor CJ, Chen K, Horvath K, et al. ESPGHAN and NASPGHAN report on the assessment of exocrine pancreatic function and pancreatitis in children. J Pediatr Gastroenterol Nutr 2015;61(1):144–53.

23. Alfaro Cruz L, Parniczky A, Mayhew A, et al. Utility of direct pancreatic function testing in children. Pancreas 2017;46(2):177–82.

24. Wali PD, Loveridge-Lenza B, He Z, et al. Comparison of fecal elastase-1 and pancreatic function testing in children. J Pediatr Gastroenterol Nutr 2012;54(2): 277–80.

25. Lankisch PG, Schmidt I, Konig H, et al. Faecal elastase 1: not helpful in diagnosing chronic pancreatitis associated with mild to moderate exocrine pancreatic insufficiency. Gut 1998;42(4):551–4.

26. Fomon SJ, Ziegler EE, Thomas LN, et al. Excretion of fat by normal full-term infants fed various milks and formulas. Am J Clin Nutr 1970;23(10):1299–313.

27. Moore DJ, Forstner GG, Largman C, et al. Serum immunoreactive cationic trypsinogen: a useful indicator of severe exocrine dysfunction in the paediatric patient without cystic fibrosis. Gut 1986;27(11):1362–8.

28. Dreiling DA Sr. An evaluation of pancreatic-function tests in the diagnosis of pancreatic disease. Trans N Y Acad Sci 1952;14(8):315–9.

29. Dreiling DA Sr. Studies in pancreatic function. V. The use of the secretin test in the diagnosis of pancreatitis and in the demonstration of pancreatic insufficiencies in gastrointestinal disorders. Gastroenterology 1953;24(4):540–55.

30. Conwell DL, Zuccaro G Jr, Vargo JJ, et al. An endoscopic pancreatic function test with synthetic porcine secretin for the evaluation of chronic abdominal pain and suspected chronic pancreatitis. Gastrointest Endosc 2003;57(1):37–40.

31. Li P, Lee KY, Chang TM, et al. Mechanism of acid-induced release of secretin in rats. Presence of a secretin-releasing peptide. J Clin Invest 1990;86(5):1474–9.

32. Li P, Lee KY, Ren XS, et al. Effect of pancreatic proteases on plasma cholecystokinin, secretin, and pancreatic exocrine secretion in response to sodium oleate. Gastroenterology 1990;98(6):1642–8.

33. Regan PT, Go VL, DiMagno EP. Comparison of the effects of cholecystokinin and cholecystokinin octapeptide on pancreatic secretion, gallbladder contraction, and plasma pancreatic polypeptide in man. J Lab Clin Med 1980;96(4):743–8.

34. Dreiling DA, Hollander F. Studies in pancreatic function; a statistical study of pancreatic secretion following secretin in patients without pancreatic disease. Gastroenterology 1950;15(4):620–7.

35. Conwell DL, Zuccaro G, Morrow JB, et al. Cholecystokinin-stimulated peak lipase concentration in duodenal drainage fluid: a new pancreatic function test. Am J Gastroenterol 2002;97(6):1392–7.

36. Stevens T, Conwell DL, Zuccaro G Jr, et al. A prospective crossover study comparing secretin-stimulated endoscopic and Dreiling tube pancreatic function testing in patients evaluated for chronic pancreatitis. Gastrointest Endosc 2008; 67(3):458–66.

37. Stevens T, Conwell DL, Zuccaro G Jr, et al. A randomized crossover study of secretin-stimulated endoscopic and dreiling tube pancreatic function test methods in healthy subjects. Am J Gastroenterol 2006;101(2):351–5.

38. Del Rosario MA, Fitzgerald JF, Gupta SK, et al. Direct measurement of pancreatic enzymes after stimulation with secretin versus secretin plus cholecystokinin. J Pediatr Gastroenterol Nutr 2000;31(1):28–32.

39. Pfefferkorn MD, Fitzgerald JF, Croffie JM, et al. Direct measurement of pancreatic enzymes: a comparison of secretagogues. Dig Dis Sci 2002;47(10):2211–6.

40. Erlanger BF, Kokowsky N, Cohen W. The preparation and properties of two new chromogenic substrates of trypsin. Arch Biochem Biophys 1961;95:271–8.

41. Delaney L, Applegate KE, Karmazyn B, et al. MR cholangiopancreatography in children: feasibility, safety, and initial experience. Pediatr Radiol 2008;38(1): 64–75.

42. Manfredi R, Lucidi V, Gui B, et al. Idiopathic chronic pancreatitis in children: MR cholangiopancreatography after secretin administration. Radiology 2002;224(3): 675–82.

43. Mensel B, Messner P, Mayerle J, et al. Secretin-stimulated MRCP in volunteers: assessment of safety, duct visualization, and pancreatic exocrine function. AJR Am J Roentgenol 2014;202(1):102–8.

44. Wathle GK, Tjora E, Ersland L, et al. Assessment of exocrine pancreatic function by secretin-stimulated magnetic resonance cholangiopancreatography and diffusion-weighted imaging in healthy controls. J Magn Reson Imaging 2014; 39(2):448–54.

45. Bian Y, Wang L, Chen C, et al. Quantification of pancreatic exocrine function of chronic pancreatitis with secretin-enhanced MRCP. World J Gastroenterol 2013; 19(41):7177–82.

46. Sanyal R, Stevens T, Novak E, et al. Secretin-enhanced MRCP: review of technique and application with proposal for quantification of exocrine function. AJR Am J Roentgenol 2012;198(1):124–32.

47. Manfredi R, Perandini S, Mantovani W, et al. Quantitative MRCP assessment of pancreatic exocrine reserve and its correlation with faecal elastase-1 in patients with chronic pancreatitis. Radiol Med 2012;117(2):282–92.

48. Bali MA, Sontou R, Arvanitakis M, et al. Evaluation of the stimulating effect of a low dose of secretin compared to the standard dose on the exocrine pancreas with MRCP: preliminary results in normal subjects (MRCP quantification of secretin stimulation). Abdom Imaging 2007;32(6):743–8.

49. Matos C, Metens T, Deviere J, et al. Pancreatic duct: morphologic and functional evaluation with dynamic MR pancreatography after secretin stimulation. Radiology 1997;203(2):435–41.

50. Bali MA, Sztantics A, Metens T, et al. Quantification of pancreatic exocrine function with secretin-enhanced magnetic resonance cholangiopancreatography: normal values and short-term effects of pancreatic duct drainage procedures in chronic pancreatitis. Initial results. Eur Radiol 2005;15(10):2110–21.

51. Trout AT, Wallihan DB, Serai S, et al. Secretin-enhanced magnetic resonance cholangiopancreatography for assessing pancreatic secretory function in children. J Pediatr 2017;188:186–91.

Current Guideline Controversies in the Management of Pancreatic Cystic Neoplasms

Christopher J. DiMaio, MD

KEYWORDS

- Pancreatic cystic lesions • Pancreatic cystic neoplasms • Pancreatic cancer
- Branch duct intraductal papillary mucinous neoplasm • Guidelines

KEY POINTS

- Most pancreatic cystic lesions are neoplastic. Branch duct intraductal papillary mucinous neoplasms (BD-IPMN) are the most common cystic lesion encountered in practice. BD-IPMN have a low, but not insignificant, long-term risk of developing cancer.
- Multiple clinical guidelines exist for the management of pancreatic cystic neoplasms. The recommendations of these guidelines are based largely on expert opinion because the available scientific data are of low quality in general.
- All guidelines emphasize that there are known cyst features, which pose an increased risk for a prevalent or future malignancy in any particular premalignant lesion. These include the presence of an intramural nodule or mass, main pancreatic duct dilation, cyst size of 3 cm or greater, and high-risk cytologic feature on fine-needle aspirate.

Pancreatic cysts represent a common, yet frustrating, entity encountered in clinical practice. The incidence of pancreatic cysts has been estimated to be between 3% and 15% in the United States with increasing prevalence with age.[1–4] The vast majority of these lesions are asymptomatic and incidentally detected on imaging studies, particularly with the increasing use of high-resolution cross-sectional imaging studies. With this increasing incidence, the last 2 decades has seen a marked increase in the understanding of their significance, namely that most of these lesions are neoplastic and may pose a risk of malignant transformation. Nevertheless, despite this increase

Conflicts of Interest: None.
Disclosures: Boston Scientific, Medtronic.
Financial Support or Sponsorship for This Manuscript: None.
Division of Gastroenterology, Icahn School of Medicine at Mount Sinai, One Gustave L. Levy Place, Box 1069, New York, NY 10029, USA
E-mail address: Christopher.DiMaio@mountsinai.org

Gastrointest Endoscopy Clin N Am 28 (2018) 529–547
https://doi.org/10.1016/j.giec.2018.05.005
1052-5157/18/© 2018 Elsevier Inc. All rights reserved.

in knowledge, much debate exists in terms of how best to manage patients who are found to have a pancreatic cyst.

Pancreatic cysts have a broad differential diagnosis. They can be categorized using various descriptors, such as neoplastic versus nonneoplastic, or mucinous versus nonmucinous, or benign versus premalignant versus malignant. Regardless of the category any particular lesion falls into, it is important for clinicians to be familiar with the most commonly encountered cystic lesions (**Table 1**).

PANCREATIC CYSTIC LESIONS
Nonneoplastic Cysts

Pancreatic pseudocysts are collections of fluid that form secondary to acute pancreatitis or pancreatic duct leaks (related to chronic pancreatitis, pancreatic surgery, or

Table 1
Epidemiology, imaging, and cyst fluid features of common pancreatic cysts

	Pseudocyst	SCA	BD-IPMN	MCN
Gender (% female)	<25%	~70%	~55%	>95%
Age (decade)	Any	6th–7th	6th–7th	4th–5th
Features				
Calcifications	No	Yes, 30%–40% central, "sunburst"	No	Yes, rare, curvilinear on rim ("eggshell")
Multifocal	Rare	No	Yes	No
Appearance	Unilocular, thick wall	Microcystic ("honeycomb" appearance) or macrocystic, or mixed	Varied: unilocular, or multicystic ("cluster of grapes"), or tubular, or mixed	Unilocular, septated
Main PD communication	Common	No	Yes (although not always demonstrable)	Rare
Main PD	Normal or irregularly dilated, stones, strictures	Normal or deviated	Normal or dilated	Normal or deviated
Cyst fluid				
Appearance	Nonmucinous, can be chocolate brown, bloody	Thin, watery, straw-colored, serosanguinous	Clear, viscous	Clear, viscous
Chemical analysis	High amylase	Very low CEA	High CEA Can have elevated amylase	High CEA

Abbreviation: PD, pancreatic duct.

Adapted from Tanaka M, Fernandez-del Castillo C, Kamisawa T, et al. Revisions of International Consensus Fukuoka Guidelines for the management of IPMN of the pancreas. Pancreatology 2017;17:741; with permission.

trauma). These cysts are nonneoplastic and carry no risk of malignant transformation. Pseudocysts may present with abdominal pain, infection, or luminal or biliary obstruction, although many can be completely asymptomatic. Traditionally, pancreatic pseudocysts were thought to be the most common type of pancreatic cystic lesion, accounting for more than 90% of all pancreatic cysts. However, this notion has been reconsidered because the development of pancreatic pseudocysts and other inflammatory collections is seen in only a minority of cases of acute or chronic pancreatitis. Furthermore, cross-sectional imaging studies note a relatively high prevalence of incidental pancreatic cysts in patients with no prior history of acute or chronic pancreatitis. As such, pancreatic pseudocysts likely account for only a small percentage of pancreatic cystic lesions.

Benign Neoplastic Cysts Without Malignant Potential

Serous cystadenomas (SCA) are neoplastic growths that are most commonly found in women. They are considered benign lesions, although there are a handful of reports of malignant transformation.[5] SCA are typically slow growing, with most lesions being asymptomatic and discovered incidentally. They can rarely grow very large and cause symptoms from mass effect, necessitating resection. However, that is more the exception rather than the rule. They are classically described as consisting of innumerable "microcysts in a honeycomb pattern." About one-third of these lesions will contain a central, calcified scar ("sunburst calcification"), which is pathognomonic for SCA.

Benign Neoplastic Cysts with Malignant Potential

Branch duct intraductal papillary mucinous neoplasm

Branch duct intraductal papillary mucinous neoplasm (BD-IPMN) is a neoplastic growth that has the potential for malignant transformation. The prevalence of BD-IPMN is estimated to be approximately 2.5%, with lesions existing in nearly 3 million people in the United States.[1,2] The past 3 decades have seen a marked increase in the diagnosis of BD-IPMN, likely secondary to increased availability and usage of high-resolution cross-sectional imaging.[4] BD-IPMN affect older men and women, typically in the sixth decade and older.

BD-IPMN, as the name implies, communicate with the main pancreatic duct as they arise from its side branches. Pathologically, BD-IPMN exhibit papillary projections lined by mucin-producing columnar epithelium. Pathologic subtypes of the papillary epithelium have been described. These subtypes include gastric, intestinal, pancreatobiliary, and oncocytic subtypes. These subtypes demonstrate variable degrees of malignant potential. All BD-IPMN exhibit some level of cytologic atypia, with at least low-grade dysplasia being found in most lesions, but can exhibit the complete range of cytologic atypia, including high-grade dysplasia and invasive cancer.

BD-IPMN can be found in any part of the pancreas. Morphologically, they have various appearances, including simple unilocular cysts, "grapelike clusters" of cysts, or a tubular appearance. They are most commonly solitary lesions, but can be multifocal in nature, ranging from a few cystic lesions throughout the pancreatic gland, or in some cases, innumerable cysts. Cyst fluid from BD-IPMN is typically clear and viscous, because the columnar epithelium produces a mucinous fluid.

Given their high prevalence and known risk for malignant transformation, BD-IPMN are perhaps the most important pancreatic cystic lesion. BD-IPMN are the most commonly encountered pancreatic cysts in clinical practice. As such, management decisions typically focus on method of evaluation, role of fine-needle aspiration (FNA), and whether surgical resection is warranted. Given the known poor prognosis related to pancreatic cancer, both patient and physician alike approach the notion of a "precancerous" lesion of the pancreas with great alarm and anxiety.

Mucinous cystic neoplasms

Another mucin-producing cyst is the mucinous cystic neoplasm (MCN). Nearly all MCN are found in women, with typical presentation occurring in middle age. Classically, MCN are located in the pancreatic body or tail. MCN are unilocular lesions, often containing septations, and occasionally have "eggshell" calcifications on the outer rim of the lesion. Pathologically, MCN are characterized by the presence of an ovarian-like stroma. The cyst wall columnar epithelium produces a clear, mucinous fluid. MCN do have malignant potential, with approximately 10% of them exhibiting high-grade dysplasia or cancer.[6]

Solid pseudopapillary neoplasms

Solid pseudopapillary neoplasms (SPN) are tumors found predominantly in young women, typically in their 20s.[7] The most common presentation is abdominal pain, although a little more than one-third of these lesions are found incidentally. Morphologically, SPN can appear solid, cystic, or mixed solid-cystic. These lesions do have malignant potential, with aggressive tumor behavior being found pathologically in about 10% of cases.[7] Surgical resection is typically associated with excellent 5-year survival.[7]

GUIDELINES FOR MANAGEMENT OF PANCREATIC CYSTIC LESIONS

Over the past 2 decades, there has been a precipitous increase in the understanding of pancreatic cysts in terms of their differential diagnosis and clinical significance of each pathologic subtype. As such, surgeons and gastroenterologists alike are much more likely to take a measured approach today in deciding which patients may benefit from surgery and which patients should be considered for surveillance. However, this approach remains far from perfect. Research in diagnostic testing in particular over the past 2 decades has helped guide the way in risk stratification for patients. However, perhaps more importantly, many of these studies have highlighted the limitations of imaging studies and endoscopic testing.

Given the uncertainty surrounding the appropriate diagnosis and management of pancreatic cysts, several guidelines have been published (**Table 2**). These guidelines are based predominantly on expert opinion, citing the relative low quality of existing data.

In 2006, the first such set of guidelines was published. Known as the Sendai guidelines (based on the meeting having occurred in Sendai, Japan), these recommendations focused entirely on the management of IPMN and MCN.[8] The group advised that all MCN should be resected, given that these lesions harbor malignant potential, the age of discovery of these lesions is in a younger cohort, thus allowing time for eventual malignant transformation, and that most of the lesions can be resected by distal pancreatectomy. The group also recommended that all main duct IPMN be resected, citing the high frequency (aggregate 70%) of high-grade dysplasia or cancer found in published surgical series.[8] In regards to BD-IPMN, the critical recommendations focused on morphologic features of the cyst. They identified several "high-risk" features for BD-IPMN. These high-risk features included the presence of symptoms, such as abdominal pain or jaundice attributable to the cyst, cyst size of 3 cm or greater, the presence of an intramural nodule, or the presence of pancreatic duct dilation of 5 mm or more. Patients exhibiting any of these features should then be considered for surgical resection, given their purported increased risk of having an incident

Table 2
Clinical guidelines for management of pancreatic cystic lesions

	Year	Cyst Types Addressed	Features Concerning for Advanced Pathologic Condition in BD-IPMN	Surveillance Imaging and Timing
Sendai	2006	IPMN, MCN	High risk • Symptoms • Cyst size ≥3 cm • Intramural nodule • Main PD ≥5 mm	MRCP and/or EUS, with type and timing depending on cyst size/features
Fukuoka	2012, 2017[a]	IPMN, MCN	High risk • Jaundice • Enhancing intramural nodule ≥5 mm • Main PD dilation ≥10 mm Worrisome • Cyst size ≥3 cm • Enhancing mural nodule <5 mm • Thickened and enhancing cyst wall • Main PD dilation 5–9 mm • Abrupt change in PD caliber with distal pancreatic atrophy • Presence of lymphadenopathy • Elevated serum CA 19-9 • Rapid growth rate >5 mm/2 y	MRCP and/or EUS, with type and timing depending on cyst size/features
European	2013	IPMN, MCN, SCA, SPPN	Absolute indications for surgery • Symptoms • Cyst size ≥4 cm • Presence of mural nodules • Main PD dilation ≥6 mm Relative indications for surgery • Rapidly increasing size • Elevated serum CA 19-9	MRCP and/or EUS, with type and timing depending on cyst size/features
AGA	2015	Asymptomatic cysts Does not make distinction among pathologic types	High risk • Cyst size ≥3 cm • Presence of solid component • Dilated main PD • HGD or cancer on cytology	MRCP and/or EUS, with type and timing depending on cyst size/features

(continued on next page)

Table 2 (continued)				
	Year	Cyst Types Addressed	Features Concerning for Advanced Pathologic Condition in BD-IPMN	Surveillance Imaging and Timing
ACG	2018	IPMN, MCN, SCA, SPPN	High risk (for mucinous cysts) • Jaundice or acute pancreatitis attributable to the cyst • Elevated CA 19-9 (when no benign cause is present) • Mural nodule or solid component within the cyst or pancreatic parenchyma • Main PD dilation >5 mm • Change in main duct with upstream atrophy • Cyst size ≥3 cm • Increase in cyst size ≥3 mm/y • HGD or cancer on cytology	MRCP and/or EUS, with type and timing depending on cyst size/features

Abbreviation: HGD, high grade dysplasia.
[a] Revisions to 2012 guidelines.

cancer already, or developing one in the future.[8] For patients who did not meet these high-risk criteria, surveillance was recommended. Methods for surveillance, such as computed tomography (CT), magnetic resonance cholangiopancreatography (MRCP), endoscopic ultrasound (EUS), or endoscopic retrograde cholangiopancreatography, as well as time interval of how often testing should be performed, were based on the size of the individual BD-IPMN.

In 2012, this group of international experts reconvened and revised the consensus guidelines. Known as the Fukuoka guidelines, this set of recommendations presented further detail particularly in regards to management of BD-IPMN.[9] These experts stratified morphologic features of BD-IPMN into 2 categories: high risk and worrisome. High-risk features include the presence of jaundice, an enhancing intramural solid component on contrast-enhanced imaging study, or the presence of main pancreatic duct dilation of 10 mm or greater. Cyst size of 3 cm or greater, which was previously considered a high-risk feature in the Sendai guidelines, was now demoted to being only a worrisome feature. Other worrisome features included presence of thickened enhanced cyst walls, nonenhancing mural nodule on contrast-enhanced cross-sectional imaging, main pancreatic duct dilation between 5 mm and 9 mm, abrupt change in caliber of the main pancreatic duct with distal pancreatic atrophy, and presence of lymphadenopathy. In 2017, the group published revisions to the Fukuoka criteria and now included the following as worrisome features: elevated serum CA 19-9 and rapid rate of cyst growth greater than 5 mm/2 years.[10] In addition, the revisions also modified the criteria for intramural solid components to be an enhancing mural nodule less than 5 mm (worrisome feature) and enhancing mural nodule ≥5 mm (high-risk feature). BD-IPMN exhibiting any high-risk feature should undergo surgical resection. BD-IPMN exhibiting worrisome features should undergo further testing with EUS, primarily to assess for high-risk features not presently seen on cross-sectional imaging. FNA was not uniformly recommended, but rather could be considered in centers with expertise in cytologic interpretation. Cysts with worrisome features who were found to have high-risk stigmata on EUS, or were found to have high-grade dysplasia or cancer on FNA, should undergo surgical resection. For BD-IPMN not meeting any of these criteria, it was recommended that lesions undergo surveillance testing, with CT or MRI with or without EUS at time intervals related to the size of the lesion (**Fig. 1**).

Following publication of the above 2 guidelines, another set of expert guidelines was published by a European contingent in 2013.[11] Acknowledging that the catch-all term "pancreatic cysts" encompasses a large list of various entities, this group focused their guidelines on the 4 most common cystic tumors: IPMN, MCN, SCA, and SPNs. The group advised against surgical resection for asymptomatic SCAs. Similar to Sendai/Fukuoka, the European guidelines recommended that surgical resection be considered for all MCN, main duct IPMN, and SPN. In regards to BD-IPMN, the group presented 2 categories of indications for surgical resection. Absolute indications for resection of BD-IPMN included presence of symptoms (eg, jaundice, acute pancreatitis), presence of mural nodules, or main pancreatic duct dilation of 6 mm or greater. Relative indications for resection were those BD-IPMN with rapidly increasing size (although this is not defined), or elevated serum CA 19-9 levels. In addition, BD-IPMN cysts measuring 4 cm or greater should also be referred for surgical resection. In BD-IPMN that do not meet any of the above criteria, a surveillance schema entailing use of MRCP or EUS was devised, with testing being performed every 6 months for the first year and then annually for years 2 to 5. Following 5 years of surveillance, the European group advocated for increased frequency of surveillance to every 6 months, citing an increased risk of malignancy in relation to the age of the lesion.

In 2015, the American Gastroenterological Association (AGA) published its own set of management guidelines for pancreatic cysts.[12] These guidelines took a slightly different tact than the other guidelines. The investigators concede that there should be concern for possible current or future malignancy in a subset of pancreatic cystic lesions. However, they note that malignant transformation is actually a rare event. As such, a more rational, evidence-based, and cost-effective approach should be devised to assess patients with an incidental pancreatic cyst. The AGA guidelines focus solely on asymptomatic cysts. Furthermore, they do not differentiate between pathologic cyst types, but rather address the various pancreatic cyst types simply as one group. High-risk features are defined as any of the following: cyst size of 3 cm or greater, presence of a solid component, or presence of a dilated main pancreatic duct. In terms of management, the AGA guidelines recommend radiographic assessment with MRCP. If 2 or more high-risk features are present, then further assessment with EUS/FNA should be pursued. Similarly, if there are significant changes in cyst morphology while under surveillance (ie, development of one or more high-risk features), then EUS/FNA should be pursued. The guidelines noted that cyst growth was not considered a statistically significant risk factor for malignancy. In addition, there are insufficient data on the relevance of increasing size of the pancreatic duct or development of a solid component in a cyst that previously did not exhibit these features. As such, the investigators cautiously recommended reassessing such patients with EUS/FNA. Surgical resection was advised for the following: any cystic lesion exhibiting 2 or more high-risk features, EUS examination revealing concerning cyst features, or FNA demonstrating high-grade dysplasia or

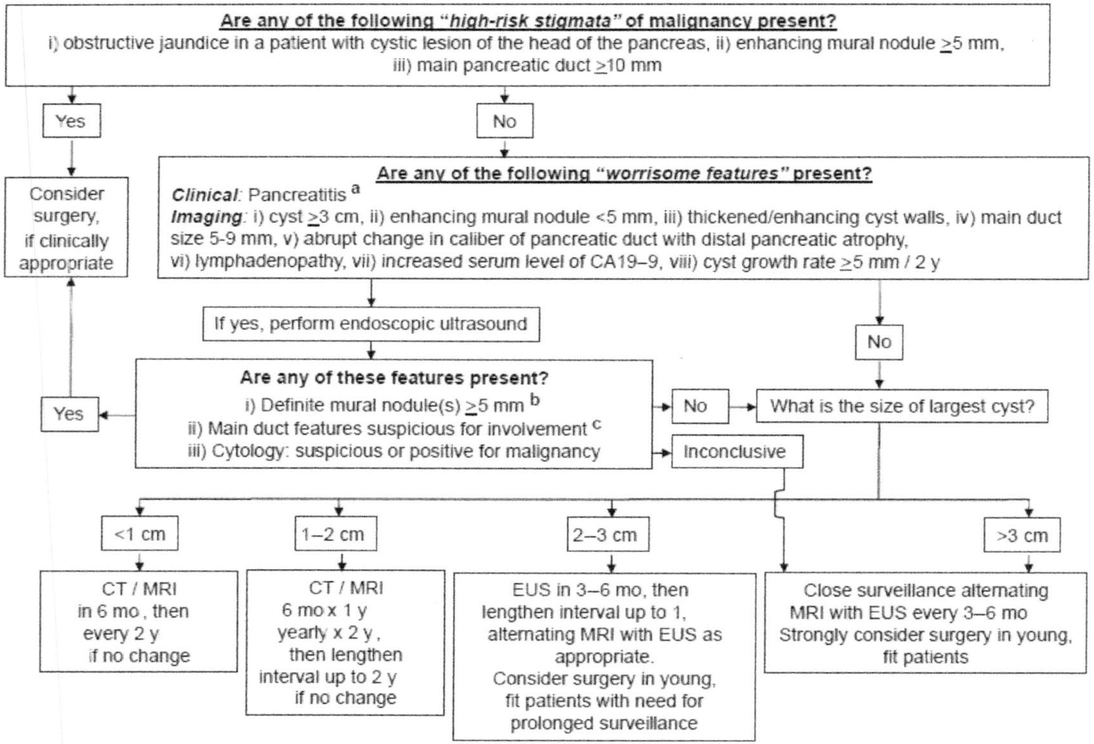
Are any of the following "high-risk stigmata" of malignancy present?
i) obstructive jaundice in a patient with cystic lesion of the head of the pancreas, ii) enhancing mural nodule ≥5 mm, iii) main pancreatic duct ≥10 mm
Yes
No
Consider surgery, if clinically appropriate
Are any of the following "worrisome features" present?
Clinical: Pancreatitis a
Imaging: i) cyst ≥3 cm, ii) enhancing mural nodule <5 mm, iii) thickened/enhancing cyst walls, iv) main duct size 5-9 mm, v) abrupt change in caliber of pancreatic duct with distal pancreatic atrophy, vi) lymphadenopathy, vii) increased serum level of CA19–9, viii) cyst growth rate ≥5 mm / 2 y
If yes, perform endoscopic ultrasound
No
Are any of these features present?
i) Definite mural nodule(s) ≥5 mm b
ii) Main duct features suspicious for involvement c
iii) Cytology: suspicious or positive for malignancy
Yes
No
What is the size of largest cyst?
Inconclusive
<1 cm
1–2 cm
2–3 cm
>3 cm
CT / MRI in 6 mo, then every 2 y if no change
CT / MRI 6 mo x 1 y yearly x 2 y, then lengthen interval up to 2 y if no change
EUS in 3–6 mo, then lengthen interval up to 1, alternating MRI with EUS as appropriate. Consider surgery in young, fit patients with need for prolonged surveillance
Close surveillance alternating MRI with EUS every 3–6 mo Strongly consider surgery in young, fit patients

Fig. 1. Revised Fukuoka guidelines (2017) on management of branch duct intraductal papillary mucinous neoplasms. [a] Pancreatitis may be an indication for surgery for relief of symptoms. [b] Differential diagnosis includes mucin. Mucin can move with change in patient position, may be dislodged on cyst lavage and does not have Doppler flow. Features of true tumor nodule include lack of mobility, presence of Doppler flow and FNA of nodule showing tumor tissue. [c] Presence of any one of thickened walls, intraductal mucin or mural nodules is suggestive of main duct involvement. In their absence main duct involvement is inconclusive. (*From* Tanaka M, Fernandez-del Castillo C, Kamisawa T, et al. Revisions of International Consensus Fukuoka Guidelines for the management of IPMN of the pancreas. Pancreatology 2017;17:741; with permission.)

cancer. For patients who do not meet these criteria, radiographic surveillance was recommended. A repeat MRCP was advised at 1 year from index examination. If no changes, then a repeat MRCP was advised 2 years later. If again no change, then repeat MRCP again in 2 years. Last, the AGA guidelines advised that if there were no significant changes in a pancreatic cyst with no high-risk features over the course of 5 years of surveillance, then surveillance imaging can be discontinued.

In 2018, the American College of Gastroenterology (ACG) published a set of clinical guidelines for the diagnosis and management of pancreatic cysts.[13] These guidelines focused on the most commonly encountered pancreatic cysts. The guidelines advised that asymptomatic cysts diagnosed as pseudocysts or SCAs do not require treatment or further evaluation. SPN on the other hand should be referred for consideration of surgical resection. In terms of management of mucinous cystic lesions (ie, BD-IPMN and MCN), the ACG guidelines followed similar recommendations as the other major guidelines in terms of identification of high-risk features, including presence of symptoms attributable to the lesion, elevated CA 19-9, presence of mural nodule or solid component, main pancreatic duct dilation greater than 5 mm, cyst size of 3 cm or greater, abrupt change in main duct diameter with associated upstream atrophy, growth of 3 mm or more per year, and presence of high-grade dysplasia or cancer on cytology. Lesions that are not resected should undergo surveillance with MRCP and/or EUS, with the modality and timing depending on cyst size and features.

GUIDELINE PERFORMANCE

Numerous studies have been published examining the performance characteristics of each of the above guidelines individually and against one another.

Studies examining the Sendai guidelines demonstrated a suboptimal performance in detecting cancer. Pelaez-Luna and colleagues[14] reviewed the outcomes of 147 patients with BD-IPMN. A total of 66 of these patients underwent surgical resection and 81 patients underwent surveillance; of these 81 patients, another 11 eventually underwent surgical resection. In examining the 77 resected patients and applying the Sendai guidelines, 16 patients had no criteria for resection, whereas 61 had at least one criterion. Cancer was found in 9/61 (15%) with at least one criterion. Overall, Sendai criteria for detecting cancer had sensitivity of 100%, specificity of 23%, positive predictive value (PPV) of 14%, and negative predictive value (NPV) of 100%. Two other studies demonstrated similar results in performance of Sendai in predicting cancer, with high sensitivities (93%–100%) and low specificities (29.8%–30%).[15,16]

A study by Sahora and colleagues[17] examined the performance of the Fukuoka criteria by retrospectively applying them to a large group of 563 patients with BD-IPMN. A total of 240 of these patients underwent surgical resection, whereas 323 underwent surveillance. In the surveillance group, 23/323 (4%) developed invasive cancer related to BD-IPMN, whereas another 21/323 (3.7%) developed pancreatic ductal adenocarcinoma. When applying the Fukuoka criteria to the cohort, 76% of resected BD-IPMN with carcinoma in situ and 95% of resected BD-IPMN with invasive cancer had high-risk stigmata or worrisome features. Nonworrisome cysts less than 3 cm in size were found to have high-grade dysplasia in 6.5%, whereas nonworrisome cysts greater than 3 cm in size were found to have high-grade dysplasia in 8.8% and 1 case with invasive cancer. In summary, the investigators stated that expectant management of BD-IPMN without high risk or worrisome features is safe, although caution should be applied to those cysts greater than 3 cm, even in the absence of worrisome features.

Kaimakliotis and colleagues[18] compared the performances of Sendai guidelines against the Fukuoka guidelines by retrospectively applying each set to a group of

194 patients who underwent surgical resection of a pancreatic cystic lesion. In regards to identifying advanced neoplasia (high-grade dysplasia or cancer), Sendai criteria had a sensitivity of 92%, specificity of 22%, PPV of 21%, and NPV of 92%. Fukuoka criteria had poorer sensitivity (55.6%) but improved specificity (73%), with similar PPV (32%) and NPV (88%) to that of Sendai. Overall, the group concluded that there was no statistically significant difference between the guidelines in terms of predicting advanced neoplasia. They further note that of these 194 patients who underwent surgery, only 18% had advanced neoplasia, and it is likely that approximately 30% would have never required surgery at all, given the final surgical pathologic condition of 57 lesions being benign, nonneoplastic, or nonpremalignant, thus demonstrating the poor accuracy of presurgical diagnostic testing. Other studies supported these findings of overall poor accuracy of both guidelines. Goh and colleagues[19] analyzed 114 mucinous cysts and demonstrated Sendai PPV of 46% and Fukuoka PPV of 62.5%. Yamada and colleagues[20] analyzed 177 patients who underwent surgical resection and demonstrated accuracy of predicting advanced pathologic condition of 35.5% for Sendai and 44.8% for Fukuoka.

The introduction of the AGA guidelines proposed a somewhat significant change in the approach to patients with pancreatic cysts. For one, this set of recommendations reserved the use of EUS in patients who had only 2 high-risk features. In addition, the guidelines recommend that practitioners cease cyst surveillance in low-risk lesions if no significant change at 5-year follow-up. These 2 aspects of the AGA guidelines were a marked change from standard practice by many physicians over the preceding 10 years.

Singhi and colleagues[21] examined the performance of the AGA guidelines in 225 patients with pancreatic cysts who had previously undergone an EUS-FNA. Diagnostic pathology was available in 41 (18%) subjects, who underwent final analysis. When applied retroactively to this group of patients, the AGA guidelines detected or predicted advanced neoplasia with a sensitivity of 62%, specificity of 79%, PPV of 57%, NPV of 82%. Furthermore, the AGA guidelines would have missed 45% of IPMN lesions exhibiting high-grade dysplasia or cancer. Last, application of these guidelines to this group would have led to unnecessary MRI surveillance in approximately 15%, who had confirmed SCA. Sahar and colleagues[22] examined the impact of the AGA guidelines recommendations regarding utilization of EUS in 125 patients. When applying the AGA threshold of 2 high-risk features to incorporate EUS, AGA guidelines had sensitivity 40% and specificity 100% in terms of identifying advanced pathologic condition. If the criteria to use EUS were lowered to those cysts having only 1 high-risk feature, then sensitivity would have increased to 80% and specificity would have increased to 95%. In addition, a more liberal approach to using EUS would have led to 11% of patients to avoid additional surveillance. Finally, with regards to the recommendation to stop surveillance after 5 years in patients with stable lesions and less than 2 high-risk features, Imbe and colleagues[23] reported that of 159 patients meeting these criteria, pancreatic cancer developed in 3 (1.9%) all after 5 years: at 84 months, 103 months, and 145 months.

Several studies compared the performance of the various guidelines against one another. Ma and colleagues[24] applied both the Fukuoka guidelines and the AGA guidelines against a group of 239 patients who underwent surgical resection for suspected mucinous pancreatic cysts. Advanced neoplasia was found in 71/239 (29.7%) of cases. In comparing performance of Fukuoka guidelines to AGA guidelines, there was no significant difference in sensitivity (28% vs 35%), specificity (96% vs 94%), PPV (both 74%), or NPV (76% vs 78%). The investigators noted that both guidelines would have missed several cases of cancer (Fukuoka 7, AGA 6) and high-grade dysplasia (Fukuoka 23, AGA 24). Sighinolfi and colleagues[25] compared Sendai, Fukuoka, and AGA guidelines against each other. This study demonstrated that based on a receiver operator curve (ROC) analysis, the Fukuoka (ROC 0.78) and AGA guidelines (ROC 0.76) were significantly more accurate than the Sendai guidelines (ROC 0.65, $P<.0001$). Last, Lekkerkerker and colleagues[26] analyzed the performance of 3 of the guidelines, Fukuoka guidelines, European guidelines, and AGA guidelines, in their ability to identify patients with advanced neoplasia who would theoretically benefit from surgical resection. This group retrospectively applied each of these guidelines to a group of 115 patients who had undergone prior surgical resection. Main outcomes studied included percentage of patients who would have had a justifiable resection in a suspected IPMN, percentage of patients who would have avoided an unnecessary resection, and number of patients who would have had a missed high-grade dysplasia or cancer. In terms of justifiable resection, all 3 criteria performed poorly: Fukuoka 54%, European 53%, AGA 59%. In terms of ability to avoid unnecessary resections, AGA (28%) was superior to Fukuoka (11%) and European (9%). However, the AGA guidelines were associated with an unreasonably high number of missed lesions with advanced neoplasia (12%), whereas Fukuoka and European guidelines would have missed none.

LIMITATIONS OF THE GUIDELINES

The various management guidelines are a helpful starting point for practitioners to broadly stratify risk in patients with a pancreatic cystic lesion and help facilitate a dialogue with their patients on the management options available. However, as noted in the above review, the various guidelines do have several weaknesses and flaws.

One major issue is that guidelines such as Sendai, Fukuoka, and the European guidelines are based on knowing what exact type of pancreatic cyst one is dealing with. These criteria provide guidance for specifically managing a branch duct IPMN, MCN, and SPN. However, current diagnostic testing for pancreatic cysts is notoriously suboptimal in confirming a true nonsurgical pathologic diagnosis. Cross-sectional imaging studies, such as contrast-enhanced CT and MRCP, are unable to adequately differentiate one cyst type from another, with one systematic review reporting CT scan accuracy of 39% to 44.7% and MRI accuracy of 39.5% to 50%.[27] Pancreatic cyst fluid analysis can provide a moderate ability to differentiate mucinous lesions from nonmucinous lesions using cyst fluid carcinoembryonic antigen concentrations, with reported pooled sensitivities of 63% and specificities of 93%.[28] Use of molecular analysis on pancreatic cyst fluid to identify KRAS and GNAS mutations have shown sensitivity of 84% to 96% and specificity of 80% to 100% for identifying mucinous lesions.[21,29–31] However, even in cases where high-grade dysplasia or cancer is present, all modalities underperform. The accuracy of MRI/MRCP to distinguish benign cysts from malignant cysts ranges from 55% to 76%.[32] EUS imaging alone has reported accuracies of 65% to 96% in determining presence of malignancy.[27] Cyst fluid cytology has poor sensitivity of detecting high-grade dysplasia or cancer, with a recent systematic review and meta-analysis reporting pooled sensitivity of 64.8%.[33]

Related to this issue is that all of the guidelines noted in this review are largely dependent on the presence and identification of cyst morphologic features: size, presence of intramural nodules, main pancreatic duct dilation, communication with the main pancreatic duct. The use of morphologic features is inherently flawed for several reasons. There can be significant interobserver variability in cyst size measurement.[34] Cyst size can be variable depending on which modality is used.[35–37] Identification of intramural nodules can be quite objective, because debris and "mucin balls" can be difficult to distinguish from a nodule. Complete visualization and assessment of the main pancreatic duct can be obscured by a large, complex cystic lesion, which may be overlying the duct or in close association to it. Depending on cyst, morphologic details can have a major impact on patient outcomes. For example, Sendai criteria identified cyst size of 3 cm or greater as a high-risk feature. As such, Sendai criteria were noted on multiple studies to have very high sensitivity for detecting advanced neoplasia, but poor specificity. However, Fukuoka criteria downgraded cyst size to a worrisome feature, and not an absolute risk factor for surgical resection. The result of this was that Fukuoka guidelines had improved specificity for advanced neoplasia (ie, fewer false positives), but significantly lower sensitivity and thus a higher chance of missing advanced neoplasia.[18]

Another major limitation in assessing the performance of one guideline against another is that they are not necessarily addressing the same lesions. For example, Sendai, Fukuoka, and European guidelines are all focused on specific pathologic subtypes, with BD-IPMN and MCN comprising the most important cysts. AGA guidelines, on the other hand, are to be applied to any pancreatic cyst, regardless of whether a mucinous lesion is suspected. Thus, caution must be taken when applying and comparing different sets of guidelines to the same set of pancreatic cystic lesions. One cannot make a fair comparison of guideline performance if, for example, BD-IPMN-oriented criteria (eg, Fukuoka) are applied to a group of unspecified pancreatic cystic lesions, and outcomes are compared with that of AGA guidelines for the same group of cysts.

Last, it should be noted that most of the data on which these guidelines are based is considered to be very low quality.[8-13] The bulk of the data was derived from retrospective case series, with associated limitations, such as heterogeneity, patient selection bias, and ultimately, an inability to apply findings to a large population of patients. There are no large, prospective, or randomized studies evaluating different management strategies for pancreatic cystic neoplasms and/or associated cancer-related outcomes.

NATURAL HISTORY AND RISK OF MALIGNANCY

Understanding the risk of malignant transformation of BD-IPMN can provide some perspective and help in counseling patients regarding best management options. Practical questions in this regard pertain to the short-term and long-term risk of malignant transformation in low-risk BD-IPMN as well as risk of malignant transformation in patients with worrisome or high-risk features.

Short-term risk of malignancy in low-risk BD-IPMN has been reported to range from 1% to 2% in up to 3 years of follow-up.[38-40] Longer-term risk, particularly after 5 years of follow-up, is of particular interest given that the AGA guidelines recommended cessation of surveillance of stable asymptomatic cysts after 5 years. A meta-analysis of 2177 patients demonstrated long-term risk of malignancy in BD-IPMN to be 3.7%, in up to 77 months of follow-up.[41] Similarly, Khannoussi and colleagues[42] reported 3.7% risk of malignancy in up to 84 months of follow-up in patients who were prospectively followed. Pergolini and colleagues[43] reported long-term outcomes in a retrospective review of 577 patients with BD-IPMN. The median follow-up in this cohort was 82 months (range: 6–329). In total, advanced pathologic condition (high-grade dysplasia or invasive cancer) developed in 20/363 (5.5%) of patients after 5 years of surveillance. In 108 patients with a cyst ≤1.5 cm, only 1 (0.9%) developed cancer. By contrast, of the 255 patients with a cyst greater than 1.5 cm, malignancy developed in 19 (7.5%) after 5 years of follow-up. Overall, these studies demonstrate that the short-term risk of malignancy in patients with low-risk BD-IPMN is low. However, the risk of malignancy appears to increase after 5 years of surveillance, especially in lesions measuring 1.5 cm or greater.

Patients with a BD-IPMN that develops a worrisome or high-risk feature should be advised to seek surgical consultation. However, in patients who choose to forego surgery or have an unfavorable risk-benefit ratio for surgery, it is essential to understand the impact of worrisome and high-risk features on their risk of developing cancer. Mukewar and colleagues[44] reported that patients with high-risk IPMN had a significantly greater 5-year risk of developing cancer, compared with those with worrisome features (49.7% vs 4.1%, P<.001). Similarly, Crippa and colleagues[45] reported that the 5-year disease-specific survival was significantly lower in those patients with high-risk IPMN (60%) compared with those with only worrisome features (96%, P<.0001). It should be noted that this latter study included those patients with main duct IPMN and mixed type branch duct and main duct IPMN. Pergolini and colleagues[43] reported that in patients followed for more than 5 years, 22% developed a worrisome or high-risk feature, and 10% of these patients subsequently developed cancer over a median time frame of 102 months.

A word of caution should be mentioned. Although the incidence of BD-IPMN has risen exponentially over the past 3 decades, the curve for IPMN-related cancers has remained flat.[4] IPMN-related cancer in general is a rare event.[46] Therefore, patients who are found to have a low-risk BD-IPMN can be given some reassurance that there is a statistically low probability of developing cancer or undergoing a prophylactic pancreatic resection. That being said, the cancer risk is not negligible. When one considers the risk of cancer in other precancerous conditions such as Barrett's esophagus (0.5% per year in nondysplastic) or colonic adenomas (up to 10% in lesions <10 mm in size) as well as the poor prognosis for patients once a diagnosis of pancreatic cancer is made, long-term surveillance of patients with low-risk BD-IPMN is very reasonable, provided the patient would be appropriate for surgery should high-risk features or advanced pathologic condition be discovered.[47–49]

FUTURE DIRECTIONS

Going forward, improvement of clinical guidelines for managing pancreatic cystic lesions would require better scientific evidence to support any recommendations. In particular, long-term, prospective studies examining the natural history of unresected BD-IPMN are sorely needed and could validate the findings from the large retrospective series. Ultimately, the key to better patient management will hinge on improving preoperative risk stratification of patients with BD-IPMN, allowing surgery to be limited to those patients who would benefit most. For example, multiple groups have developed and reported nomograms to predict malignancy in patients with BD-IPMN.[50,51]

Another strategy to improve preoperative risk stratification would be to identify other patient-related and cyst-related risk factors for cancer.

BD-IPMN growth rate may be associated with higher risk of advanced pathologic condition. In a multicenter, retrospective study of 284 patients with low-risk BD-IPMN, Kwong and colleagues[52] reported that growth rate of 2 to 5 mm/y was associated with an increased risk of malignancy, when compared with those subjects with growth rate less than 2 mm/y. They also noted that all malignant BD-IPMN grew by at least 10 mm before cancer diagnosis. Similarly, Kolb and colleagues[53] analyzed 189 patients with low-risk BD-IPMN and found that growth rate was significantly greater in those lesions that developed worrisome features, compared with those who did not (2.84 mm/y vs 0.23 mm/y, P<.001). Han and colleagues[54] reported that larger BD-IPMN, particularly those 2 cm and greater in size, showed significantly faster growth rates and were more likely to develop main pancreatic duct dilation and cyst wall thickening compared with smaller lesions.

One potential subgroup of patients with BD-IPMN who may be at higher risk for malignant transformation are those patients with a strong family history of pancreatic cancer. Canto and colleagues[55] found that BD-IPMN were found in more than 50% of asymptomatic, high-risk individuals aged 60 to 69 undergoing pancreatic cancer screening. The same group demonstrated that precursor lesions are of a higher grade in patients with a strong family history of pancreatic cancers.[56] However, a recent study demonstrated that individuals with a pancreatic cyst and a family history of pancreatic ductal adenocarcinoma do not have an increased 5-year risk of cancer, compared with those individuals with a pancreatic cyst but no family history of pancreatic cancer.[57] Further studies may be needed to clarify the impact of family history on risk of cancer formation in BD-IPMN.

Last, patients with BD-IPMN who also have a genetic syndrome associated with increased risk of pancreatic cancer, such as Peutz-Jeghers syndrome, BRCA mutations, and Lynch syndrome, may have a higher risk of malignant transformation in their cystic lesion. Further investigation is needed to clarify this theory.

As discussed in previous sections, current nonsurgical diagnostic modalities for pancreatic cystic lesions in general are mostly inadequate in their ability to obtain a pathologic diagnosis of any particular cystic lesion, or to stratify premalignant lesions as having high-risk pathologic condition or low-risk pathologic condition. As a result, many patients may undergo surgical resection, only to discover that the cyst had low risk pathologic condition or had no potential for malignant transformation at all. Advances in endoscopic imaging and tissue acquisition may allow for more definitive preoperative diagnosis of pancreatic cystic lesions.

Confocal laser endomicroscopy (CLE) is a novel imaging modality allowing for real-time, in vivo microscopic imaging of the gastrointestinal mucosa. Small-diameter CLE probes that can be advanced through a 19-gauge FNA needle can be used to perform needle-based CLE (nCLE). The use of nCLE allows for visualization of the pancreatic cyst wall and identification of various features of the epithelial lining and associated vascular patterns. Specific epithelial and vascular features have been identified for a variety of pancreatic cystic lesions. For example, BD-IPMN are characterized by the presence of papillary projections with a vascular core, whereas SCAs are noted to have a dense fernlike pattern of vessels described as a superficial vascular network.[58] Other epithelial and vascular patterns have been described for MCNs, cystic neuroendocrine tumor, and pancreatic pseudocysts.[58] Published clinical data show promise that this endoscopic tool can provide a diagnosis for pancreatic cysts. Mucinous cystic lesions can be detected with a sensitivity of 80%, specificity of 100%, and accuracy of 89%, whereas SCAs can be detected with sensitivity of 69%, specificity of 100%, and accuracy of 87%.[59,60] The largest prospective trial to date has shown that for the diagnosis of mucinous lesions, nCLE (91%) is superior to both EUS morphology (47%, $P<.05$) and cyst fluid CEA levels (71%, $P<.01$).[61]

Through-the-needle microforceps are a novel tool allowing for direct biopsies of the pancreatic cyst wall. These miniature biopsy forceps can be inserted through a 19-gauge FNA needle. Mittal and colleagues[62] described their experience in 27 patients and a reported a diagnostic yield in 88.9% of cases. Basar and colleagues[63] reported a similar cyst tissue acquisition yield of 90%, and that microforceps biopsy was far superior to cyst fluid cytology for providing a specific cyst diagnosis (35.7% vs 4.8%, $P = .001$).

The development of novel cyst fluid biomarkers that can distinguish lesions with low-risk pathologic condition from those with advanced pathologic condition would also allow for better preoperative risk stratification of patients. A variety of DNA-based, micro-RNA-based, and protein-based biomarkers have been identified that have the potential to discern between nonneoplastic pancreatic cysts and mucinous cysts as well as discerning mucinous cysts with low-risk pathologic condition from those with advanced neoplasia.[64] Combining composite molecular markers with clinical features could also improve classification of pancreatic cysts and possibly impact clinical care. Springer and colleagues[29] performed a multicenter, retrospective study of 130 patients with resected pancreatic cystic neoplasms. Cyst fluid was analyzed to detect the presence or absence of a variety of molecular markers. When these results were combined with clinical features, cyst types were able to be classified with 90% to 100% sensitivity and 92% to 98% specificity. Furthermore, the molecular marker panel correctly identified 67 of the 74 patients who did not require surgery, and would have reduced the number of unnecessary operations by 91%.

SUMMARY

Pancreatic cystic lesions are a common clinical entity, a subset of which poses a potentially significant health risk to patients. Multiple expert guidelines have been published. Variances exist among these different guidelines with regards to specific recommendations pertaining to evaluation, indications for surgery, and surveillance intervals. No one guideline appears to perform optimally. However, they all do highlight the importance of identification of high-risk features in precancerous cystic lesions such as the presence of solid nodular components, main pancreatic duct dilation, cyst size, and high-risk cytologic features on FNA sampling. The identification of other patient-related and cyst-related risk factors as well as advances in pancreatic cyst wall tissue sampling and cyst fluid biomarker development will certainly lead to improvements in identifying which patients would benefit most from surgical resection.

REFERENCES

1. Laffan TA, Horton KM, Klein AP, et al. Prevalence of unsuspected pancreatic cysts on MDCT. AJR Am J Roentgenol 2008;191:802–7.
2. De Jong K, Nio CY, Hermans JJ, et al. High prevalence of pancreatic cysts detected by screening magnetic resonance imaging examinations. Clin Gastroenterol Hepatol 2010;8:806–11.
3. Sohn TA, Yeo CJ, Camern JL, et al. Intraductal papillary mucinous neoplasms of the pancreas. An updated experience. Ann Surg 2004;239:788–99.
4. Klibansky DA, Reid-Lombardo KM, Gordon SR, et al. The clinical relevance of the increasing incidence of intraductal papillary mucinous neoplasm. Clin Gastroenterol Hepatol 2012;10:555–8.
5. Jals B, Rebours V, Malleo G, et al. Serous cystic neoplasm of the pancreas: a multinational study of 2622 patients under the auspices of the International Association of Pancreatology and European Pancreatic Club (European Study Group on Cystic Tumors of the Pancreas). Gut 2016;65:305–12.
6. Park JW, Jang JY, Kang MJ, et al. Mucinous cystic neoplasm of the pancreas: Is surgical resection recommended for all surgically fit patients? Pancreatology 2014;14:131–6.
7. Law JK, Ahmed A, Singh VK, et al. A systematic review of solid-pseudopapillary neoplasms: are these rare lesions? Pancreas 2014;43:331–7.

8. Tanaka M, Chari S, Adsay V, et al. International consensus guidelines for management of intraductal papillary mucinous neoplasms and mucinous cystic neoplasms of the pancreas. Pancreatology 2006;6:17–32.
9. Tanaka M, Fernandez-del Castillo C, Adsay V, et al. International consensus guidelines 2012 for the management of IPMN and MCN of the pancreas. Pancreatology 2012;12:183–97.
10. Tanaka M, Fernandez-del Castillo C, Kamisawa T, et al. Revisions of international consensus Fukuoka guidelines for the management of IPMN of the pancreas. Pancreatology 2017;17:738–53.
11. Del Chiaro M, Verbeke C, Salvia R, et al. European experts consensus statement on cystic tumors of the pancreas. Dig Liver Dis 2013;45:703–11.
12. Vege SS, Ziring B, Jain R, et al. American Gastroenterological Association Institute guideline on the diagnosis and management of asymptomatic neoplastic pancreatic cysts. Gastroenterology 2015;148:819–22.
13. Elta GH, Enestvedt BK, Sauer BG, et al. ACG clinical guideline: diagnosis and management of pancreatic cysts. Am J Gastroenterol 2018;113(4):464–79.
14. Pelaez-Luna M, Chari ST, Smyrk TC, et al. Do consensus indications for resection in branch duct intraductal papillary mucinous neoplasm predict malignancy? A study of 147 patients. Am J Gastroenterol 2007;102(8):1759–64.
15. Tang RS, Weinberg B, Dawson DW, et al. Evaluation of the guidelines for management of pancreatic branch-duct intraductal papillary mucinous neoplasm. Clin Gastroenterol Heptaol 2008;6:815–9.
16. Nagai K, Doi R, Ito T, et al. Single-institution validation of the international consensus guidelines for treatment of branch duct intraductal papillary mucinous neoplasms of the pancreas. J Hepatobiliary Pancreat Surg 2009;16:353–8.
17. Sahora K, Mino-Kenudson M, Brugge W, et al. Branch duct intraductal papillary mucinous neoplasms: does cyst size change the tip of the scale? A critical analysis of the revised international consensus guidelines in a large single-institutional series. Ann Surg 2013;258:466–75.
18. Kaimakliotis P, Riff B, Pourmand K, et al. Sendai and Fukuoka consensus guidelines identify advanced neoplasia in patients with suspected mucinous cystic neoplasms of the pancreas. Clin Gastroenterol Hepatol 2015;13:1808–15.
19. Goh BK, Thng CH, Tan DM, et al. Evaluation of the Sendai and 2012 international consensus guidelines based on cross-sectional imaging findings performed for the initial triage of mucinous cystic lesions of the pancreas: a single institution experience with 114 surgically treated patients. Am J Surg 2014;208:202–9.
20. Yamada S, Fujii T, Murotani K, et al. Comparison of the international consensus guidelines for predicting malignancy in intraductal papillary mucinous neoplasms. Surgery 2016;159:878–84.
21. Singhi AD, Zeh HJ, Brand RE, et al. American Gastroenterological Association guidelines are inaccurate in detecting pancreatic cysts with advanced neoplasia: a clinicopathologic study of 225 patients with supporting molecular data. Gastrointest Endosc 2016;83:1107–17.
22. Sahar N, Razzak A, Kanji ZS, et al. New guidelines for use of endoscopic ultrasound for evaluation and risk stratification of pancreatic cystic lesions may be too conservative. Surg Endosc 2018;32(5):2420–6.
23. Imbe K, Nagata N, Hisada Y, et al. Validation of the American Gastroenterological Association guidelines on management of intraductal papillary mucinous neoplasms: more than 5 years of follow-up. Eur Radiol 2018;28:170–8.
24. Ma GK, Goldberg DS, Thiruvengadam N, et al. Comparing American Gastroenterological Association guidelines with Fukuoka consensus guidelines as

predictors of advanced neoplasia in patients with suspected pancreatic cystic neoplasms. J Am Coll Surg 2016;223:729–37.

25. Sighinolfi M, Quan SY, Lee Y, et al. Fukuoka and AGA criteria have superior diagnostic accuracy for advanced cystic neoplasms than Sendai criteria. Dig Dis Sci 2017;62:626–32.

26. Lekkerkerker SJ, Besselink MG, Busch OR, et al. Comparing 3 guidelines on the management of surgically removed pancreatic cysts with regard to pathological outcome. Gastrointest Endosc 2017;85:1025–31.

27. Tirkes T, Alsen AM, Cramer HM, et al. Cystic neoplasms of the pancreas; findings on magnetic resonance imaging with pathological, surgical, and clinical correlation. Abdom Imaging 2014;39:1088–101.

28. Thornton GD, McPhail MJ, Nayagam S, et al. Endoscopic ultrasound guided fine needle aspiration for the diagnosis of pancreatic cystic neoplasms: a meta-analysis. Pancreatology 2013;13:48–57.

29. Springer S, Wang Y, Dal Molin M, et al. A combination of molecular markers and clinical features improve the classification of pancreatic cysts. Gastroenterology 2015;149:1501–10.

30. Rosenbaum MW, Jones M, Dudley JC, et al. Next-generation sequencing adds value to the preoperative diagnosis of pancreatic cysts. Cancer Cytopathol 2016;125:41–7.

31. Jones M, Zheng Z, Wang J, et al. Impact of next-generation sequencing on the clinical diagnosis of pancreatic cysts. Gastrointest Endosc 2016;82:140–8.

32. Jones MJ, Buchanan AS, Neal CP, et al. Imaging of indeterminate pancreatic cystic lesions: a systematic review. Pancreatology 2013;13:436–42.

33. Suzuki R, Thosani N, Annangi S, et al. Diagnostic yield of EUS-FNA-based cytology distinguishing malignant and benign IPMNs: a systematic review and meta-analysis. Pancreatology 2014;14:380–4.

34. Dunn DP, Brook OR, Brook A, et al. Measurement of pancreatic cystic lesions on magnetic resonance imaging; efficacy of standards in reducing inter-observer variability. Abdom Radiol (NY) 2016;41:500–7.

35. Boos J, Brook A, Chingkoe CM, et al. MDCT vs MRI for incidental pancreatic cysts: measurement variability and impact on clinical management. Abdom Radiol (NY) 2017;42:521–30.

36. Maimone S, Agrawal D, Pollack MJ, et al. Variability in measurements of pancreatic cyst size among EUS, CT, and magnetic resonance imaging. Gastrointest Endosc 2010;71:945–50.

37. Du C, Chai NL, Linghu EQ, et al. Comparison of endoscopic ultrasound, computed tomography and magnetic resonance imaging in assessment of detailed structures of pancreatic cystic neoplasms. World J Gastroenterol 2017;23:3184–92.

38. Gaujoux S, Brennan MF, Gonen M, et al. Cystic lesions of the pancreas: changes in the presentation and management of 1,424 patients at a single institution over a 15-year time period. J Am Coll Surg 2011;212:590–600.

39. Del Chiaro M, Ateeb Z, Hansson MR, et al. Survival analysis and risk for progression of intraductal papillary mucinous neoplasia of the pancreas (IPMN) under surveillance: a single-institution experience. Ann Surg Oncol 2017;24: 1120–6.

40. Moris M, Raimondo M, Woodward TA, et al. International intraductal papillary mucinous neoplasms registry: long-term results based on the new guidelines. Pancreas 2017;46:306–10.

41. Crippa S, Capurso G, Cammà C, et al. Risk of pancreatic malignancy and mortality in branch-duct IPMNs undergoing surveillance: a systematic review and meta-analysis. Dig Liver Dis 2016;48:473–9.

42. Khannoussi W, Vullierme MP, Rebours V, et al. The long term risk of malignancy in patients with branch duct intraductal papillary mucinous neoplasms of the pancreas. Pancreatology 2012;12:198–202.

43. Pergolini I, Sahora K, Ferrone CR, et al. Long-term risk of pancreatic malignancy in patients with branch duct intraductal papillary mucinous neoplasm in a referral center. Gastroenterology 2017;153:1284–94.

44. Mukewar S, de Pretis N, Aryal-Khanal A, et al. Fukuoka criteria accurately predict risk for adverse outcomes during follow-up of pancreatic cysts presumed to be intraductal papillary mucinous neoplasms. Gut 2017;66:1811–7.

45. Crippa S, Bassi C, Salvia R, et al. Low progression of intraductal papillary mucinous neoplasms with worrisome features and high-risk stigmata undergoing non-operative management: a mid-term follow up analysis. Gut 2017;66: 495–506.

46. Gardner TB, Glass LM, Smith KD, et al. Pancreatic cyst prevalence and the risk of mucin-producing adenocarcinoma in US adults. Am J Gastroenterol 2013;108: 1546–50.

47. Shaheen NJ, Falk GW, Iyer PG, et al. ACG clinical guideline: diagnosis and management of Barrett's esophagus. Am J Gastroenterol 2016;111:30–50.

48. Butterfly LF, Chase MP, Pohl H, et al. Prevalence of clinically important histology in small adenomas. Clin Gastroenterol Hepatol 2006;4:343–8.

49. Lieberman D, Moravec M, Holub J, et al. Polyp size and advanced histology in patients undergoing colonoscopy screening: implications for CT colonography. Gastroenterology 2008;135:1100–5.

50. Attiyeh MA, Fernandez-del Castillo C, Al Efishat M, et al. Development and validation of a multi-institutional preoperative nomogram for predicting grade of dysplasia in intraductal papillary mucinous neoplasm (IPMNs) of the pancreas: a report from the pancreatic surgery consortium. Ann Surg 2018;267:157–63.

51. Jang JY, Park T, Lee S, et al. Proposed nomogram predicting the individual risk of malignancy in the patients with branch duct type intraductal papillary mucinous neoplasms of the pancreas. Ann Surg 2017;266:1062–8.

52. Kwong WT, Lawson RD, Hunt G, et al. Rapid growth rates of suspected pancreatic cyst branch duct intraductal papillary mucinous neoplasms predict malignancy. Dig Dis Sci 2015;60:2800–6.

53. Kolb JM, Argiriadi P, Lee K, et al. Higher growth rate of branch duct intraductal papillary mucinous neoplasms associates with worrisome features. Clin Gastroenterol Hepatol 2018. [Epub ahead of print].

54. Han Y, Lee H, Kang JS, et al. Progression of pancreatic branch duct intraductal papillary mucinous neoplasm associates with cyst size. Gastroenterology 2018; 154:576–84.

55. Canto MI, Hruban RH, Fishman EK, et al. Frequent detection of pancreatic lesions in asymptomatic high-risk individuals. Gastroenterology 2012;142:796–804.

56. Shi C, Klein AP, Goggins M, et al. Increased prevalence of precursor lesions in familial pancreatic cancer patients. Clin Cancer Res 2009;15:7737–43.

57. Mukewar SS, Sharma A, Phillip N, et al. Risk of pancreatic cancer in patients with pancreatic cysts and family history of pancreatic cancer. Clin Gastroenterol Hepatol 2018;16(7):1123–30.

58. Napoleon B, Lemaistre AL, Pujol B, et al. In vivo characterization of pancreatic cystic lesions by needle-based confocal laser endomicroscopy (nCLE):

proposition of a comprehensive nCLE classification confirmed by an external retrospective evaluation. Surg Endosc 2016;30:2603–12.

59. Nakai Y, Iwashita T, Park DH, et al. Diagnosis of pancreatic cysts: EUS-guided, through-the-needle confocal laser-induced endomicroscopy and cystoscopy trial: DETECT study. Gastrointest Endosc 2015;81:1204–14.

60. Napoleon B, Lemaistre AI, Pujol B, et al. A novel approach to the diagnosis of pancreatic serous cystadenoma: needle-based confocal laser endomicroscopy. Endoscopy 2015;47:26–32.

61. Napoleon B, Pujol B, Palazzo M, et al. Needle-based confocal laser endomicoscopy (nCLE) for the diagnosis of pancreatic cystic lesions: preliminary results of the first prospective multicenter study. Gastroenterology 2017;152:S132–3.

62. Mittal C, Obuch JC, Hammad H, et al. Technical feasibility, diagnostic yield, and safety of microforceps biopsies during EUS evaluation of pancreatic cystic lesions (with video). Gastrointest Endosc 2018;87(5):1263–9.

63. Basar O, Yuksel O, Yang D, et al. Feasibility and safety of micro-forceps biopsy in the diagnosis of pancreatic cysts. Gastrointest Endosc 2018;88(1):79–86.

64. Singh H, McGrath K, Singhi AD. Novel biomarkers for pancreatic cysts. Dig Dis Sci 2017;62:1796–807.

The Use of Biomarkers in the Risk Stratification of Cystic Neoplasms

Jeremy H. Kaplan, MD, Tamas A. Gonda, MD*

KEYWORDS

- Pancreatic cysts • Biomarkers • Molecular diagnosis
- Intraductal papillary mucinous neoplasm (IPMN) • Mucinous neoplasm • Malignancy

KEY POINTS

- Distinguishing mucinous cysts from nonmucinous cysts is essential to diagnosing pancreatic cysts.
- A combination of DNA markers, amylase, and oncogene testing can be used to diagnose pancreatic cyst subtypes.
- Cyst fluid DNA markers and oncogenes may be used to stratify pancreatic cysts by their malignant potential.

BACKGROUND

Introduction

The frequent use of cross-sectional imaging has led to the identification of an increasing number of pancreatic cysts. The incidence of pancreatic cysts rises with age and is now estimated to be present in approximately 2% of adults.[1] Although a majority of these lesions are benign, 15% are cyst types known to be precursor lesions for invasive carcinoma, thus requiring further monitoring.[2] Given the high morbidity and mortality associated with pancreatic cancer, there is a significant interest in risk stratifying benign pancreatic cysts based on malignant potential. Currently, surgical resection is the only therapeutic intervention, and this is associated with considerable morbidity and mortality rates. This makes accurate biopsy or fluid sampling–based evaluation of these cysts essential.

Disclosures: None.
Funding/Conflicts of Interest: There was no grant support or other financial support for this article. All authors declare no conflicts of interest.
Division of Digestive and Liver Diseases, Department of Medicine, Columbia University, 161 Fort Washington Avenue, New York, NY 10032, USA
* Corresponding author.
E-mail address: tg2214@cumc.columbia.edu

Gastrointest Endoscopy Clin N Am 28 (2018) 549–568
https://doi.org/10.1016/j.giec.2018.05.006
1052-5157/18/© 2018 Elsevier Inc. All rights reserved.

giendo.theclinics.com

Although a majority of cysts identified in the pancreas are neoplastic, many of these lesions are not associated with a significant malignancy risk. These include predominantly serous cystadenomas (SCAs) and other benign pancreatic or peripancreatic cysts. There are also cysts that are identified in the pancreas adjacent to a solid mass or as a consequence of cystic degeneration of either adenocarcinomas or neuroendocrine tumors. Mucinous cysts, including mucinous cyst neoplasms (MCNs) and intraductal papillary mucinous neoplasms (IPMNs), represent the majority of neoplastic premalignant cysts identified in the pancreas. A retrospective study of 851 individuals undergoing surgical resection of pancreatic cystic neoplasms over 33 years demonstrated that IPMNs are the most common subtype of cyst, followed by mucinous cystic neoplasms (MCNs), serous cystic neoplasms, and cystic neuroendocrine neoplasms.[3] Most diagnostic strategies approach pancreatic cysts by first attempting to recognize mucinous cysts and subsequently risk stratify suspected MCNs or IPMNs based on malignancy risk. In this article, this strategy is followed in presenting the utility of biomarkers.

In most studies of cystic biomarkers, a dichotomy is made between mucinous and nonmucinous cysts. Clinically, however, the distinction of greatest importance is between cysts with malignant potential, cysts without malignant potential, and malignancies. With this understanding, this article takes the approach of first discussing the role of biomarkers in distinguishing mucinous from nonmucinous cysts. Thereafter, the use of biomarkers for the risk stratification of cysts based on their malignant potential is discussed.

Nonmucinous Cysts

Of the nonmucinous cysts, SCAs are the most commonly encountered.[4] These cysts are typically found incidentally but may cause abdominal pain if large enough. Although not true cysts, pancreatic pseudocysts (PCs) are also common and often associated with pancreatitis.[4] Most importantly, SCAs and PCs have no malignant potential.[5] Non-neoplastic pancreatic cysts include a variety of rare cysts that do not frequently cause symptoms and pose no danger. They include true cysts (or benign epithelial cysts), retention cysts that may occur in the setting of ductal obstruction, and lymphoepithelial cysts. The lymphoepithelial cysts are lined by mature keratinized squamous epithelium surrounded by lymphoid tissue. Resection is rarely required.[6] Similarly, congenital cysts and squamoid cyst of ducts have virtually no malignant potential.[7]

Rare cystic tumors occurring as a result of degenerative/necrotic changes in solid tumors include cystic ductal adenocarcinomas, cystic endocrine neoplasia, and solid pseudopapillary tumor (SPT). SPTs are a rare but important cyst type because, despite variable degrees of aggressiveness, they are all considered malignant.[7] SPTs represent less than 10% of all pancreatic cysts and occur almost exclusively in young women. Identification is important because resection is usually curative.[8]

Mucinous Cysts

Mucinous cysts are further subdivided into MCNs, including mucinous cystadenomas and cystadenocarcinomas and intraductal papillary MCNs (IPMNs). MCNs and IPMNS harbor malignant potential and, therefore, require diagnosis and appropriate management.[9] Surgical removal of a premalignant MCN or IPMN confers a 5-year survival of nearly 100%. With the development of invasive carcinoma, however, survival drops to under 60%.[10]

Guideline-Based Management of Intraductal Papillary Mucinous Cystic Neoplasm

With the understanding that IPMNs are the cyst type with the most variable course, great efforts have been made to create guidelines based on clinical features for the management of these benign cysts. An international consensus guideline was created in Fukuoka, Japan, in 2012 and modified in 2017. IPMNs are divided into 3 cyst types, including main duct IPMN, branch duct (BD)-type IPMN, and mixed-type IPMN, based on imaging and/or histology. The risk stratification of these cysts and the recommended management is based on the presence of high-risk stigmata and worrisome features.[11] The presence of any high-risk stigmata comes with a recommendation for surgical intervention. The features and clinical factors that lead to this designation are obstructive jaundice in a patient with a cystic pancreatic head mass, enhanced solid component within the cyst, and/or a main pancreatic duct size of greater or equal to 10 mm. Dilation of the main pancreatic duct is concerning because the frequency of malignancy in such patients is approximately 60%.

The Fukuoka guidelines report a mean frequency of invasive carcinoma and high-grade dysplasia in main duct IPMN of 61.6%. As such, surgical resection is strongly recommended for all surgically fit patients with a main pancreatic duct greater than 10 mm, jaundice, or mural nodules.[12] Risk stratification, however, of BD-IPMNS is more challenging because of the greater range of malignant potential. The presence of mural nodules on CT conferred an odds ratio of 19.3. Multivariate analysis found that cyst size greater than 3 cm was also an independent risk factor for the presence of malignancy BD-IPMN.[13]

Nonetheless, the Fukuoka guidelines designate a range of other features as worrisome, requiring further risk stratification using endoscopic ultrasound (EUS) and surveillance.[12] With that comes a range of potential parameters that may be used for risk stratification. To date, there is extensive debate about the role of fluid markers for further examination of these cysts. There remains a paucity of guidelines regarding the use of these biomarkers and their application in surveillance. It is here that fluid markers may help in risk stratifying these lesions. A subsequent study demonstrated, however, that Fukuoka-negative cysts confer a 5-year risk of pancreatic cancer of under 2% regardless of cyst size. The notion that cysts with high-risk stigmata have the highest risk of malignant transformation was validated by the study's finding of a approximately 50% risk of pancreatic cancer at 3 years and 5 years.[14]

The American Gastroenterological Association has also released guidelines regarding the management of pancreatic cysts. In their 2015 guidelines, surgery is recommended in surgically fit patients with proved high-grade dysplasia or imaging features suggestive of malignancy.[15] These imaging features were highlighted in a technical review that same year and included cyst size greater than 3 cm, solid component associated with the cyst, and a dilated pancreatic duct.[16] They do not specifically address the role of fluid biomarkers in risk stratification of IPMNs.

A more recent set of guidelines was released from the American College of Radiology in 2017. In their management algorithm, the first set of important variables is the size of the lesion, presence of main pancreatic duct communication, and patient age.[17] They further embrace the Fukuoka nomenclature of "worrisome features" and "high-risk stigmata." They recommend the assumption that a cyst is mucinous unless there are definitive features of alternative histology or if biopsy proves otherwise.

The Role of Endoscopic Ultrasound and Fine-Needle Aspiration in the Diagnosis of Pancreatic Cysts

Despite the importance of classifying pancreatic cysts for risk stratification, preoperative diagnosis for cyst type may be incorrect in 20% to 30% of patients, highlighting the importance of further tests to increase accuracy.[18,19] Initially developed in the 1980s, EUS has proved valuable in the evaluation of pancreatic cysts. EUS morphology alone carries a diagnostic accuracy of 40% to 96%. As a single test, the accuracy of EUS in distinguishing mucinous from nonmucinous cysts is only 51%.[20] EUS, however, provides the opportunity for fine-needle aspiration (FNA), which can be done under real-time guidance. The fluid sampled through this procedure can be used for cytologic, molecular, and/or biochemical testing. Additionally, the cyst wall can be biopsied, which may increase diagnostic yield by as much as 37%.[21] The use of EUS to categorize pancreatic lesions has been revolutionary. It may be marked, however, by low interobserver agreement.[22]

Studies dating back to the early 2000s have explored the utility of EUS-FNA cytology. EUS-FNA is known to be safe, with a mortality rate less than 0.05% and morbidity rate of under 5%.[23] In principle, cytology should provide an accurate diagnosis of mucinous neoplasms and exclude malignancy. Diagnostic yield is hindered, however, by the relatively low cellular content of cyst fluid, resulting in a disappointingly low sensitivity of 54%. Yield is increased if the needle is moved back and forth repeatedly.[24] Other techniques proposed to increase diagnostic yield include use of the Moray microforceps and cytology brushes.[25,26] Despite a high specificity of 93%, the potential miscategorization of cysts as nonmucinous limits the utility of cytology.[27] Other limitations include distinguishing the cellular contents in the cyst from gastrointestinal contaminants. Ultimately, the most useful role of cytology is in diagnosing invasive malignancy; however, its role in determining the degree of dysplasia in the cyst tissue is limited.[28]

Cyst fluid markers become important when lesions cannot be reliably subtyped and cancer cannot be ruled out. Most commonly, this applies to pancreatic cysts with equivocal imaging. Most diagnostic uncertainty is centered on pancreatic cysts less than 2.5 cm in size.[17] Although guidelines exist for the risk stratification based on imaging, it may be difficult to determine the relationship between the cyst and the pancreatic duct, and whether mural nodules are present. Although cyst size is associated with an increased risk of harboring high-grade dysplasia and invasive cancer, there is no size cutoff to predict risk and size alone is not sufficient to indicate surgery.[29,30]

THE USE OF BIOMARKERS IN DIAGNOSING CYST TYPE
Fluid Amylase

In cases of EUS-FNA cytology that is indeterminate, there may be utility in sampling the fluid for various biomarkers. One of the earlier ideas was to test the fluid for amylase. The presence of a high fluid amylase indicates communication between a cyst and the ductal system.[4] Consequently, cyst fluid–rich in amylase indicates ductal disruption, as seen in a pseudocyst, suggesting the presence of a communication between the cyst and ducts, which is present in IPMN. With a specificity of 98% a fluid amylase of less than 250 U/L essentially rules out communication with the duct.[31] Unfortunately, amylase alone cannot distinguish between MCN and IPMN.[21] This limitation is significant because it is recommended that MCNs undergo resection, whereas IPMNS may be monitored.[11] Furthermore, low cyst fluid amylase does not rule out malignancy nor can it be used to risk stratify for premalignant potential.[32] In differentiating between IPMN and pseudocyst, the clinical history is invaluable. A preceding episode of pancreatitis favors a diagnosis of pseudocyst. The IPMNs, however, occasionally may cause pancreatitis.[33]

Tumor Markers

Carcinoembryonic antigen (CEA) is a marker of mucin production and has been proposed as a way of differentiating cysts lined with mucinous epithelium, including

MCNs and IPMNs, from those cysts lacking a mucinous epithelial lining (SCA and pseudocyst).[4] In doing so, the aim is to rule out lesions with premalignant potential. The challenge with using CEA to differentiate mucinous from nonmucinous cysts is attempting to set an appropriate cutoff value. A pooled analysis of 332 CEA concentrations in cyst fluid of PC, SCA, and MCN demonstrated a positive predictive value of 94% in diagnosis of mucinous cystadenoma and mucinous cystadenocarcinoma when a CEA cutoff was set at greater than 800 ng/mL. The negative predictive value was 75%, however, signifying that several premalignant cysts may be missed.[31] Reducing the CEA cutoff to greater than 192 gives a likelihood ratio of 4.37, suggesting a good predictor of mucinous cysts.[27] In these earlier studies, mucinous cysts were characterized as mucinous cystadenomas and mucinous cystadenocarcinomas. Although guidelines continue to suggest a CEA cutoff of 192 ng/mL to 200 ng/mL, there is no recommendation for its use as a single test to diagnose a mucinous cyst type.[12]

Given the challenge in setting a CEA cutoff to risk stratify benign cysts by categorization, several studies have examined coupling CEA with endosonographic findings. A combination of cyst morphology, CEA, and cytology may predict 91% of mucinous lesions. This is at the cost, however, of a specificity of 31%.[20] Morphologic criteria for mucinous cysts in that study included macrocystic septations or adjacent mass. Although no single marker is sufficient to differentiate mucinous from nonmucinous cysts, CEA is the most accurate.[34,35] Like amylase, however, CEA cannot be used to differentiate MCN from IPMN. Potentially, the greatest utility of CEA as a single marker is of predicting a nonmucinous tumor because a CEA less than 5 rules out mucinous tumors in based on a positive predictive value of 94% for identification of SCA and PC.[31]

Other tumor markers that have been examined for the potential in distinguishing varying types of cysts include cancer antigen (CA) 72-4, CA 125, and CA 15-3. All are inferior to cyst fluid CEA in distinguishing mucinous from nonmucinous cysts.[20,31]

von Hippel-Lindau and Vascular Endothelial Growth Factor in the Diagnosis of Serous Cystadenoma

The recognition that SCAs occur in more than 15% of patients with von Hippel-Lindau syndrome spurred interest in the use of this biomarker to diagnose this benign cyst type.[36] SCAs characteristically appear on cross-sectional imaging as multiple small microcysts with central calcification. On EUS, honeycombing is often seen.[37] If a diagnosis cannot be reached based on imaging characteristics alone, fluid sampling for VHL can be performed. Mutations are seen in up to 75% of SCAs.[38] VHL has been reported to have up to 100% sensitivity in the diagnosis of SCA.[1] Recently it was noted that VEGF-A is very elevated in SCA fluid. VEGF-A alone has a 100% sensitivity and 83.7% specificity for distinguishing SCN from other cystic lesions when a threshold is set at greater than 5000 pg/mL.[39] Ultimately, SCA can often be diagnosed using a combination of radiologic features, low CEA, and potentially VEGF-A levels.

DNA Markers for Mucinous Lesions

Whereas cellular content may be difficult to obtain, DNA shed from the epithelial lining of pancreatic cysts is more abundant. DNA is also a relatively stable molecule, making any evaluation more plausible. Mutations of interest include KRAS and GNAS, among others. KRAS is a proto-oncogene located on chromosome arm 12p and encodes a membrane-bound guanosine triphosphate–binding protein. It is involved in cell proliferation, survival, and motility as well as signal transduction. GNAS is an oncogene involved with G protein production One of the earlier studies to identify the role of pancreatic cyst fluid DNA analysis in evaluating pancreatic cysts was performed by Khalid and colleagues.[40] The multicenter Pancreatic Cyst DNA Analysis (PANDA) study evaluated cyst fluid from 113 patients with different cyst types for genetic markers. The investigators concluded that KRAS fluid mutations were helpful in the diagnosis of mucinous cysts, with a specificity of 95% and sensitivity of 45%. A meta-analysis of 6 studies examined the ability of KRAS to differentiate mucinous and nonmucinous cysts. Specificity was close to 1.0, with pooled sensitivity estimates closer to 0.5. These data suggest that a mutation in KRAS is useful in identifying mucinous lesions but may miss cases.[41]

In 2011, Wu and colleagues[42] sought to determine the sequences of 169 presumptive cancer genes in the cyst fluids of 19 IPMNs. In doing so they identified mutations in KRAS and GNAS as common. Although KRAS was known to be associated with multiple epithelial tumors, GNAS was previously only rarely seen in these masses.[43] The presence of mutations in the oncogene GNAS has proved an effective way of differentiating IPMN from MCN and SCN. In a sample of 147 cysts, GNAS mutations were found in 61% of IPMNs but 0% of SCN and MCNs.[42] A subsequent study of 25 cysts again noted that GNAS mutations were found only in IPMNs and added that KRAS mutations were also limited to IPMNs alone.[44]

Combined cytopathology and mutation analysis of KRAS and GNAS together may increase sensitivity and specificity for the diagnosis of IPMN to 92% and 50%, respectively.

A summary of various biomarkers and their sensitivity and specificity for the diagnosis of pancreatic cyst type is found in **Table 1**.

THE USE OF BIOMARKERS IN DETECTING PROGRESSION IN BENIGN PANCREATIC NEOPLASMS
Tumor Markers

Beyond its role in the subtyping of pancreatic cysts, CEA levels have also been evaluated in assessing cysts for malignant transformation and risk stratifying cysts for dysplasia. Data have been fairly mixed. A study of 54 fluid tests evaluated in patients with confirmed MCNs resected over a 24-year period demonstrated that CEA levels were significantly higher in cysts with low-grade dysplasia than in cysts with high-grade dysplasia. High levels of CEA were also seen in patients with malignancy.[32] Numerous other studies, however, have demonstrated that CEA levels do not correlate with an increased probability of malignancy in mucinous cysts.[20,31,56] Based on these data, CEA alone should not be used to evaluate mucinous cysts for degree of dysplasia nor to rule out malignancy.

DNA Markers

The recognition that DNA mutations occur in parallel to pancreatic carcinogenesis has raised the prospect of using certain molecular changes to risk stratify benign pancreatic lesions.[57] Mutations of interest include KRAS, GNAS, and SMAD4, among others.

The use of KRAS as a biomarker of particular interest stems from its presence in more than 90% of pancreatic adenocarcinomas.[58] KRAS is also seen in a significant number of patients with pancreatitis likely because of the high prevalence of pancreatic intraepithelial neoplasia in chronic pancreatitis.[59] For the accuracy of tests of KRAS mutations in differentiating malignant from benign cysts, however, the pooled sensitivity averaged 0.59, with a specificity of 0.78. More significant is the finding that when paired with loss of heterozygosity tests, KRAS mutations accurately differentiate malignant from benign cysts with a poled specificity of 0.69 and sensitivity of

Table 1
The use of biomarkers for identification of cyst type

Gene		Sensitivity	Specificity
KRAS[40–42,45–47]	Combined vs nonmucinous	33–86	80–100
KRAS[40,41,48,49]	Mucinous vs nonmucinous	11–59	78–100
GNAS[44,47,50]	Mucinous	27–81	84–100
KRAS and GNAS[47]	Mucinous vs nonmucinous (include MCN, PanNET, SCA, retention cysts, PC, lymphoepithelial cyst)	65	100
LOH[41,49,51]	Mucinous vs nonmucinous	43–70	68–100
Elevated DNA[40,46,49]	Mucinous vs nonmucinous	29–45	68–100
Molecular markers + clinical features (BRAF, CDKN2A, CTNNB1, GNAS, KRAS, NRAS, PIK3CA, RNF43, SMAD4, TP53, VHL)[52]	Cyst type in patients with SCA, MCN, IPMN tissue vs fluid	90–100	92–98
CEA >192[20,46,47,53]	Mucinous cyst from nonmucinous Fluid/surgical path	73–78	65–84
CEA >800 ng/mL[31]	Mucinous vs nonmucinous	48	98
CEA <5 ng/mL[31]	SCA or pseudocyst	50	95
MUC5AC and endorepellin panel[54]	Mucinous vs nonmucinous	92	94
MicroRNA 21[55]	Cyst fluid samples, including cystic precursors (IPMN, SCA, benign)	76	80
VEGF-A >8500 pg/mL[39]	SCA	100	97

Abbreviation: LOH, loss of heterozygosity.

0.89. Like mutations in *KRAS,* however, loss of heterozygosity alone is relatively insensitive in differentiating mucinous from nonmucinous cysts.[41] The finding that KRAS mutations are equally abundant in IPMNs with all grades of dysplasia suggests that these mutations are an early event in neoplastic transformation.[42,60]

GNAS mutations are commonly found in both IPMNS alone and IPMNS associated with pancreatic ductal adenocarcinoma (PDAC) rather than in PDAC alone, which highlights their early role in oncogenesis.[61] The presence of GNAS mutation, however, has not been found to correlate with the degree of dysplasia.[62] *GNAS* mutations may be found less frequently in IPMNS that progress to distinct pancreatic adenocarcinoma.[63] Conversely, a more recent mutation analysis of 126 patients with pancreatic adenocarcinoma suggested that activating mutations in *GNAS* and *KRAS* cooperatively promote pancreatic tumorigenesis.[64] As such, *GNAS* alone cannot be used to detect transformation but may have a role in multimarker panels and in combination with *KRAS*. With combined cytopathology and mutation analysis of KRAS and GNAS, malignancy can accurately be predicted in 80% of IPMNs using this analysis.[65,66]

Telomerase

With the understanding that telomere shortening is a crucial event in the development of many human cancers, telomere expression in IPMN has been evaluated in cyst progression. Telomere shortening has been associated with IPMN progression. This is believed related to the up-regulation of human telomerase reverse transcriptase expression, which is clearly higher in pancreatic adenocarcinoma compared with samples from patients with chronic pancreatitis and patients without pancreas cancer.[67] Telomerase activity measured in surgically aspirated cyst fluid samples form 219 patients who subsequently underwent resection demonstrated a marked increase in telomerase activity in cysts with high-grade dysplasia and/or associated invasive cancer. A multivariate analysis in this study demonstrated that telomerase activity independently predicted the presence of invasive cancer/high-grade dysplasia, making it a potentially useful diagnostic study.[68]

Hedgehog Signaling Pathway and Other Tumor Suppressor Genes

Like telomerase activity, sonic hedgehog (SHH) is associated with dysplastic transformation. SHH expression differs, however, in that it is absent in pancreatitis, potentially making it more specific for cyst progression.[69,70] In IPMN, SHH expression has been reported in 46.2% of low grade, 35.7% of intermediate-grade, 80% of high-grade, and 84.6% of invasive carcinomas.[71] This suggests that the presence of SHH in IPMN should raise concern for progression toward malignancy.

Tumor suppressor genes have also been evaluated as markers of cyst progression. p53 is a well-known gene involved in protecting against mutation accumulation by DNA damage by inducing apoptosis.[72] In IPMN tissue, degree of dysplasia is directly correlated with p53, with close to 40% mutations in high-grade dysplasia.[73] Similarly, CDKN2A/p16 are involved with regulation of the cell cycle. Loss of either p53 or p16 genes is associated with carcinogenesis in IPMN lesions.[74,75] Like p53 mutations, however, the loss of these 2 genes may occur early in transformation, but is not uniformly present, limiting its diagnostic utility.

Next-Generation Sequencing and Molecular Panels

Given the limited utility of single markers or imaging for the identification of cyst type and premalignant potential, researchers have started to evaluate panels, which have included several biomarkers. Recently, next-generation sequencing (NGS) has presented the opportunity to rapidly detect mutations in a select panel of genes impli-cated in the development of cancer.[76] When coupled with imaging, such molecular tested has been demonstrated to change the diagnosis in a significant number of cases of pancreatic cysts.[59] Combination panels have been developed that identify multiple mutations within cyst fluid and can identify the cyst subtype, with a sensitivity of 90% to 100% and specificity of 92% to 95%. Markers examined included BRAF, CDKN2A, CTNNB1, GNAS, KRAS, NRAS, PIK3CA, RNF43, SMAD4, TP53, and VHL.[52] A study of 626 pancreatic cyst fluid sample from 595 patients reported a 10-day turnaround and cost of $750, making this test a reasonable option for catego-rizing cyst type.[38] When correlated with surgical specimens matched to the fluid sam-ples, NGS detection of KRAS and/or GNAS mutations had 100% sensitivity and 96% specificity for IPMN. In conjunction with alterations in TP53, PIK3CA, and/or PTEN, this particular panel had 88% sensitivity and 97% specificity for IPMNS with advanced neoplasia. This marks a significant improvement over endosonographic findings of main pancreatic duct dilation and a mural nodule, which has a sensitivity under 50% in this same group of patients.

Another multicenter study evaluated the use of integrated molecular pathology (IMP) to assess the malignant potential of pancreatic cysts.[77] The IMP combines mo-lecular analysis with first-line tests results, including cytology, imaging, and fluid chemistry. A total of 492 patients were studied retrospectively and their clinical outcome was correlated with previous IMP diagnosis versus international consensus guidelines from International Consensus Guidelines Meeting in Sendai, Japan, 2012. IMP more accurately determined the malignant potential of pancreatic cysts with the IMP demonstrating a specificity of 90.6 for the assessing malignant potential compared with 46.2 for the Sendai model.

Epigenetics

In addition to the recognition that DNA mutations have a role in tumorigenesis, there has been increased research into associated epigenetic factors. One potentially prom-ising focus has been on DNA methylation. Early research into the topic noted that CpG island methylation was present in high-grade IPMNs.[78] A subsequent study of 164 pa-tients who had undergone surgical resection and concomitant fluid aspiration of a pancreatic cyst demonstrated that an assay for 7 genes, including SOX17, PTCHD2, BNIP3, FOXE1, SLIT2, EYA4, and SFRP, were effective at discriminating between cases with invasive cancer/high-grade dysplasia versus all other cysts.[79] When coupled with cytology, accuracy was further increased.

Another epigenetic marker is microRNA. miR-21 was found effective at differenti-ating premalignant mucinous cysts from malignant cysts in 40 surgically resected pancreatic cysts. Expression was also increased in miR-21 and miR-17-3p.[55] Further studies are needed, however, to validate these preliminary data.

Monoclonal Antibodies as Biomarkers

Further efforts to subtype IPMNs have led to efforts to find other markers that are spe-cific to each histotype. More than 30 years ago, Das and colleagues,[79] developed a murine monoclonal antibody, mAb Das-1, which reacts specifically with normal colonic epithelium. Between 1990 and 2010, the investigators group examined tissue from pathologically confirmed IPMNs.[80] Separately, they gathered lesional fluid from a cohort of 38 patients with IPMN. They then evaluated mAb Das-1 expression with immunohistochemistry and Western blot. The results demonstrated that mAb Das-1 is overexpressed in pancreatic cyst fluid from high-risk and malignant IPMNs compared with low-risk lesions. They were ultimately able to differentiate high-risk and malignant lesions from low-risk lesions, with sensitivity of 85% and specificity of 95%, which marks a vast improvement over existing tests, including CEA. Further studies are needed to validate these figures.

Targeted Protein-Based Biomarkers

The identification of subtypes of IPMN almost 20 years ago raised interest in using this subtyping to risk stratify for cancer progression. A consensus meeting in 2005 established 4 subtypes of IPMN, which include gastric, intestinal, pancreatobiliary, and oncocytic.[81] Intestinal type is most similar to villous adenomas, with a majority harboring carcinoma in situ. The pancreatobiliary type most closely resembles neoplasms of the biliary tract and is associated with a more aggressive clinical course. The gastric and intestinal subtypes are most common and confer the most favorable prognosis.[82] They are also most frequently associated with BD-IPMNs. Pancreatobilliary and oncocytic IPMNs are less frequent and more associated with main duct IPMN and confer the worst prognosis. Differentiating between these subtypes is most commonly assessed through immunohistochemical mucins (MUC) expression. Although data are limited, with the advent of tissue biopsy, mucins subtypes have generated interest.

Mucins—heavily glycosylated high-molecular-weight glycoproteins—are involved with lubrication, moisturization, and protection of duct lining.[83] Their implication in carcinogenesis and tumor invasion raises the possibility of their use in evaluating IPMNs.[84–86] Varying levels of MUCs may correspond with levels of dysplasia, whereas the gastric subtype frequently expresses MUC5AC but not MUC1 or MUC2. The intestinal subtype usually expresses MUC2.[82] On the other hand, invasive ductal adenocarcinomas frequently overexpress MUC1 but demonstrate an absence of MUC2. Similarly, MUC4 levels seem directly correlated with degree of dysplasia in cysts.[87]

In addition to cyst fluid sampling, there is a possibility of sampling the cyst wall, septations, and/or mural nodules using a microforceps device that passes through the endoscope.[25] This confers the advantage of increasing cellular yield. Limited case reports have demonstrated that use of this device is safe and successfully guided therapy.[88]

BLOOD, SALIVA, AND STOOL BIOMARKERS

It is well established that hematogenous spread of disease is present across various cancer types. Traditional teaching, however, is that such dissemination occurs in late-stage disease. More recent analyses of circulating epithelial cells (CECs) bring that notion into question. Several patients undergoing pancreatectomy for chronic pancreatitis go on to develop PDAC despite surgical pathology, showing only precancerous pancreatic intraepithelial neoplasia.[89] A subsequent blinded prospective study of 3 cohorts, including a control group with no cancer history; a group with known precancerous cystic lesions (eg, IPMN or MCN), all of whom did not qualify for surgery by guidelines; and a group with known pancreatic adenocarcinoma, was conducted to further examine this topic. A majority (78%) of patients with PDAC had CECs, which are also known as circulating tumor cells. A smaller number (40%) of patients with cystic pancreatic lesions had detectable CECs.[90] A significant difference in CECs was seen across the 3 groups.[90] In a more recent study of 26 patients undergoing resection of IPMNs, 19 without an associated malignancy demonstrated that CECs were significantly more likely found in patients with IPMNS with high-grade dysplasia.[91] These studies suggest that CECs may eventually be helpful in risk categorizing premalignant pancreatic neoplastic lesions.

Table 2
The use of biomarkers in risk stratifying lesions of malignant potential

Gene	Clinical Scenario	Sensitivity	Specificity
KRAS[41,46,48,96]	Cyst fluid vs pathology (malignant = CIS, IC)	20–91	56–97
KRAS + LOH[46]	Comparison of malignant and benign cysts	50	96
LOH[41,97]	Adenomas, carcinomas, borderline tumors	75–100	50–83
GNAS[65]	Cytopathology alone in IPMN	55	100
Elevated DNA[40,46,49]	Cyst fluid vs path (malignant = CIS, IC)	40–83	78–93
TP53/SMAD4 concentration (duodenal aspirate)[98]	Pancreatic juice from controls, PDAC, IPMN	32	100
Plec-1[99]	49 tissue samples IPMNs with HGD, LGD, PDAC and cyst fluidBenign vs malignant IPMN	84	83
CA19-9 + CA24-2 + CEA[100]	87 patients with surgical resection (4 LGD, 34 IGD, 16 HGD, 33 IC)	71	88
CEA >109.9[101]	504 patients with cyst fluid samples	63	63
CEA >200[102]	Diagnosis of malignant IPMN (HGD and IC) in EUS-FNA cyst fluid and surgical resection of IPMN	52	42
DNA methylation of MUC1, MUC2, MUC4[103]	Pancreatic juice in various lesions paired with pancreatic tissue from PDAC	80	87
Pancreatic ductal lavage cytology: MUC1, MUC2, MUC5AC, MUC6[104]	Lavage and cell block samples in BD-IPMN	92	100
MUC1 mRNA[105]	Pancreatic juice PDAC, 7 IC/HGD, 2 IGD, 7 LGD, 5 CP	89	71
CEA >192 + PGE2 >0.5[106]	Cyst fluid IPMN and tissue path with LGD/IGD, HGD, IC, IPMN	78	100

Abbreviations: CIS, cancer in situ; CP, chronic pancreatitis; HGD, high-grade dysplasia; IC, invasive carcinoma; IGD, intermediate-grade dysplasia; LGD, low-grade dysplasia; LOH, loss of heterozygosity.

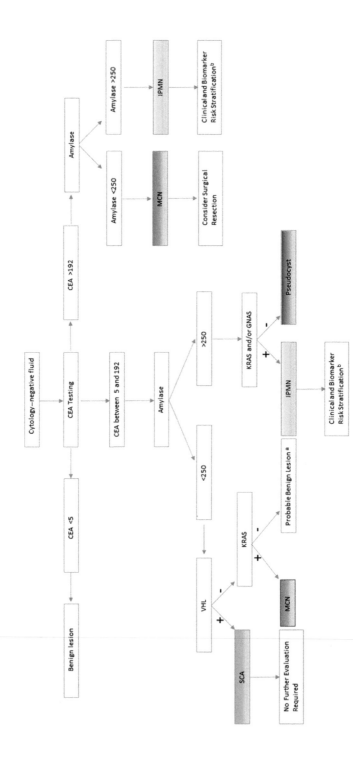

Fig. 1. Proposed algorithm for pancreatic cyst diagnosis and management. [a] Consider molecular panel if suspicion for mucinous lesion remains. [b] Stratification based on guidelines.

Along those same lines, there has been some suggestion that the same mutations seen in pancreatic tissues like *GNAS* and *KRAS* alterations may be seen in the blood. A single study demonstrated that a tumor-derived fraction of circulating cell-free DNA (cfDNA) isolated from blood samples contains many of these mutations and the total amount of cfDNA can discriminate between patients without pancreatic lesions and those with Fukuoka-negative BD-IPMN or pancreatic cancer.[92] A subsequent proof-of-concept study demonstrated the potential clinical utility of circulating exosomal DNA for the identification of KRAS and TP53 mutations in patients with pancreas-associated pathologies, including PDAC, chronic pancreatitis, and IPMN.[93] Exosomes are vesicles produced by tumor cells, which may be involved with the transfer of materials implicated in progression of disease. cfDNA and exosomes analysis holds the promise of a less invasive method of differentiating high-risk IPMN from low-risk IPMN and detecting subclinical cancer of the pancreas.

With the promising results seen in NGS panels, there has been increased interest in sequencing of fluid taken from other places. More specifically, pancreatic juice drawn from the duodenum may be used for similar mutation analyses. NGS performed on pancreatic juice taken from 19 patients who underwent endoscopic retrograde cholangiopancreatography prior to pancreatic resection proved able to diagnose malignant IPMN using the *TP53* mutation.[94] In this study, 52 cancer-related genes were examined. In the future, increased sequencing depth and the addition of more appropriate target genes may improve sensitivity and specificity.

Stool testing for detection of colorectal neoplasia has proved useful for its noninvasive value and high sensitivity. Similar studies in pancreatic cancer are limited. A stool study that examined 9 target genes, including *BMP3*, *NDRG4*, *EYA4*, *UCHL1*, *MDF1*, *Vimentin*, *CNTNAP2*, *SFRP2*, and *TFPI2*, proved useful. AT 90% specificity, methylated *BMP3* alone detected 51% of pancreatic cancers, mutant *KRAS* detected 50%, and combination detected 67%.[95] Further studies in patients with premalignant neoplasms are needed to assess whether stool studies have any role in risk stratification.

A summary of various biomarkers and their sensitivity and specificity for risk stratifying lesions of malignant potential is found in **Table 2**.

SUMMARY

Although the management of cystic lesions is guided by both clinical presentation and radiologic criteria, there is an emerging role to incorporate cyst fluid biomarkers in their evaluation. This review divides the use of these markers into diagnostic biomarkers (those that are used to identify neoplasms with malignant potential) and biomarkers used to stratify malignancy risk. **Fig. 1** presents an algorithmic approach to incorporate some of the best understood genetic and biochemical markers in the evaluation of cyst fluid aspirates from intermediate-risk lesions. The authors expect this field will continue to evolve in the direction of the use of combination of marker panels because most biomarkers studies thus far have insufficient accuracy but strongly correlate with the biology of changes in a subset of cysts. The authors also anticipate that future guidelines will continue to define the clinical subgroups where biomarkers have the greatest impact and that the guidelines will increasingly rely on these biomarkers.

REFERENCES

1. De Jong K, Nio CY, Hermans JJ, et al. High prevalence of pancreatic cysts detected by screening magnetic resonance imaging examinations. Clin Gastroenterol Hepatol 2010;8(9):806–11.

2. Al-Haddad M, El Hajj II, Eloubeidi MA. Endoscopic ultrasound for the evaluation of cystic lesions of the pancreas. JOP 2010;11(4):299–309.

3. Valsangkar NP, Morales-Oyarvide V, Thayer SP, et al. 851 resected cystic tumors of the pancreas: a 33-year experience at the Massachusetts General Hospital. Surgery 2012;152(3 Suppl 1):S4–12.

4. Brugge WR, Lauwers GY, Sahani D, et al. Cystic neoplasms of the pancreas. N Engl J Med 2004;351(12):1218–26.

5. Thiruvengadam N, Park WG. Systematic review of pancreatic cyst fluid biomarkers: the path forward. Clin Transl Gastroenterol 2015;6:e88.

6. Classification of pancreatic cysts - UpToDate [Internet]. Available at: https://www.uptodate.com/contents/classification-of-pancreatic-cysts. Accessed January 10, 2018.

7. Adsay NV. Cystic neoplasia of the pancreas: pathology and biology. J Gastrointest Surg 2008;12(3):401–4.

8. Klimstra DS, Wenig BM, Heffess CS. Solid-pseudopapillary tumor of the pancreas: a typically cystic carcinoma of low malignant potential. Semin Diagn Pathol 2000;17(1):66–80.

9. ASGE Standards of Practice Committee, Muthusamy VR, Chandrasekhara V, et al. The role of endoscopy in the diagnosis and treatment of cystic pancreatic neoplasms. Gastrointest Endosc 2016;84(1):1–9.

10. Suzuki Y, Atomi Y, Sugiyama M, et al. Cystic neoplasm of the pancreas: a Japanese multiinstitutional study of intraductal papillary mucinous tumor and mucinous cystic tumor. Pancreas 2004;28(3):241–6.

11. Tanaka M, Fernández-del Castillo C, Adsay V, et al. International consensus guidelines 2012 for the management of IPMN and MCN of the pancreas. Pancreatology 2012;12(3):183–97.

12. Tanaka M, Fernández-Del Castillo C, Kamisawa T, et al. Revisions of international consensus Fukuoka guidelines for the management of IPMN of the pancreas. Pancreatology 2017;17(5):738–53.

13. Kim TH, Song TJ, Hwang J-H, et al. Predictors of malignancy in pure branch duct type intraductal papillary mucinous neoplasm of the pancreas: a nationwide multicenter study. Pancreatology 2015;15(4):405–10.

14. Mukewar S, de Pretis N, Aryal-Khanal A, et al. Fukuoka criteria accurately predict risk for adverse outcomes during follow-up of pancreatic cysts presumed to be intraductal papillary mucinous neoplasms. Gut 2017;66(10):1811–7.

15. Vege SS, Ziring B, Jain R, et al, Clinical Guidelines Committee, American Gastroenterology Association. American gastroenterological association institute guideline on the diagnosis and management of asymptomatic neoplastic pancreatic cysts. Gastroenterology 2015;148(4):819–22 [quize: 12].

16. Scheiman JM, Hwang JH, Moayyedi P. American gastroenterological association technical review on the diagnosis and management of asymptomatic neoplastic pancreatic cysts. Gastroenterology 2015;148(4):824–48.e22.

17. Megibow AJ, Baker ME, Morgan DE, et al. Management of incidental pancreatic cysts: a white paper of the ACR incidental findings committee. J Am Coll Radiol 2017;14(7):911–23.

18. Cho CS, Russ AJ, Loeffler AG, et al. Preoperative classification of pancreatic cystic neoplasms: the clinical significance of diagnostic inaccuracy. Ann Surg Oncol 2013;20(9):3112–9.

19. Correa-Gallego C, Ferrone CR, Thayer SP, et al. Incidental pancreatic cysts: do we really know what we are watching? Pancreatology 2010;10(2–3):144–50.

20. Brugge WR, Lewandrowski K, Lee-Lewandrowski E, et al. Diagnosis of pancreatic cystic neoplasms: a report of the cooperative pancreatic cyst study. Gastroenterology 2004;126(5):1330–6.
21. Rogart JN, Loren DE, Singu BS, et al. Cyst wall puncture and aspiration during EUS-guided fine needle aspiration may increase the diagnostic yield of mucinous cysts of the pancreas. J Clin Gastroenterol 2011;45(2):164–9.
22. Ahmad NA, Kochman ML, Brensinger C, et al. Interobserver agreement among endosonographers for the diagnosis of neoplastic versus non-neoplastic pancreatic cystic lesions. Gastrointest Endosc 2003;58(1):59–64.
23. Wang KX, Ben QW, Jin ZD, et al. Assessment of morbidity and mortality associated with EUS-guided FNA: a systematic review. Gastrointest Endosc 2011; 73(2):283–90.
24. Hong S-KS, Loren DE, Rogart JN, et al. Targeted cyst wall puncture and aspiration during EUS-FNA increases the diagnostic yield of premalignant and malignant pancreatic cysts. Gastrointest Endosc 2012;75(4):775–82.
25. Shakhatreh MH, Naini SR, Brijbassie AA, et al. Use of a novel through-the-needle biopsy forceps in endoscopic ultrasound. Endosc Int Open 2016;4(4): E439–42.
26. Sendino O, Fernández-Esparrach G, Solé M, et al. Endoscopic ultrasonography-guided brushing increases cellular diagnosis of pancreatic cysts: a prospective study. Dig Liver Dis 2010;42(12):877–81.
27. Thornton GD, McPhail MJW, Nayagam S, et al. Endoscopic ultrasound guided fine needle aspiration for the diagnosis of pancreatic cystic neoplasms: a meta-analysis. Pancreatology 2013;13(1):48–57.
28. Maker AV, Lee LS, Raut CP, et al. Cytology from pancreatic cysts has marginal utility in surgical decision-making. Ann Surg Oncol 2008;15(11):3187–92.
29. Jang JY, Park T, Lee S, et al. Validation of international consensus guidelines for the resection of branch duct-type intraductal papillary mucinous neoplasms. Br J Surg 2014;101(6):686–92.
30. Del Chiaro M, Verbeke C, Salvia R, et al. European experts consensus statement on cystic tumours of the pancreas. Dig Liver Dis 2013;45(9):703–11.
31. Van der Waaij LA, van Dullemen HM, Porte RJ. Cyst fluid analysis in the differential diagnosis of pancreatic cystic lesions: a pooled analysis. Gastrointest Endosc 2005;62(3):383–9.
32. Scourtas A, Dudley JC, Brugge WR, et al. Preoperative characteristics and cytological features of 136 histologically confirmed pancreatic mucinous cystic neoplasms. Cancer 2017;125(3):169–77.
33. Jang JW, Kim M-H, Jeong SU, et al. Clinical characteristics of intraductal papillary mucinous neoplasm manifesting as acute pancreatitis or acute recurrent pancreatitis. J Gastroenterol Hepatol 2013;28(4):731–8.
34. Cizginer S, Turner BG, Bilge AR, et al. Cyst fluid carcinoembryonic antigen is an accurate diagnostic marker of pancreatic mucinous cysts. Pancreas 2011;40(7): 1024–8.
35. Allen PJ, Qin L-X, Tang L, et al. Pancreatic cyst fluid protein expression profiling for discriminating between serous cystadenoma and intraductal papillary mucinous neoplasm. Ann Surg 2009;250(5):754–60.
36. Neumann HP, Dinkel E, Brambs H, et al. Pancreatic lesions in the von Hippel-Lindau syndrome. Gastroenterology 1991;101(2):465–71.
37. Sakorafas GH, Smyrniotis V, Reid-Lombardo KM, et al. Primary pancreatic cystic neoplasms revisited. Part I: serous cystic neoplasms. Surg Oncol 2011 Jun; 20(2):e84–92.

38. Singhi AD, McGrath K, Brand RE, et al. Preoperative next-generation sequencing of pancreatic cyst fluid is highly accurate in cyst classification and detection of advanced neoplasia. Gut 2017. https://doi.org/10.1136/gutjnl-2016-313586.

39. Carr RA, Yip-Schneider MT, Dolejs S, et al. Pancreatic cyst fluid vascular endothelial growth factor A and carcinoembryonic antigen: a highly accurate test for the diagnosis of serous cystic neoplasm. J Am Coll Surg 2017. https://doi.org/10.1016/j.jamcollsurg.2017.05.003.

40. Khalid A, Zahid M, Finkelstein SD, et al. Pancreatic cyst fluid DNA analysis in evaluating pancreatic cysts: a report of the PANDA study. Gastrointest Endosc 2009;69(6):1095–102.

41. Guo X, Zhan X, Li Z. Molecular analyses of aspirated cystic fluid for the differential diagnosis of cystic lesions of the pancreas: a systematic review and meta-analysis. Gastroenterol Res Pract 2016;2016:3546085.

42. Wu J, Matthaei H, Maitra A, et al. Recurrent GNAS mutations define an unexpected pathway for pancreatic cyst development. Sci Transl Med 2011;3(92):92ra66.

43. Wood LD, Parsons DW, Jones S, et al. The genomic landscapes of human breast and colorectal cancers. Science 2007;318(5853):1108–13.

44. Siddiqui AA, Kowalski TE, Kedika R, et al. EUS-guided pancreatic fluid aspiration for DNA analysis of KRAS and GNAS mutations for the evaluation of pancreatic cystic neoplasia: a pilot study. Gastrointest Endosc 2013;77(4):669–70.

45. Nikiforova MN, Khalid A, Fasanella KE, et al. Integration of KRAS testing in the diagnosis of pancreatic cystic lesions: a clinical experience of 618 pancreatic cysts. Mod Pathol 2013;26(11):1478–87.

46. Winner M, Sethi A, Poneros JM, et al. The role of molecular analysis in the diagnosis and surveillance of pancreatic cystic neoplasms. JOP 2015;16(2):143–9.

47. Singhi AD, Nikiforova MN, Fasanella KE, et al. Preoperative GNAS and KRAS testing in the diagnosis of pancreatic mucinous cysts. Clin Cancer Res 2014;20(16):4381–9.

48. Talar-Wojnarowska R, Pazurek M, Durko L, et al. A comparative analysis of K-ras mutation and carcinoembryonic antigen in pancreatic cyst fluid. Pancreatology 2012;12(5):417–20.

49. Sawhney MS, Devarajan S, O'Farrel P, et al. Comparison of carcinoembryonic antigen and molecular analysis in pancreatic cyst fluid. Gastrointest Endosc 2009;69(6):1106–10.

50. Kanda M, Knight S, Topazian M, et al. Mutant GNAS detected in duodenal collections of secretin-stimulated pancreatic juice indicates the presence or emergence of pancreatic cysts. Gut 2013;62(7):1024–33.

51. Shen J, Brugge WR, Dimaio CJ, et al. Molecular analysis of pancreatic cyst fluid: a comparative analysis with current practice of diagnosis. Cancer 2009;117(3):217–27.

52. Sasaki S, Yamamoto H, Kaneto H, et al. Differential roles of alterations of p53, p16, and SMAD4 expression in the progression of intraductal papillary-mucinous tumors of the pancreas. Oncol Rep 2003;10(1):21–5.

53. Nagula S, Kennedy T, Schattner MA, et al. Evaluation of cyst fluid CEA analysis in the diagnosis of mucinous cysts of the pancreas. J Gastrointest Surg 2010;14(12):1997–2003.

54. Sinha J, Cao Z, Dai J, et al. A gastric glycoform of MUC5AC is a biomarker of mucinous cysts of the pancreas. PLoS One 2016;11(12):e0167070.
55. Hong S-M, Omura N, Vincent A, et al. Genome-wide CpG island profiling of intraductal papillary mucinous neoplasms of the pancreas. Clin Cancer Res 2012; 18(3):700–12.
56. Farrell JJ, Fernández-del Castillo C. Pancreatic cystic neoplasms: management and unanswered questions. Gastroenterology 2013;144(6):1303–15.
57. Hruban RH, Adsay NV, Albores-Saavedra J, et al. Pancreatic intraepithelial neoplasia: a new nomenclature and classification system for pancreatic duct lesions. Am J Surg Pathol 2001;25(5):579–86.
58. Eser S, Schnieke A, Schneider G, et al. Oncogenic KRAS signalling in pancreatic cancer. Br J Cancer 2014;111(5):817–22.
59. Jones M, Zheng Z, Wang J, et al. Impact of next-generation sequencing on the clinical diagnosis of pancreatic cysts. Gastrointest Endosc 2016;83(1): 140–8.
60. Kitago M, Ueda M, Aiura K, et al. Comparison of K-ras point mutation distributions in intraductal papillary-mucinous tumors and ductal adenocarcinoma of the pancreas. Int J Cancer 2004;110(2):177–82.
61. Hosoda W, Sasaki E, Murakami Y, et al. GNAS mutation is a frequent event in pancreatic intraductal papillary mucinous neoplasms and associated adenocarcinomas. Virchows Arch 2015;466(6):665–74.
62. Tan MC, Basturk O, Brannon AR, et al. GNAS and KRAS mutations define separate progression pathways in intraductal papillary mucinous neoplasm-associated carcinoma. J Am Coll Surg 2015;220(5):845–54.e1.
63. Ideno N, Ohtsuka T, Matsunaga T, et al. Clinical significance of GNAS mutation in intraductal papillary mucinous neoplasm of the pancreas with concomitant pancreatic ductal adenocarcinoma. Pancreas 2015;44(2):311–20.
64. Zhou L, Baba Y, Kitano Y, et al. KRAS, BRAF, and PIK3CA mutations, and patient prognosis in 126 pancreatic cancers: pyrosequencing technology and literature review. Med Oncol 2016;33(4):32.
65. Bournet B, Vignolle-Vidoni A, Grand D, et al. Endoscopic ultrasound-guided fine-needle aspiration plus KRAS and GNAS mutation in malignant intraductal papillary mucinous neoplasm of the pancreas. Endosc Int Open 2016;4(12): E1228–35.
66. Heestand GM, Kurzrock R. Molecular landscape of pancreatic cancer: implications for current clinical trials. Oncotarget 2015;6(7):4553–61.
67. Hashimoto Y, Murakami Y, Uemura K, et al. Telomere shortening and telomerase expression during multistage carcinogenesis of intraductal papillary mucinous neoplasms of the pancreas. J Gastrointest Surg 2008;12(1):17–28.
68. Hata T, Dal Molin M, Suenaga M, et al. Cyst fluid telomerase activity predicts the histologic grade of cystic neoplasms of the pancreas. Clin Cancer Res 2016; 22(20):5141–51.
69. Zheng Z, Liebers M, Zhelyazkova B, et al. Anchored multiplex PCR for targeted next-generation sequencing. Nat Med 2014;20(12):1479–84.
70. Springer S, Wang Y, Dal Molin M, et al. A combination of molecular markers and clinical features improve the classification of pancreatic cysts. Gastroenterology 2015;149(6):1501–10.
71. Al-Haddad MA, Kowalski T, Siddiqui A, et al. Integrated molecular pathology accurately determines the malignant potential of pancreatic cysts. Endoscopy 2015;47(2):136–42.

72. Ohuchida K, Mizumoto K, Fujita H, et al. Sonic hedgehog is an early developmental marker of intraductal papillary mucinous neoplasms: clinical implications of mRNA levels in pancreatic juice. J Pathol 2006;210(1):42–8.

73. Satoh K, Kanno A, Hamada S, et al. Expression of Sonic hedgehog signaling pathway correlates with the tumorigenesis of intraductal papillary mucinous neoplasm of the pancreas. Oncol Rep 2008;19(5):1185–90.

74. Jang K-T, Lee KT, Lee JG, et al. Immunohistochemical expression of Sonic hedgehog in intraductal papillary mucinous tumor of the pancreas. Appl Immunohistochem Mol Morphol 2007;15(3):294–8.

75. Hong SM, Park JY, Hruban RH, et al. Molecular signatures of pancreatic cancer. Arch Pathol Lab Med 2011;135(6):716–27.

76. Abe K, Suda K, Arakawa A, et al. Different patterns of p16INK4A and p53 protein expressions in intraductal papillary-mucinous neoplasms and pancreatic intraepithelial neoplasia. Pancreas 2007;34(1):85–91.

77. Wada K. p16 and p53 gene alterations and accumulations in the malignant evolution of intraductal papillary-mucinous tumors of the pancreas. J Hepatobiliary Pancreat Surg 2002;9(1):76–85.

78. Das KM, Sakamaki S, Vecchi M, et al. The production and characterization of monoclonal antibodies to a human colonic antigen associated with ulcerative colitis: cellular localization of the antigen by using the monoclonal antibody. J Immunol 1987;139(1):77–84.

79. Das KK, Xiao H, Geng X, et al. mAb Das-1 is specific for high-risk and malignant intraductal papillary mucinous neoplasm (IPMN). Gut 2014;63(10):1626–34.

80. Ryu JK, Matthaei H, Dal Molin M, et al. Elevated microRNA miR-21 levels in pancreatic cyst fluid are predictive of mucinous precursor lesions of ductal adenocarcinoma. Pancreatology 2011;11(3):343–50.

81. Furukawa T, Klöppel G, Volkan Adsay N, et al. Classification of types of intraductal papillary-mucinous neoplasm of the pancreas: a consensus study. Virchows Arch 2005;447(5):794–9.

82. Tulla KA, Maker AV. Can we better predict the biologic behavior of incidental IPMN? A comprehensive analysis of molecular diagnostics and biomarkers in intraductal papillary mucinous neoplasms of the pancreas. Langenbecks Arch Surg 2017;403(2):151–94.

83. Maker AV, Carrara S, Jamieson NB, et al. Cyst fluid biomarkers for intraductal papillary mucinous neoplasms of the pancreas: a critical review from the international expert meeting on pancreatic branch-duct-intraductal papillary mucinous neoplasms. J Am Coll Surg 2015;220(2):243–53.

84. Hollingsworth MA, Strawhecker JM, Caffrey TC, et al. Expression of MUC1, MUC2, MUC3 and MUC4 mucin mRNAs in human pancreatic and intestinal tumor cell lines. Int J Cancer 1994;57(2):198–203.

85. Yonezawa S, Goto M, Yamada N, et al. Expression profiles of MUC1, MUC2, and MUC4 mucins in human neoplasms and their relationship with biological behavior. Proteomics 2008;8(16):3329–41.

86. Yonezawa S, Sato E. Expression of mucin antigens in human cancers and its relationship with malignancy potential. Pathol Int 1997;47(12):813–30.

87. Maker AV, Katabi N, Gonen M, et al. Pancreatic cyst fluid and serum mucin levels predict dysplasia in intraductal papillary mucinous neoplasms of the pancreas. Ann Surg Oncol 2011;18(1):199–206.

88. Chen AL, Misdraji J, Brugge WR, et al. Acinar cell cystadenoma: a challenging cytology diagnosis, facilitated by moray® micro-forceps biopsy. Diagn Cytopathol 2017;45(6):557–60.
89. Sakorafas GH, Sarr MG. Pancreatic cancer after surgery for chronic pancreatitis. Dig Liver Dis 2003;35(7):482–5.
90. Rhim AD, Thege FI, Santana SM, et al. Detection of circulating pancreas epithelial cells in patients with pancreatic cystic lesions. Gastroenterology 2014; 146(3):647–51.
91. Poruk KE, Valero V, He J, et al. Circulating epithelial cells in intraductal papillary mucinous neoplasms and cystic pancreatic lesions. Pancreas 2017;46(7): 943–7.
92. Berger AW, Schwerdel D, Costa IG, et al. Detection of hot-spot mutations in circulating cell-free DNA from patients with intraductal papillary mucinous neoplasms of the pancreas. Gastroenterology 2016;151(2):267–70.
93. Yang S, Che SPY, Kurywchak P, et al. Detection of mutant KRAS and TP53 DNA in circulating exosomes from healthy individuals and patients with pancreatic cancer. Cancer Biol Ther 2017;18(3):158–65.
94. Takano S, Fukasawa M, Kadokura M, et al. Next-generation sequencing revealed TP53 mutations to be malignant marker for intraductal papillary mucinous neoplasms that could be detected using pancreatic juice. Pancreas 2017;46(10):1281–7.
95. Kisiel JB, Yab TC, Taylor WR, et al. Stool DNA testing for the detection of pancreatic cancer: assessment of methylation marker candidates. Cancer 2012; 118(10):2623–31.
96. Khalid A, McGrath KM, Zahid M, et al. The role of pancreatic cyst fluid molecular analysis in predicting cyst pathology. Clin Gastroenterol Hepatol 2005;3(10): 967–73.
97. Schoedel KE, Finkelstein SD, Ohori NP. K-Ras and microsatellite marker analysis of fine-needle aspirates from intraductal papillary mucinous neoplasms of the pancreas. Diagn Cytopathol 2006;34(9):605–8.
98. Yu J, Sadakari Y, Shindo K, et al. Digital next-generation sequencing identifies low-abundance mutations in pancreatic juice samples collected from the duodenum of patients with pancreatic cancer and intraductal papillary mucinous neoplasms. Gut 2017;66(9):1677–87.
99. Bausch D, Mino-Kenudson M, Fernández-Del Castillo C, et al. Plectin-1 is a biomarker of malignant pancreatic intraductal papillary mucinous neoplasms. J Gastrointest Surg 2009;13(11):1948–54 [discussion: 1954].
100. You L, Ma L, Zhao WJ, et al. Emerging role of tumor markers and biochemistry in the preoperative invasive assessment of intraductal papillary mucinous neoplasm of the pancreas. Clin Chim Acta 2016;454:89–93.
101. Ngamruengphong S, Bartel MJ, Raimondo M. Cyst carcinoembryonic antigen in differentiating pancreatic cysts: a meta-analysis. Dig Liver Dis 2013;45(11): 920–6.
102. Kucera S, Centeno BA, Springett G, et al. Cyst fluid carcinoembryonic antigen level is not predictive of invasive cancer in patients with intraductal papillary mucinous neoplasm of the pancreas. JOP 2012;13(4):409–13.
103. Yokoyama S, Kitamoto S, Higashi M, et al. Diagnosis of pancreatic neoplasms using a novel method of DNA methylation analysis of mucin expression in pancreatic juice. PLoS One 2014;9(4):e93760.
104. Sai JK, Nobukawa B, Matsumura Y, et al. Pancreatic duct lavage cytology with the cell block method for discriminating benign and malignant branch-duct type

intraductal papillary mucinous neoplasms. Gastrointest Endosc 2013;77(5): 726–35.

105. Shimamoto T, Tani M, Kawai M, et al. MUC1 is a useful molecular marker for malignant intraductal papillary mucinous neoplasms in pancreatic juice obtained from endoscopic retrograde pancreatography. Pancreas 2010;39(6): 879–83.

106. Yip-Schneider MT, Carr RA, Wu H, et al. Prostaglandin E2: a pancreatic fluid biomarker of intraductal papillary mucinous neoplasm dysplasia. J Am Coll Surg 2017;225(4):481–7.

Interventional Endoscopic Ultrasonography in the Pancreas

Jeffrey Michael Adler, MD, MSc, Amrita Sethi, MD, MSc*

KEYWORDS

- Pancreatic fluid collections (PFC) • Endoscopic transmural drainage
- EUS-Guided access • EUS-Guided pancreatic duct intervention (EUS-PDI)
- Rendezvous procedures

KEY POINTS

- The use of endoscopic ultrasonography (EUS) has greatly expanded the capabilities of therapeutic endoscopists to treat a variety of benign pancreatic disease.
- EUS facilitates the localization of inflammatory pancreatic fluid collections and may provide some key safety advantages over conventional endoscopic transmural drainage.
- Skillful application of EUS may allow for access into the pancreatic duct to provide therapy when other routes are not a possibility.

INTRODUCTION

Endoscopic ultrasonography (EUS) has become indispensable in the treatment of nonmalignant conditions of the pancreas. It is frequently used in the treatment of inflammatory pancreatic fluid collections (PFCs), and to facilitate access to the pancreatic duct when a transpapillary or transanastomotic approach is not technically feasible (see Amit H. Sachdev and Frank G. Gress article's, "Celiac Plexus Block and Neurolysis," in this issue). This article reviews the evidence and current state of the art in EUS-guided techniques for these indications.

Disclosure Statement: J.M. Adler has nothing to disclose. A. Sethi is a consultant for Olympus and Boston Scientific.
Division of Digestive and Liver Disease, Department of Medicine, Columbia University Medical Center, New York Presbyterian Hospital, 630 West 168th Street, Box 83, P&S3-401, New York, NY 10032, USA
* Corresponding author.
E-mail address: as3614@cumc.columbia.edu

Gastrointest Endoscopy Clin N Am 28 (2018) 569–578
https://doi.org/10.1016/j.giec.2018.06.003

ENDOSCOPIC ULTRASONOGRAPHY FOR THE TREATMENT OF PANCREATIC FLUID COLLECTIONS
Background

Encapsulated inflammatory fluid collections of the pancreas manifest in 1 of 2 varieties: pancreatic pseudocysts (PP) and walled-off necrosis (WON).[1] Pancreatic pseudocysts represent collections of fluid without a solid component surrounded by an inflammatory wall, and in general form in communication with the pancreatic duct. They may develop as a delayed complication of acute pancreatitis or in the context of chronic pancreatitis. In contrast, WON represents an organized collection of necrotic debris arising as a sequelae of necrotizing acute pancreatitis.

Most PPs arising from acute pancreatitis resolve spontaneously, whereas those associated with chronic pancreatitis often persist.[2–4] The decision to treat PPs is usually based on whether they are symptomatic (eg, causing abdominal symptoms, infected, leading to gastric outlet obstruction, or impairing biliary drainage),[5] although at times there may be special indications for treatment for asymptomatic collections.[6]

Once the decision is made to treat an inflammatory fluid collection, endoscopic therapy is preferred over percutaneous catheter or surgical drainage on the basis of higher treatment success rates and lower costs and morbidity.[7,8] One of the principal endoscopic approaches used to drain these collections relies on transmural access[a], which is facilitated by the use of endosonography.

History and Present Application of Endoscopic Ultrasonography in the Treatment of Inflammatory Fluid Collections of the Pancreas

Early experience with endoscopic transmural drainage of PFCs did not use endosonography, and relied almost exclusively on a visible luminal bulge to target the site for intervention (conventional transmural drainage [CTD]).[9,10] It was not until the early 2000s that EUS was explored for this indication (EUS-guided transmural drainage [EUD])[b][11] and despite growing experience and prospective study, it was not clear that routine use of this technology was necessarily advantageous.[12] This would later be explored in 2 randomized controlled trials comparing CTD with EUD for PPs. In both studies, technical success was greater with EUD (94%–100%) compared with CTD (33%–72%).[13,14]

There was also a nontrivial frequency of crossover to EUD from CTD groups in these 2 studies. Overall 28% (n = 8 of 29) to 60% (n = 9 of 15) of patients randomized to CTD could not be successfully treated with esophagogastroduodenoscopy alone due to the absence of an identifiable luminal compression or "bulge," but were successfully treated after crossing-over to the EUS-guided method. Similarly, meta-analysis including these 2 trials (and 2 additional nonrandomized prospective studies) found overall higher technical success with EUD compared with CTD.[15] On the other hand, short-term and long-term clinical outcomes (ie, clinical and radiologic resolution

---

[a] An alternative endoscopic method for treating PPs relies on retrograde pancreatography and transpapillary drainage (TPD). This is sometimes considered for small (ie, <5–6 cm) PPs communicating with the main pancreatic duct, and is probably most successful in cases of partial duct disruption and where a pancreatic duct stent can be positioned to bridge the duct disruption.[32,45] Furthermore, although there has been conflicting evidence, it is not convincing that combining TPD with transmural drainage improves outcomes in the treatment of PPs.[46] Transpapillary drainage is not considered to be an appropriate option for treating WON.

[b] An echoendoscope may be used to identify an underlying fluid collection in the absence of luminal compression, and identify intervening vasculature, as well as properties and contents of the collection. Transmural access may be performed under direct EUS guidance. Alternatively, the echoendoscope may be used just to localize and mark an entry site with biopsy forceps or ink.

at 1 to 6 months after intervention, respectively) were not significantly different. This is likely because the main advantage of EUD is in achieving *initial* access.[5] The subsequent methods that affect drainage and influence final resolution are otherwise very similar. In terms of the treatment of WON, there have been no similar randomized trials comparing EUD with CTD; however, the same general principles for EUS-guided localization likely still apply.

One potential limitation of EUD relates to the smaller working channel of typical therapeutic echoendoscopes (ie, 3.7–3.8 mm) in comparison with the standard duodenoscope (ie, 4.2 mm) often selected for CTD. Consequently, in the 2 randomized trials cited previously, larger-sized stents were used in cases in which CTD was performed (10 Fr vs 7 Fr; theoretically, larger-sized stents might improve drainage success). That is not to say that 10-Fr stents cannot be passed through therapeutic echoendoscopes,[16] but it can be difficult depending on the scope angle, and when using a "double-wire"[c] technique as was the case in these 2 trials. This issue, however, may become less relevant in the current era of lumen apposing covered self-expanding metal stents (LACSEMS), which is covered more later in this article. These are large-bore dumbbell-shaped stents that are easily deployed over a single wire through a therapeutic echoendoscope, or alternatively free hand using the cautery-tip version, and have been very successful in the treatment of PPs.[17]

Echoendosonography also can be used to help identify intervening vessels between the gastrointestinal lumen and the wall of the fluid collection.[18] Intuitively, this might be expected to reduce the risk of major bleeding; however, this has not been fully supported in the evidence.[12,19] One explanation may be in the overall infrequency of major bleeding complications in these studies. In the randomized trial by Varadarajulu and colleagues,[13] there were only 2 major bleeding complications, and in the trial by Park and colleagues[14] there were only 3 minor bleeding events. Furthermore, no significant difference in the risk of major complications was detected in meta-analysis.[15] However, the apparent equivalent risk of bleeding complications with CTD and EUS should be interpreted with caution, especially for unique patient populations with portal hypertension or bleeding tendencies. First, in the trial by Varadarajulu and colleagues, the bleeding events were only noted in the CTD group, and were attributed to the presence of gastric collaterals or intervening vessels not seen on standard endoscopy. Second, patients with suspected portal hypertension or bleeding tendencies all underwent EUD, and therefore an adverse event comparison with CTD under these circumstances cannot be made.

Given the risk of inadvertently puncturing vessels, it has been discussed that a noncautery assisted or "cold needle" entry technique might be safer when not using EUS guidance.[20] The rationale is that if a vessel is pierced, the cold needle could simply be withdrawn and the vessel allowed to tamponade. Additionally, if the collection is altogether missed during CTD, the cold needle could be removed without major concern for a clinically significant perforation. A limitation of cold access is the potential difficulty in entering a thick-walled inflammatory fluid collection, a challenge that may be made greater with the tangential orientation created by EUS guidance. However, this is not typically a hindrance, and EUS-guided cold needle access remains technically successful in the vast majority of cases.[21]

After the collection is accessed, the tract is usually dilated, and 1 or more stents are inserted. One potentially unresolved issue is whether the dilation step presents a

---

[c] Double-wire technique involves maintaining 2 separate wires through the transmural tract to avoid the technical challenge of having to recannulate after the first stent is deployed.

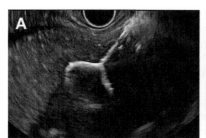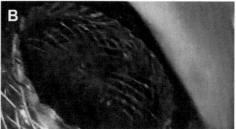

Fig. 1. (*A*) Endosonographic image of LACSEMS within internal flange opening within fluid collection. (*B*) Endoscopic image of LACSEMS with flange opening within stomach.

particular risk of bleeding or perforation. An alternative is a single-step cautery-assisted access system designed with a preloaded stent that does not require dilation.[22] One such device that has gained considerable traction has been the cautery-assisted LACSEMS.[23,24] The LACSEMS itself is a dumbbell-shaped stent with flanges that help anchor the device, and a large internal bore that allows for rapid drainage and passage of an endoscope for debridement if needed **Fig. 1**. The cautery-assisted access and delivery system that has more recently become available can easily penetrate thick walls, and simplifies the access and deployment process to a few steps.[25–27] One other advantage when using these devices with EUS guidance is that fluoroscopy is not routinely required. Technical success with these devices has approached 98%, with similarly high clinical success rates depending on the type of underlying fluid collection.[28] However, despite these apparent advantages, it still remains unclear whether these stents actually improve clinical outcomes, are worth their cost, or have an acceptable short-term and delayed safety record.[29,30]

ENDOSCOPIC ULTRASONOGRAPHY–GUIDED PANCREATIC DUCT INTERVENTION WHEN A TRANSPAPILLARY OR TRANSANASTOMOTIC APPROACH IS NOT TECHNICALLY FEASIBLE
Background

Difficulties with pancreatic duct intervention in benign pancreatic disease, through conventional transpapillary or transpancreaticoenteric route, can occur due to intraductal strictures, disrupted ducts, obstructive stones, and anastomotic strictures. Endosonography is also a powerful tool that can be used to gain access to the pancreatic duct when this cannot be accomplished via these conventional approaches (ie, direct transpapillary or transanastomotic cannulation[d]). Endoscopic ultrasonography–guided pancreatic duct intervention (EUS-PDI) need not be viewed as a new therapy per se, but as a novel and advanced method for accessing the pancreatic duct so that more familiar interventions can be performed. Therefore, the indications for performing EUS-PDI are not far from those that would warrant conventional endoscopic retrograde pancreatography (ERP).[31] However, currently EUS-PDI is still generally reserved for cases in which ERP has failed. One exception may be in the treatment of disconnected pancreatic syndrome (DPDS), in which ERP may more likely be futile. These are scenarios in which a surgical remnant or an isolated segment of residual pancreas persists[e] with an intact duct that continues to secrete

---

[d] For example, postsurgical pancreatico-enteric anastomoses.

[e] For example, a persistent pancreatic tail that persists after acute necrosis of the body and/or head of the pancreas.

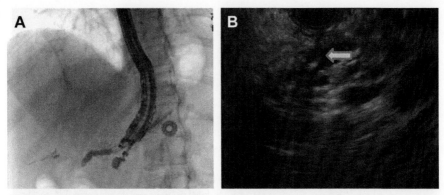

Fig. 2. (*A*) Fluoroscopic image of EUS-guided transgastric pancreatic duct access. Pancreatogram performed by injecting contrast through needle. (*B*) Endosonographic image of needle entering pancreatic duct (*arrow*). (*Courtesy of* [A] Uzma D. Siddiqui, MD, Center for Endoscopic Research and Therapeutics (CERT) University of Chicago.)

pancreatic fluid into a space no longer in continuity with the bowel. As opposed to partial duct leaks that may be bridged with conventional ERP, it may not be possible to access the remnant duct in DPDS with a transpapillary approach. In these cases, EUS guidance may be used to enter into the disconnected duct, and a transmural pathway (typically transgastric) for drainage into the bowel reestablished and maintained with an endoprosthesis.[32,33]

Techniques

The technical approaches described for EUS-guided pancreatic duct drainage include EUS-guided antegrade and EUS-guided rendezvous pancreatic duct access.[34,35] The procedure in both methods begins in a similar fashion. First, a linear echoendoscope is used to target a site for transmural pancreatic duct entrance with either a 19-guage or 22-guage needle (**Fig. 2**). Once the pancreatic duct is entered, a guidewire is advanced through the needle into the duct (**Fig. 3**). The 19-gauge needle can accommodate both 0.035-inch and 0.025-inch wires, whereas the 22-guage needle can accept only an 0.018-inch wire.[f] At this point, the antegrade and rendezvous procedures diverge. In the antegrade approach, the entire procedure is completed through the transmural tract into the pancreatic duct maintained by the wire. If a stent is deployed, it is positioned across the transmural tract so that it drains into either the stomach or small bowel (depending on where the needle puncture was made). The intraductal portion of the stent may be positioned angulated either toward the head or tail of the pancreas[g] (**Fig. 4**).

In a rendezvous procedure, transmural access of the pancreatic duct and pancreatogram are quickly followed by attempts to advance the wire through the duct and across the papilla or pancreatic anastomosis. The echoendoscope is then exchanged for either a side-viewing or straight-viewing endoscope. The wire is recaptured from its exit from the papilla or anastomosis, pulled through the scope, and the procedure

---

[f] Currently there are no wires on the market that can be advanced through a 25-guage needle.

[g] In some cases, it may be desirable to deploy a transpapillary or transanastamotic stent. This may still be accomplished via the antegrade approach if the wire can be positioned across the papilla or anastomotic orifice.

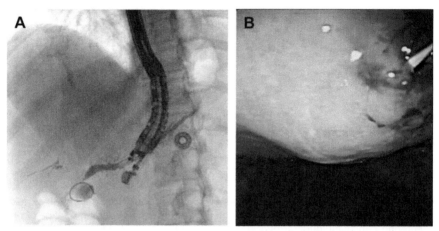

Fig. 3. (*A*) Guidewire passed through needle into pancreatic duct and coiled in small bowel. (*B*) Endoscopic image of wire passing through gastric wall into pancreatic duct. (*Courtesy of* [*A*] Uzma D. Siddiqui, MD, Center for Endoscopic Research and Therapeutics (CERT) University of Chicago.)

completed from the more conventional position. The particular method selected (ie, antegrade approach vs rendezvous) and interventions performed are usually at the discretion of the treating interventionalist, and often dictated by individual patient factors. Antegrade and rendezvous techniques have been described to drain the minor papilla as well, through transgastric or transduodenal approaches.[36]

If the anatomy prevents passage of the wire across the papilla or anastomosis, but a transpapillary or transanastamotic approach is still preferred, a small amount of methylene blue may be injected into the pancreatic duct under EUS guidance.[37] Direct cannulation can then be pursued by searching for excretion of the dye from the expected site of the papilla or pancreatic anastomosis. With this technique, caution should be

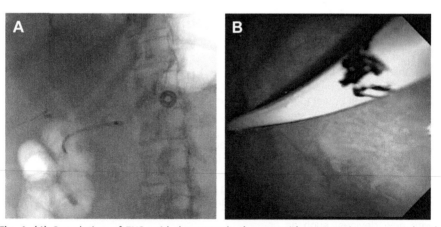

Fig. 4. (*A*) Completion of EUS-guided antegrade therapy with pancreatic stent angulated toward the head of the pancreas and crossing pancreatic duct orifice into small bowel. (*B*) Endoscopic image of stent passing through stomach wall into pancreatic duct. (*Courtesy of* [*A*] Uzma D. Siddiqui, MD, Center for Endoscopic Research and Therapeutics (CERT) University of Chicago.)

exercised to avoid over pressurizing the pancreatic ducts with any injectant, given the potential risk of acute pancreatitis. Direct access with fine-needle aspiration into the jejunal limb through a pancreaticojejunostomy via transgastric pancreatic duct access has also been described when the length of the duct would not accommodate a transmural stent.[38]

Once the pancreatic duct has been accessed, individualized therapeutic interventions may be performed with instruments common to pancreaticobiliary care. For example, dilating catheters and balloons may be selected, as well as appropriately sized plastic straight or pigtail stents. There also has been some successful experience with fully covered self-expanding metal stents,[39] although use of these is less common. Uncovered metal stents should not be used because of the potential for leakage within the tract between the duct and gastrointestinal wall.

Outcomes

Outcomes regarding EUS-PDI have been largely in the form of large case series and have quite variable technical and clinical success rates likely due to large variabilities in sample size, indication, anatomy, techniques used, and equipment available at the time of study.[40] Technical success rates in 2 of the earlier single-center studies with sample sizes of 45 to 84 patients ranged from 59% to 74%, and with clinical success rates of 78% to 85%.[41,42] Adverse events rates ranged from 6% to 18%. A more recent multicenter experience of 80 patients demonstrated a technical success rate of 89% and clinical success rate of 81%, with a 20% adverse event rate.[35] Reported adverse events include abdominal pain requiring hospitalization, pancreatitis, intra-abdominal abscesses, pancreatic duct leaks, perforation, and bleeding.

Although satisfactory outcomes of the EUS-PDI in experience or registry data may confirm feasibility and safety of this technique, valuable comparative data are still lacking regarding an algorithmic approach to patients with pancreatic ductal disease and altered anatomy. Currently, it remains a second-line approach when conventional methods of ductal access fail. One recent study retrospectively compared EUS-guided drainage versus enteroscopy-assisted endoscopic retrograde cholangiopancreatography (e-ERCP) in patients with altered anatomy.[43] Sixty-six patients (40 EUS-ERP vs 35 e-ERCP) were included and technical (92.5% vs 20%) and clinical (87.5% vs 23.1%) success rates were significantly higher in the EUS-ERP group. These remarkable differences were at the cost of a significantly higher adverse event rate in the EUS-ERP group (35.0% vs 2.9%) although no serious adverse events were noted.

SUMMARY

Endosonography has clearly established itself as a game-changing technology with regard to the diagnosis and therapeutic management of benign pancreatic disease. Interventional EUS in particular has revolutionized the way we manage the sequelae of pancreatitis and postsurgical changes. EUS-guided PFC drainage, both in its early techniques as well as advances in equipment, has shifted endoscopic management of pseudocysts and WON to the first line in management algorithms, while leaving conventional open surgical approaches to be last-resort salvage options. As experience with new devices, such as cautery-enhanced LACSEMS, builds, algorithmic approaches and standardization of methods may start to take shape.

EUS-guided access also has significantly impacted the way we can tackle challenging pancreatic ducts with minimally invasive methods of drainage that avoid cumbersome surgical interventions. Although success rates are less than other

EUS-guided interventions, such as PFC drainage, advances in techniques and equipment will hopefully allow for improvement. The rising technical success seen with these types of procedures are encouraging,[35,44] and with appropriate patient selection and expertise, it may in the future become suitable as a first-line option.[43] For now, however, these types of procedures are typically reserved for those with specialized training in major referral centers.

REFERENCES

1. Banks PA, Bollen TL, Dervenis C, et al. Classification of acute pancreatitis–2012: revision of the Atlanta classification and definitions by international consensus. Gut 2013;62(1):102–11.
2. Cheruvu CV, Clarke MG, Prentice M, et al. Conservative treatment as an option in the management of pancreatic pseudocyst. Ann R Coll Surg Engl 2003;85(5): 313–6.
3. Gouyon B, Levy P, Ruszniewski P, et al. Predictive factors in the outcome of pseudocysts complicating alcoholic chronic pancreatitis. Gut 1997;41(6):821–5.
4. Bourliere M, Sarles H. Pancreatic cysts and pseudocysts associated with acute and chronic pancreatitis. Dig Dis Sci 1989;34(3):343–8.
5. ASGE Standards of Practice Committee, Muthusamy VR, Chandrasekhara V, Acosta RD, et al. The role of endoscopy in the diagnosis and treatment of inflammatory pancreatic fluid collections. Gastrointest Endosc 2016;83(3):481–8.
6. Lerch MM, Stier A, Wahnschaffe U, et al. Pancreatic pseudocysts: observation, endoscopic drainage, or resection? Dtsch Arztebl Int 2009;106(38):614–21.
7. Keane MG, Sze SF, Cieplik N, et al. Endoscopic versus percutaneous drainage of symptomatic pancreatic fluid collections: a 14-year experience from a tertiary hepatobiliary centre. Surg Endosc 2016;30(9):3730–40.
8. Gurusamy KS, Pallari E, Hawkins N, et al. Management strategies for pancreatic pseudocysts. Cochrane Database Syst Rev 2016;(4):CD011392.
9. Cremer M, Deviere J, Engelholm L. Endoscopic management of cysts and pseudocysts in chronic pancreatitis: long-term follow-up after 7 years of experience. Gastrointest Endosc 1989;35(1):1–9.
10. Sahel J, Bastid C, Pellat B, et al. Endoscopic cystoduodenostomy of cysts of chronic calcifying pancreatitis: a report of 20 cases. Pancreas 1987;2(4):447–53.
11. Giovannini M, Pesenti C, Rolland AL, et al. Endoscopic ultrasound-guided drainage of pancreatic pseudocysts or pancreatic abscesses using a therapeutic echo endoscope. Endoscopy 2001;33(6):473–7.
12. Kahaleh M, Shami VM, Conaway MR, et al. Endoscopic ultrasound drainage of pancreatic pseudocyst: a prospective comparison with conventional endoscopic drainage. Endoscopy 2006;38(4):355–9.
13. Varadarajulu S, Christein JD, Tamhane A, et al. Prospective randomized trial comparing EUS and EGD for transmural drainage of pancreatic pseudocysts (with videos). Gastrointest Endosc 2008;68(6):1102–11.
14. Park DH, Lee SS, Moon SH, et al. Endoscopic ultrasound-guided versus conventional transmural drainage for pancreatic pseudocysts: a prospective randomized trial. Endoscopy 2009;41(10):842–8.
15. Panamonta N, Ngamruengphong S, Kijsirichareanchai K, et al. Endoscopic ultrasound-guided versus conventional transmural techniques have comparable treatment outcomes in draining pancreatic pseudocysts. Eur J Gastroenterol Hepatol 2012;24(12):1355–62.

16. Seifert H, Faust D, Schmitt T, et al. Transmural drainage of cystic peripancreatic lesions with a new large-channel echo endoscope. Endoscopy 2001;33(12): 1022–6.

17. Itoi T, Binmoeller KF, Shah J, et al. Clinical evaluation of a novel lumen-apposing metal stent for endosonography-guided pancreatic pseudocyst and gallbladder drainage (with videos). Gastrointest Endosc 2012;75(4):870–6.

18. Sriram PV, Kaffes AJ, Rao GV, et al. Endoscopic ultrasound-guided drainage of pancreatic pseudocysts complicated by portal hypertension or by intervening vessels. Endoscopy 2005;37(3):231–5.

19. Varadarajulu S, Wilcox CM, Tamhane A, et al. Role of EUS in drainage of peripancreatic fluid collections not amenable for endoscopic transmural drainage. Gastrointest Endosc 2007;66(6):1107–19.

20. Monkemuller KE, Baron TH, Morgan DE. Transmural drainage of pancreatic fluid collections without electrocautery using the Seldinger technique. Gastrointest Endosc 1998;48(2):195–200.

21. Varadarajulu S, Tamhane A, Blakely J. Graded dilation technique for EUS-guided drainage of peripancreatic fluid collections: an assessment of outcomes and complications and technical proficiency (with video). Gastrointest Endosc 2008;68(4):656–66.

22. Kruger M, Schneider AS, Manns MP, et al. Endoscopic management of pancreatic pseudocysts or abscesses after an EUS-guided 1-step procedure for initial access. Gastrointest Endosc 2006;63(3):409–16.

23. Yoo J, Yan L, Hasan R, et al. Feasibility, safety, and outcomes of a single-step endoscopic ultrasonography-guided drainage of pancreatic fluid collections without fluoroscopy using a novel electrocautery-enhanced lumen-apposing, self-expanding metal stent. Endosc Ultrasound 2017;6(2):131–5.

24. Anderloni A, Orellana F, Jovani M, et al. Endoscopic ultrasound-guided drainage of a pancreatic pseudocyst with a novel lumen-apposing metal stent on an electrocautery-enhanced delivery system. Dig Liver Dis 2015;47(10):e17.

25. Adler DG, Taylor LJ, Hasan R, et al. A retrospective study evaluating endoscopic ultrasound-guided drainage of pancreatic fluid collections using a novel lumen-apposing metal stent on an electrocautery enhanced delivery system. Endosc Ultrasound 2017;6(6):389–93.

26. Patil R, Ona MA, Papafragkakis C, et al. Endoscopic ultrasound-guided placement of AXIOS stent for drainage of pancreatic fluid collections. Ann Gastroenterol 2016;29(2):168–73.

27. Shah RJ, Shah JN, Waxman I, et al. Safety and efficacy of endoscopic ultrasound-guided drainage of pancreatic fluid collections with lumen-apposing covered self-expanding metal stents. Clin Gastroenterol Hepatol 2015;13(4): 747–52.

28. Siddiqui AA, Adler DG, Nieto J, et al. EUS-guided drainage of peripancreatic fluid collections and necrosis by using a novel lumen-apposing stent: a large retrospective, multicenter U.S. experience (with videos). Gastrointest Endosc 2016; 83(4):699–707.

29. Bang JY, Hasan M, Navaneethan U, et al. Lumen-apposing metal stents (LAMS) for pancreatic fluid collection (PFC) drainage: may not be business as usual. Gut 2017;66(12):2054–6.

30. Bang JY, Hasan MK, Navaneethan U, et al. Lumen-apposing metal stents for drainage of pancreatic fluid collections: when and for whom? Dig Endosc 2017;29(1):83–90.

31. Fujii-Lau LL, Levy MJ. Endoscopic ultrasound-guided pancreatic duct drainage. J Hepatobiliary Pancreat Sci 2015;22(1):51–7.
32. Varadarajulu S, Rana SS, Bhasin DK. Endoscopic therapy for pancreatic duct leaks and disruptions. Gastrointest Endosc Clin N Am 2013;23(4):863–92.
33. Will U, Fueldner F, Goldmann B, et al. Successful transgastric pancreaticography and endoscopic ultrasound-guided drainage of a disconnected pancreatic tail syndrome. Therap Adv Gastroenterol 2011;4(4):213–8.
34. Itoi T, Yasuda I, Kurihara T, et al. Technique of endoscopic ultrasonography-guided pancreatic duct intervention (with videos). J Hepatobiliary Pancreat Sci 2014;21(2):E4–9.
35. Tyberg A, Sharaiha RZ, Kedia P, et al. EUS-guided pancreatic drainage for pancreatic strictures after failed ERCP: a multicenter international collaborative study. Gastrointest Endosc 2017;85(1):164–9.
36. Attam R, Arain M, Trikudanathan G, et al. EUS-guided pancreatic duct access and wire placement to facilitate dorsal duct cannulation after failed ERCP. Gastrointest Endosc 2015;81(5):1260.
37. Elmunzer BJ, Piraka CR. EUS-guided methylene blue injection to facilitate pancreatic duct access after unsuccessful ERCP. Gastroenterology 2016;151(5):809–10.
38. Uche-Anya EN, Packey CD, Khan AS, et al. EUS-guided pancreatic duct puncture for difficult cannulation of stenosed pancreaticojejunostomy. Dig Dis Sci 2018;63(1):268–9.
39. Oh D, Park DH, Cho MK, et al. Feasibility and safety of a fully covered self-expandable metal stent with antimigration properties for EUS-guided pancreatic duct drainage: early and midterm outcomes (with video). Gastrointest Endosc 2016;83(2):366–73.e2.
40. Will U, Reichel A, Fueldner F, et al. Endoscopic ultrasonography-guided drainage for patients with symptomatic obstruction and enlargement of the pancreatic duct. World J Gastroenterol 2015;21(46):13140–51.
41. Will U, Fuldner F, Reichel A, et al. EUS-guided drainage of the pancreatic duct (EUPD)–promising therapeutic alternative to surgical intervention in case of symptomatic retention of the pancreatic duct and unsuccessful ERP. Zentralbl Chir 2014;139(3):318–25.
42. Fujii LL, Topazian MD, Abu Dayyeh BK, et al. EUS-guided pancreatic duct intervention: outcomes of a single tertiary-care referral center experience. Gastrointest Endosc 2013;78(6):854–64.e1.
43. Chen YI, Levy MJ, Moreels TG, et al. An international multicenter study comparing EUS-guided pancreatic duct drainage with enteroscopy-assisted endoscopic retrograde pancreatography after Whipple surgery. Gastrointest Endosc 2017;85(1):170–7.
44. Itoi T, Kasuya K, Sofuni A, et al. Endoscopic ultrasonography-guided pancreatic duct access: techniques and literature review of pancreatography, transmural drainage and rendezvous techniques. Dig Endosc 2013;25(3):241–52.
45. Dumonceau JM, Delhaye M, Tringali A, et al. Endoscopic treatment of chronic pancreatitis: European Society of Gastrointestinal Endoscopy (ESGE) Clinical Guideline. Endoscopy 2012;44(8):784–800.
46. Yang D, Amin S, Gonzalez S, et al. Transpapillary drainage has no added benefit on treatment outcomes in patients undergoing EUS-guided transmural drainage of pancreatic pseudocysts: a large multicenter study. Gastrointest Endosc 2016;83(4):720–9.

Celiac Plexus Block and Neurolysis: A Review

Amit H. Sachdev, MD*, Frank G. Gress, MD

KEYWORDS

- Chronic pancreatitis • Pancreatic cancer • Treatment • Endoscopic ultrasound
- Celiac plexus block • Celiac plexus neurolysis • Celiac ganglia

KEY POINTS

- Pain is often associated with chronic pancreatitis and pancreatic cancer.
- Often times opioids are used to treat pain; however, the use of opioids is frequently difficult because of the adverse effects associated with these medications.
- Endoscopic ultrasound-guided celiac plexus block and celiac plexus nuerolysis are safe and effective modalities used to alleviate pain associated with chronic pancreatitis and pancreatic cancer, respectively.
- Although used interchangeably, celiac plexus block is a transient interruption of the plexus by local anesthetic, while celiac plexus neurolysis is prolonged interruption of the transmission of pain from the celiac plexus using chemical ablation such as alcohol or phenol.
- The techniques also vary.

INTRODUCTION

Abdominal pain related to chronic pancreatitis and pancreatic cancer is often times extremely disabling.[1–4] Endoscopic ultrasound (EUS)-guided celiac plexus block (CPB) is used to reduce pain associated with chronic pancreatitis. EUS-guided celiac plexus neurolysis (CPN) is typically used to reduce pain associated with pancreatic cancer.[5] Initially, pain associated with chronic pancreatitis and pancreatic cancer is managed medically. Medical management from pancreatic cancer pain begins with nonopioid drugs. Often times, more powerful opioid medications are needed, because non-narcotic medications are inadequate for pain relief and are associated with a variety of adverse effects including nausea and constipation. If patients have refractory pain or cannot tolerate increasing amounts of opioid medications, EUS-guided celiac plexus block and neurolysis play an important role. Celiac plexus block (CPB), a temporizing treatment, most commonly refers to the

Division of Digestive and Liver Diseases, Columbia University Medical Center, 161 Fort Washington Avenue, New York, NY 10032, USA
* Corresponding author.
E-mail address: ahs2173@cumc.columbia.edu

Gastrointest Endoscopy Clin N Am 28 (2018) 579–586
https://doi.org/10.1016/j.giec.2018.06.004
1052-5157/18/© 2018 Elsevier Inc. All rights reserved.

injection of a steroid and a long-acting local anesthetic into the celiac plexus. In contrast, CPN generally refers to injection of alcohol or phenol, agents with more permanent effect.

This article discusses the history of EUS-guided celiac plexus block and nuerolysis, the anatomy of the celiac plexus, the indications, contraindications, preprocedural evaluation and technique, associated complications, and the efficacy of EUS-guided CPB and CPN.

HISTORY OF CELIAC PLEXUS BLOCK AND CELIAC PLEXUS NEUROLYSIS

The initial technique for performing CPN was described in 1914 by Kappis and colleagues[6] and was an intraoperative procedure. Since that time, CPB and CPN have been conducted under radiographic, fluoroscopic, ultrasound, and computed tomography (CT) approaches.[7–9] The first case of EUS-guided CPB/CPN in pancreatic cancer was described in 1996 by Faigel and colleagues[10] and Wiersema and colleagues.[11,12] The first case of EUS-guided CPB in patients with pain related to chronic pancreatitis was described in 1999 by Gress and colleagues.[13] Since then, numerous medium-sized prospective and retrospective studies have been performed and have shown that CPB/CPN is beneficial in alleviating pain. The advantage of the EUS approach is the fine orientation of the needle above or lateral to the celiac trunk and the real-time performance of the procedure under Doppler control of vessel interposition. In addition, the technique is easy, requiring only 2 to 3 minutes immediately after the staging or sampling of an inoperable pancreatic tumor. Better results can be expected owing to the better orientation of the needle, compared with the US or CT approach, and the real-time accomplishment of the procedure.[14]

ANATOMY OF THE CELIAC PLEXUS

The celiac plexus is a network of ganglia that relays preganglionic sympathetic and parasympathetic efferent fibers and visceral sensory afferent fibers to the upper abdominal viscera. The celiac plexus transmits the sensation of pain from the pancreas. The visceral sensory afferent fibers transmit nociceptive impulses from the liver, gallbladder, pancreas, spleen, adrenal glands, kidneys, distal esophagus, and bowel to the level of the distal transverse colon. Located in the retroperitoneum just inferior to the celiac trunk and along the bilateral anterolateral aspects of the aorta, between the levels of T12-L1 disc space and L2, the celiac plexus can easily be reached by several different approaches.

The plexus contains 1 to 5 large ganglia, which receive sympathetic fibers from the 3 splanchnic nerves. Although the terms celiac plexus and sphlancnic nerves are often used interchangeably, it is important to note that they are distinct structures.[15] The splanchnic nerves are located above and posterior to the diaphragm and anterior most often to the twelfth thoracic vertebra. The celiac plexus is located below and anterior to the diaphragm and surrounds the origin of the celiac trunk. The greater (T5–T9), lesser (T10–T11), and least (T12) are preganglionic in nature, and traverse the posterior mediastinum and enter the abdomen through the crura of the diaphragm above L1.[15] Parasympathetic fibers from the vagus nerve provide autonomic supply to the liver, pancreas, gallbladder, stomach, spleen, kidneys, adrenal glands, omentum, small bowel, and large bowel to the level of the splenic flexure, as well as the blood vessels of the abdomen.

INDICATIONS

CPB is indicated for management of pain associated with chronic pancreatitis. CPN (according to the National Comprehensive Cancer Network [NCCN] guidelines) is indicated for pain associated with chronic pancreatitis and pancreatic cancer.[5] Pain is a common symptom reported in up to 90% of patients with advanced pancreatic cancer, and it is a major issue in the management of these patients.[5] CPN is especially beneficial when patients have intolerable adverse effects of opioid therapy such as drowsiness, somnolence, confusion, delirium, dry mouth, anorexia, constipation, nausea, and vomiting, or if an analgesic ceiling is seen because of neurotoxicity.[16]

CONTRAINDICATIONS

Absolute contraindications for CPB and CPN are a lack of patient cooperation, platelet count less than 50,000, or coagulopathy. Relative contraindications for CPB and CPN are altered anatomy from prior surgery and congenital abnormalities. EUS-CPN should be considered an adjunct method to standard pain management. Studies have shown that it moderately reduces pain in pancreatic cancer, without completely eliminating it. Nearly all patients need to continue opioid use, often at a constant dose. The effect on quality of life is controversial, and survival is not influenced.

Contraindications specific to CPB and CPN include bowel obstruction in the face of increased peristalsis from unopposed parasympathetic activity resulting from the block. Patients taking disulfiram are not good candidates, because they can get tachycardia, nausea, vomiting, and headache because of accumulation of acetaldehyde, as the alcohol is not able to be broken down.

Patients with drug-seeking behavior and physical dependence may be appropriate for CPB and CPN in order to limit the use of opioid medications for their pain control, but it is critical that patients are carefully selected.

PREPROCEDURE WORKUP AND EVALUATION

Appropriate patient selection and communication are two of the most important aspects that of preprocedural assessments in patients undergoing CPB and CPN. Basic laboratory evaluation that should be performed prior to the procedure includes a complete blood cell count, coagulation panel, and abdominal CT scan.

Patients should be questioned about allergies and the use of anticoagulants. Oral anticoagulants must be stopped for the appropriate time frame and long-acting opioids should be continued. Patients should take nothing by mouth for 6 hours, which enables sedation to be given safely. If the patient is being considered for neurolysis following a successful block, immediately following local anesthetic administration, breakthrough medications may be held to allow a higher pain score for adequate evaluation of the block. If the neurolysis will be performed at a later date, short-acting agents for breakthrough might be held in the periprocedural period to avoid confounding.

CELIAC PLEXUS BLOCK AND NEUROLYSIS TECHNIQUE

Prior to the procedure, the patient should be placed in the left lateral position. Patients should get preprocedural hydration with normal saline (typically 500–1000 mL) to minimize the risk of hypotension. During the procedure, the patient should be continually monitored. Noninvasive blood pressure monitoring and pulse oximetry along with electrocardiogram (ECG) monitoring should be performed.

In order to perform both procedures, the endosonographer will need a curved linear array echoendoscope. A 20 gauge EUS-guided spray needle is frequently used. For anesthesia, either general anesthesia with propofol, or deep intravenous sedation with 2 to 4 mg of midazolam can be used. Some endosonographers recommend antibiotic prophylaxis, which is thought to help avoid formation of retroperitoneal abscess. Alcohol is also considered a bactericidal agent.

CPB is generally performed with the unilateral approach. Generally 20 mL of 0.25% bupivacaine followed by 40 mg of triamcinolone for injection on each side of the celiac plexus is used in the bilateral approach or 80 mg on 1 side in the unilateral approach.

Two approaches are currently used for EUS-CPN. The classic approach, known as the central technique, involves injection of the agent at the base of the CA. In the second approach, the bilateral technique, the neurolytic agent is injected on both sides of the CA. For CPN, 20 mL of 0.25% bupivacaine followed by 98% dehydrated ethyl alcohol for injection into the celiac plexus. The amount of ethanol that is injected varies. In most cases performed, 10 to 20 mL of alcohol is used.

When identifying the celiac axis, visualization is best through the posterior lesser curvature of the gastric fundus, which permits identification of the aorta, which appears in a longitudinal plane. The aorta is traced distally to the celiac trunk, which is the first major branch below the diaphragm. Studies have shown that the celiac plexus can be recognized directly as a discrete structure, although this remains controversial. Color Doppler is used to confirm the vascular nature of the adjacent structures (**Fig. 1**).

Prior to injecting into the celiac plexus, the needle is flushed with 3 cc of normal saline to remove any tissue acquired during insertion. An aspiration test is performed to rule out vessel penetration prior to each injection. This is a critical step in this process, as direct injection into a blood vessel can be deadly. Before withdrawing the needle, it should be flushed with 3 mL normal saline to prevent seeding of the needle track with alcohol, which may produce transient severe postprocedure pain.

In some cases, EUS-guided direct celiac ganglia neurolysis is used. This technique was developed by Levy and colleagues in 2008, and the celiac ganglia is identified usually between the aorta and the left adrenal gland. Ethanol is then injected into the gangia.[17] One study compared the results when 10 or 20 mL alcohol injection were used during intraganglia or central injection, and no difference in pain alleviation was noted (**Fig. 2**).[18]

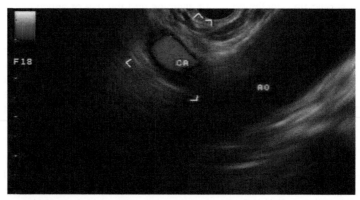

Fig. 1. Doppler evaluation of the celiac artery. The descending aorta is usually located 35 cm from the incisors. The celiac artery takeoff or trunk is usually located 40 to 50 cm from the incisors.

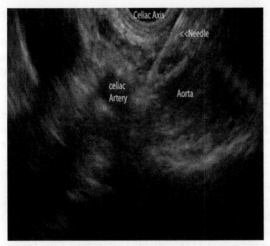

Fig. 2. Endoscopic ultrasound image showing the position of the EUS needle above the celiac ataxias. The origin of the celiac axis just above the celiac artery takeoff from the aorta is seen.

COMPLICATIONS

Serious complications from CPB and CPN are rare. The 2 most common complications are diarrhea and orthostatic hypotension.[13,19] These may be seen in up to 38% and 44% of patients, respectively, whether performed by EUS or percutaneous approaches.[20] They are transient complications. Postprocedure diarrhea is related to blockade of the sympathetic innervation to the abdominal viscera, and results from unopposed parasympathetic stimulation. Hypotension occurs due the dilation of the splanchnic vasculature and can be treated with intravenous hydration. Intravenous fluid bolus prior to the procedure can help prevent hypotension from occurring.

Other complications that can occur include empyema,[21] retroperitoneal abscess,[22] hematuria caused by needles piercing the kidney, intravascular injection, which can cause local anesthetic toxicity or increased blood alcohol levels, neurolysis, and pneumothorax. Infections and infarction of the liver or spleen[23] and peritonitis are also risks associated with this procedure. Other complications include pulmonary embolism.[24] Studies have shown that major complications occur in less than 1% of patients.[25]

POSTPROCEDURE FOLLOW-UP

After the procedure, the patient's vital signs should be monitored (temperature, blood pressure, and heart rate) for at least 2 hours. Individual institutions should consider formulating protocols for preprocedure, postprocedure observation, and follow-up. Referral to higher-volume centers should be considered if institutional experience is limited.

EFFICACY

Studies have shown that there is variability in the efficacy in regards to pain relief associated with CPB and CPN. Although CPB and CPN are considered safe procedures, the long-term efficacy of CPB and CPN has been limited in terms of duration of pain relief, and the effects on quality of life are controversial depending on the study.

Most studies evaluating percutaneous CPB for controlling pain from chronic pancreatitis have been small retrospective case series and have reported marginal benefit. A meta-analysis of EUS-guided CPB and CPN reported response rates of 59% in chronic pancreatitis and 80% in pancreatic cancer; however, most of these patients continued to take analgesic medications.[18]

The average length of relief for patients with CPB is approximately 3 months in most studies, and CPB is therefore seen as a temporizing measure. It is important to note that only 60% of patients with CPB report relief of pain after EUS-CPB.[26] In 1 study, younger patients and patients with prior pancreatic surgery were less likely to respond. The reasons for this are unclear. Studies have shown, however, that repeated EUS-CPB in a single patient can be safe, and that response to the first EUS-CPB is associated with response to subsequent blocks.[27] In fact, in this study, patients had up to 10 blocks with pain relief and without serious adverse events, although most patients in this study received 4 blocks total.

In a large meta-analysis of 1145 patients undergoing CPN for palliation of cancer pain (63% of whom had pancreatic cancer) good or excellent pain relief was noted in 70% to 90% of patients 3 months after the procedure.[20] One randomized control trial comparing central versus bilateral technique for CPN showed no difference in duration of pain relief or reduction in pain medications.[28] The type of technique showing the best response is still controversial depending on the study.[29] CPN in pancreatic cancer had no survival benefit in 2 large randomized control trials.[28,30] Studies have also looked at the effective of using phenol instead of alcohol in the procedure. Further studies need to be conducted; however, initial studies suggest that phenol-gylcerol is an alternative agent that may be able to provide pain relief for patients with pancreatic cancer.[31]

The timing of performing EUS-guided CPN also matters. Studies have shown that pain reduction and narcotic use after early (at the time of initial diagnostic and staging EUS) EUS-CPN can reduce pain and moderate morphine consumption in patients with painful, inoperable pancreatic cancers.

A recent randomized trial also suggested that CPB might be superior to CPN for patients with pancreatic cancer.[32] The positive response rate at day 7 and the complete response rate were higher in the ganglia neurolysis group (75.5% vs 45.5% and 50% vs 18.2%, respectively).

Further research needs to be conducted on the long-term benefits of CPB versus CPN for patients with pancreatic cancer.

SUMMARY

EUS-guided CPB and CPN are relatively safe and effective procedures that can be used to reduce pain associated with pancreatitis and pancreatic cancer. Further studies need to be conducted to make more reliable conclusions about the benefits of these procedures.

REFERENCES

1. Cornman-Homonoff J, Holzwanger DJ, Lee KS, et al. Celiac plexus block and neurolysis in the management of chronic upper abdominal pain. Semin Intervent Radiol 2017;34:376–86.
2. Yasuda I, Wang HP. Endoscopic ultrasound-guided celiac plexus block and neurolysis. Dig Endosc 2017;29:455–62.

3. Yeager MP, Colacchio TA, Yu CT, et al. Morphine inhibits spontaneous and cyto-kine- enhanced natural killer cell cytotoxicity in volunteers. Anesthesiology 1995; 83:500–8.

4. Chernish SM, Davidson JA, Brunelle RL, et al. Response of normal subjects to a single 2-milligram dose of glucagon administered intramuscularly. Arch Int Phar-macodyn Ther 1975;218:312–27.

5. Caraceni A, Portenoy RK. Pain management in patients with pancreatic carci-noma. Cancer 1996;78:639–53.

6. Kappis M. Erfahrungen mit local anasthetic bic bauchoperationen. Vehr Dtsch Gesellsch Chir 1914;43:87–9.

7. Yan BM, Myers RP. Neurolytic celiac plexus block for pain control in unresectable pancreatic cancer. Am J Gastroenterol 2007;102:430–8.

8. Wang PJ, Shang MY, Qian Z, et al. CT-guided percutaneous neurolytic celiac plexus block technique. Abdom Imaging 2006;31:710–8.

9. Carroll I. Celiac plexus block for visceral pain. Curr Pain Headache Rep 2006;10: 20–5.

10. Faigel DO, Veloso KM, Long WB, et al. Endosonography-guided celiac plexus in-jection for abdominal pain due to chronic pancreatitis. Am J Gastroenterol 1996; 91:1675.

11. Levy MJ, Wiersema MJ. EUS-guided celiac plexus neurolysis and celiac plexus block. Gastrointest Endosc 2003;57:923–30.

12. Hoffman BJ. EUS-guided celiac plexus block/neurolysis. Gastrointest Endosc 2002;56:S26–8.

13. Gress F, Schmitt C, Sherman S, et al. A prospective randomized comparison of endoscopic ultrasound- and computed tomography-guided celiac plexus block for managing chronic pancreatitis pain. Am J Gastroenterol 1999;94:900–5.

14. Fusaroli P, Jenssen C, Hocke M, et al. EFSUMB guidelines on interventional ultra-sound (INVUS), part V. Ultraschall Med 2016;37:77–99.

15. Ward EM, Rorie DK, Nauss LA, et al. The celiac ganglia in man: normal anatomic variations. Anesth Analg 1979;58:461–5.

16. Kaufman M, Singh G, Das S, et al. Efficacy of endoscopic ultrasound-guided ce-liac plexus block and celiac plexus neurolysis for managing abdominal pain associated with chronic pancreatitis and pancreatic cancer. J Clin Gastroenterol 2010;44:127–34.

17. Levy MJ, Topazian MD, Wiersema MJ, et al. Initial evaluation of the efficacy and safety of endoscopic ultrasound-guided direct Ganglia neurolysis and block. Am J Gastroenterol 2008;103:98–103.

18. Puli SR, Reddy JB, Bechtold ML, et al. EUS-guided celiac plexus neurolysis for pain due to chronic pancreatitis or pancreatic cancer pain: a meta-analysis and systematic review. Dig Dis Sci 2009;54:2330–7.

19. Wiersema MJ, Wiersema LM. Endosonography-guided celiac plexus neurolysis. Gastrointest Endosc 1996;44:656–62.

20. Eisenberg E, Carr DB, Chalmers TC. Neurolytic celiac plexus block for treatment of cancer pain: a meta-analysis. Anesth Analg 1995;80:290–5.

21. Muscatiello N, Panella C, Pietrini L, et al. Complication of endoscopic ultrasound-guided celiac plexus neurolysis. Endoscopy 2006;38:858.

22. Ahmed HM, Friedman SE, Henriques HF, et al. End-organ ischemia as an unfore-seen complication of endoscopic-ultrasound-guided celiac plexus neurolysis. Endoscopy 2009;41(Suppl 2):E218–9.

23. Jang HY, Cha SW, Lee BH, et al. Hepatic and splenic infarction and bowel ischemia following endoscopic ultrasound-guided celiac plexus neurolysis. Clin Endosc 2013;46:306–9.
24. Petersen EW, Pohler KR, Burnett CJ, et al. Pulmonary embolism: a rare complication of neurolytic alcohol celiac plexus block. Pain Physician 2017;20:E751–3.
25. Lillemoe KD, Cameron JL, Kaufman HS, et al. Chemical splanchnicectomy in patients with unresectable pancreatic cancer. A prospective randomized trial. Ann Surg 1993;217:447–55 [discussion: 456–7].
26. LeBlanc JK, DeWitt J, Johnson C, et al. A prospective randomized trial of 1 versus 2 injections during EUS-guided celiac plexus block for chronic pancreatitis pain. Gastrointest Endosc 2009;69:835–42.
27. Sey MS, Schmaltz L, Al-Haddad MA, et al. Effectiveness and safety of serial endoscopic ultrasound-guided celiac plexus block for chronic pancreatitis. Endosc Int open 2015;3:E56–9.
28. LeBlanc JK, Al-Haddad M, McHenry L, et al. A prospective, randomized study of EUS- guided celiac plexus neurolysis for pancreatic cancer: one injection or two? Gastrointest Endosc 2011;74:1300–7.
29. Leblanc JK, Rawl S, Juan M, et al. Endoscopic ultrasound-guided celiac plexus neurolysis in pancreatic cancer: a prospective pilot study of safety using 10 mL versus 20 mL alcohol. Diagn Ther Endosc 2013;2013:327036.
30. Wyse JM, Carone M, Paquin SC, et al. Randomized, double-blind, controlled trial of early endoscopic ultrasound-guided celiac plexus neurolysis to prevent pain progression in patients with newly diagnosed, painful, inoperable pancreatic cancer. J Clin Oncol 2011;29:3541–6.
31. Ishiwatari H, Hayashi T, Yoshida M, et al. Phenol-based endoscopic ultrasound-guided celiac plexus neurolysis for East Asian alcohol-intolerant upper gastrointestinal cancer patients: a pilot study. World J Gastroenterol 2014;20:10512–7.
32. Doi S, Yasuda I, Kawakami H, et al. Endoscopic ultrasound-guided celiac ganglia neurolysis vs. celiac plexus neurolysis: a randomized multicenter trial. Endoscopy 2013;45:362–9.

The Role of Genetics in Pancreatitis

Aws Hasan, MD[a], Dagmara I. Moscoso, MS[b], Fay Kastrinos, MD, MPH[c],*

KEYWORDS

- Hereditary pancreatitis • Familial pancreatitis • Genetic evaluation
- Genetic variants associated with pancreatitis • PRSS1 • SPINK1 • CFTR

KEY POINTS

- Genetic risk assessment for individuals with suspected hereditary and familial pancreatitis provides an opportunity to discover a causative cause for disease.
- Early identification of hereditary pancreatitis, through genetic evaluation and testing, and proper management in gene mutation carriers requires a multidisciplinary approach in order to be complete and most effective.
- Continued advances in genomic technologies with complete genotyping can establish additional associations between complex genetic causes and environment interactions that may provide personalized management and preventive strategies for pancreatitis in the future.

INTRODUCTION

Individuals with recurrent acute and chronic pancreatitis (CP) may have an inherited predisposition to the development of the disease. Pancreatitis in the setting of a significant family history of the disease can be classified as hereditary or familial pancreatitis. Hereditary pancreatitis (HP) has been defined as either 2 or more individuals within a family exhibiting pancreatitis for 2 or more generations or pancreatitis linked to the inheritance of a pathogenic mutation in the cationic trypsinogen PRSS1 (protease serine 1) gene.[1] Most HP cases are related to acute pancreatitis or CP in an autosomal dominant pattern of inheritance, although additional cases have been attributed to autosomal recessive inheritance.[2,3] On the other hand, familial pancreatitis (FP) is a broader term used to describe families in which pancreatitis occurs with a greater

Disclosure Statement: No disclosures.
[a] Department of Internal Medicine, Columbia University Medical Center, 630 West 168 Street, New York, NY, 10032, USA; [b] Division of Digestive and Liver Diseases, Columbia University Medical Center, 630 West 168 Street, New York, NY, 10032, USA; [c] Division of Digestive and Liver Diseases, Columbia University Medical Center, Herbert Irving Comprehensive Cancer Center, 161 Fort Washington Avenue, Suite 862, New York, NY, 10032, USA
* Corresponding author.
E-mail address: fk18@columbia.edu

Gastrointest Endoscopy Clin N Am 28 (2018) 587–603
https://doi.org/10.1016/j.giec.2018.06.001
1052-5157/18/© 2018 Elsevier Inc. All rights reserved.

giendo.theclinics.com

incidence than expected by chance alone in the general population.[4–6] Familial pancreatitis may or may not be caused by a genetic defect.

In 1952, Comfort and Steinberg were the first to describe HP as recurrent acute pancreatitis (RAP) and CP that tends to run in families.[7] In 1996, facilitated by advancements in molecular genetics, Whitcomb and colleagues[8–10] discovered that HP was caused by a gain-of-function mutation in the cationic trypsinogen gene, which consequently revolutionized the understanding of the mechanism of disease. This finding supported the trypsin-dependent theory where gain-of-function mutations result in trypsinogen or trypsin that is degradation resistant. In addition, premature trypsin activation may provide an alternate mechanism leading to RAP, with a subset of these patients then progressing to CP. Additional genes have been identified in those individuals with personal and family history of pancreatitis, and genetic testing is a useful risk assessment tool to determine whether an individual has an underlying pathogenic variant and increased risk of developing pancreatitis.[11,12] It is important to also recognize and consider relevant environmental factors and exposures and their potential impact on the clinical manifestations in individuals with a genetic predisposition to the development of pancreatitis.

In this chapter, the authors closely examine the specific genes implicated in pancreatitis, investigate the role of genetic testing for diagnosis, and describe the impact of genetic testing results on clinical management.

GERMLINE VARIANTS ASSOCIATED WITH PANCREATITIS

There are several germline genetic alterations that have been associated with the development of pancreatitis. Since its discovery in 1996, *PRSS1* and additional genes have been implicated in HP as either disease causing or modifiers of disease. These include serine protease inhibitor Kazal type 1 (*SPINK 1*) and cystic fibrosis transmembrane conductance regulator (*CFTR*) genes. Both carry a 1% penetrance in comparison to 80% or higher penetrance reported with *PRSS1* gene mutations.[2,3] In addition, many HP cases seem to have a complex multigene and multifactorial cause, including gene–environment interactions between various pathogenic gene variants that affect trypsin regulation, such as calcium-sensing receptor (*CASR*), chymotrypsin C (*CTRC*), and claudin-2 (*CLDN2*) (**Fig. 1, Table 1**).[1,4–6,13]

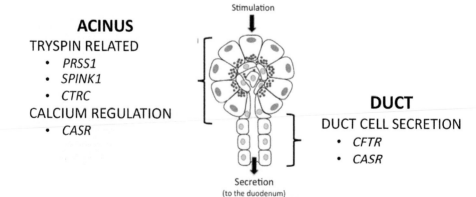

Fig. 1. Genetic variants that affect trypsinogen activation in pancreatic acinar cells and ducts. (*Adapted from* Solomon S, Whitcomb DC. Genetics of pancreatitis: an update for clinicians and genetic counselors. Curr Gastroenterol Rep 2012;14(2):112–7; with permission.)

Table 1
Pathogenic gene variants associated with pancreatitis

Risk of Pancreatitis	Inheritance Pattern	Pathogenic Gene (Variant)	Molecular/Functional Consequence
High	Autosomal dominant	*PRSS1* (R122H,N29I)	Protein resistant to degradation
	Autosomal dominant with low penetrance or multigenic	*PRSS1* (A16V)	Protein partially resistant to degradation
Moderate	Autosomal dominant with low penetrance or multigenic	*SPINK1* (c.27delC, p.Tyr54His)	Severe loss of protein function
	Autosomal dominant with low penetrance or multigenic	*CTRC* (p.K247_R254del24, p.R254W, p.Ala73Thr)	
	Autosomal recessive or multigenic	*CFTR* (p.F508del, c.del_exon2, 3 p.G551D)	
Mild	Autosomal recessive or multigenic	*CFTR* (p.R75Q)	Selective loss of protein function
	Autosomal recessive or multigenic	*SPINK1* (p.N34S)	
Modifiers	Complex	*PRSS1* (c.−408T >C)	Altered expression of protein
	Complex	*CLDN2* (c.−275 to 1293G >A)	
	Complex	*CTRC* (c.180C >T)	

Adapted from LaRusch J, Solomon S, Whitcomb DC. Pancreatitis overview 2014. In: Adam MP, Ardinger HH, Pagon RA, et al, editors. GeneReviews [Internet]. Seattle (WA): University of Washington, Seattle; 1993–2018. Available at: https://www.ncbi.nlm.nih.gov/ books/NBK190101/; with permission.

PRSS1

HP caused by mutations in the *PRSS1* gene is inherited in an autosomal dominant manner that causes RAP or CP across all ages. Pathogenic variants in *PRSS1* are present in more than 60% of large families with pancreatitis affecting several generations.[1] Although more than 35 *PRSS1* mutations are currently recognized, the most common disease-causing variants are R122H, N29I, and A16V. The 2 missense mutations, R122H and N29I, make up nearly 90% of *PRSS1*-related HP cases, where each accounts for nearly 65% and 25% of cases, respectively.[8,9,13,14]

Mechanism of action

The HP locus was mapped to chromosome 7q35, which contains the *PRSS1* gene.[8] The *PRSS1* gene encodes the cationic form of trypsinogen, which is a zymogen precursor to trypsin. Trypsin is the most abundant digestive enzyme secreted by the pancreas and activates other zymogens in the small intestine. In the healthy state, pancreatic acinar and ductal cells have mechanisms, such as autolysis, to protect against premature or excessive trypsin activation. If activated in the wrong location, trypsin can initiate an immune response as seen in pancreatitis, and the primary defense against pancreatitis development is proper control of trypsin activity. Pathogenic *PRSS1* mutations cause prematurely activated or degradation-resistant trypsin that promotes increased autoactivation of mutant trypsinogens and higher intrapancreatic trypsin activity.[4,15,16] Nearly all of the pathogenic *PRSS1* variants associated with HP occur at trypsin's regulatory regions that contain calcium-binding sites for activation or autolysis and whose conformation is dictated by calcium concentration. The trypsinogen-activating peptide, which is stabilized under high calcium concentration, cleaves trypsinogen to yield active trypsin and with low calcium levels, trypsin lysis occurs.

Epidemiology and prevalence

The prevalence of HP has been explored in several European, population-based studies. In a series of 112 families recruited from the European Registry of Hereditary Pancreatitis and Pancreatic Cancer (EUROPAC) study across 14 countries, the distribution of PRSS1 mutations was explored in addition to correlations between genotype and phenotype.[2] Among 418 individuals with HP (defined as having 2 first-degree relatives [FDR] or ≥3 second-degree relatives [SDR] in 2 or more generations with RAP and or CP), germline mutations were detected in 327 (78%), 72 (17%) were negative, and 19 (5%) did not undergo testing. In a national survey study conducted in France, the prevalence of HP was 0.3/100,000 persons and determined among individuals with (1) CP and family history of RAP, (2) CP in 2 FDR, (3) CP in 3 or more SDRs, or (4) a known PRSS1 gene mutation.[17] Of the eligible 200 individuals with HP, 135 (68%) were PRSS1 carriers of which 93% had clinical or morphologic signs of HP (penetrance). Similar to previous findings, the R122H variant was most frequently detected than other variants. Despite having a significant family history of pancreatitis, 32% did not carry a germline mutation in PRSS1, which suggests that additional germline alterations may contribute to the development of pancreatitis.

Variable prevalence estimates have been reported and genotypic variation may differ among diverse populations. In a Danish population-based cohort of individuals with pancreatitis of unknown origin diagnosed by age 30 years, PRSS1 mutations were detected in 18/122 (15%) of individuals and the prevalence rate of HP was 57/100,000 for symptomatic HP patients and 0.13/100,000 for PRSS1 carriers.[18] The overall penetrance for PRSS1 mutations was 77%, of which penetrance of R122H-associated HP was 86% and 55% for A16V-associated HP. In contrast to other reports, the A16V variant was the second most frequent germline variant as opposed to N29I, because there were no N29I mutation carriers identified. Additional germline mutations associated with pancreatitis were identified in SPINK1 (n = 15) and CFTR (n = 9) and 11 individuals carried 2 or more germline mutations (SPINK-PRSS1 [n = 6], CFTR-SPINK1 [n = 4], CFTR-PRSS1 [n = 1]), yielding an overall mutation prevalence of 38% (46/122).

Clinical manifestations

The age of onset for PRSS1-related HP ranges from 10 to 12 years.[1,2,4,17] The clinical presentation of acute pancreatitis due to pathogenic PRSS1 gene mutations is not significantly different from non-PRSS1–related cases[19,20] and occurs in 69% of carriers with increases in the pancreatic enzymes, amylase, and lipase. The disease progresses to CP by a median age of 22 to 25 years and calcifications are prevalent in 61% of carriers with CP.[21] Exocrine and endocrine pancreatic insufficiency with diabetes mellitus occurs in 34% and 26% at a median age of 29 and 38 years, respectively (**Fig. 2**).[2,17]

In the EUROPAC study of HP cases, patients with R122H variants displayed a slightly younger age of symptom onset at 10 years, which is 4 to 5 years earlier compared with N29I carriers or those lacking a mutation.[2] Carriers of the R122H gene variant are also reported to have a more severe presentation of pancreatitis, and aggregate levels of exocrine and endocrine failure have been significantly higher compared with other forms of CP. However, not all studies report differences in clinical and morphologic data based on the specific type of gene alteration but do concur with

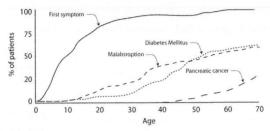

Fig. 2. Time to symptom development and associated clinical manifestations in hereditary pancreatitis. (*From* Shelton CA, Whitcomb DC. Hereditary pancreatitis. pancreapedia: exocrine pancreas knowledge base, 2016. Available at: https://www.pancreapedia.org/reviews/hereditary-pancreatitis. Accessed May 30, 2018; with permission.)

the median age of symptom onset of 10 years and that females had earlier symptom onset at 11 years compared with 15 years for males.[17] Among the Danish population-based cohort of HP patients, an average delay of 11.5 years was noted from symptom onset to diagnosis, which confirms findings from earlier studies.[2,18]

Serine Protease Inhibitor Kazal Type 1

Soon after the discovery of *PRSS1* as a causative mutation of HP, the *SPINK1* gene was recognized as another contributor of the pathogenesis of inherited pancreatitis. *SPINK1* is a trypsin inhibitor that was first identified in 1948, but its association with CP was not appreciated until 2000.[22] HP with an autosomal recessive pattern of inheritance occurs in individuals who carry homozygous or compound heterozygous alterations in the *SPINK1* gene.

Mechanism of action
The *SPINK1* gene is located on chromosome 5q32 and encodes a strong trypsin inhibitor. This protects the pancreas against premature trypsinogen activation and inhibits up to 20% of intrapancreatic trypsin.[22] *SPINK1* is regulated as an acute phase reactant and is expressed in pancreatic acinar cells during inflammation; upregulation of *SPINK1* expression during an acute inflammatory response provides feedback inhibition of trypsin to prevent inappropriate trypsinogen activation and pancreatic injury. Pathogenic *SPINK1* mutations lower levels of trypsin inhibitor and thereby increase susceptibility to pancreatitis (see **Fig. 1**).[16,23,24]

Epidemiology and prevalence
SPINK1 variants are common among the general population with a prevalence of nearly 2%.[25] Although ongoing studies continue to identify new gene mutations in *SPINK1*, the N34S variant is the most common high-risk haplotype reported globally and is prevalent in the United States, Europe, and India; a second pathogenic alteration, the IVS3+2T >C splice variant, is most common in Japan, Korea, and China.[26–30]

Less than 1% of heterozygous *SPINK1* carriers develop CP in the absence of additional contributing factors.[1,24,26] Most individuals who carry a single pathogenic variant are often healthy, thereby suggesting a multifactorial cause for the development of pancreatitis. Unlike *PRSS1* mutations, alterations in *SPINK1* can modify the presentation of pancreatitis in carriers by either lowering the threshold of initiating pancreatitis or worsening the severity of pancreatitis caused by other genetic or environmental factors (see **Table 1**). Among individuals with idiopathic CP, the frequency

Table 2	
Phenotypic expression of gene variants associated with pancreatitis	
Gene Variant	**Phenotype**
PRSS1	Hereditary pancreatitis
SPINK1/SPINK1	Familial pancreatitis
$CFTR^{sev}/CFTR^{sev}$	Cystic fibrosis
$CFTR^{sev}/CFTR^{m-v}$	Atypical cystic fibrosis
$CFTR^{bicarb}/CFTR^{any}$	Pancreatitis/sinus/CBAVD
$CFTR^{any}/SPINK1$	Recurrent acute pancreatitis/chronic pancreatitis
CTRC/SPINK1	Recurrent acute pancreatitis/chronic pancreatitis
CASR/SPINK1	Recurrent acute pancreatitis/chronic pancreatitis

Abbreviations: CBAVD, congenital bilateral absence of the vas deferens; $CFTR^{any}$, CFTR variant in any Class or bicarbonate conductance disrupting variant; $CFTR^{bicarb}$, CFTR gene variant that is bicarbonate conductance disrupting; $CFTR^{m-v}$, mild to variable CFTR mutations in Class IV; $CFTR^{sev}$, severe CFTR mutations in Class I–III.

of SPINK1 mutations is up to 25% and can occur with heterozygous, compound heterozygous, or homozygous genotypes.[1] In a population-based cohort of individuals with pancreatitis of unknown origin diagnosed by age 30 years in Denmark, 25/122 (20%) had SPINK1 mutations, of which the majority carried the N34S variant (N = 24) and only 1 carried the P55S variant.[18]

Clinical manifestations

Inheritance of 2 pathogenic variants (whether homozygous or compound heterozygous) in SPINK1 leads to autosomal recessive pancreatitis and may phenotypically be similar to PRSS1 mutation carriers. When compared with individuals without SPINK1 mutations, the overall odds ratio of developing pancreatitis was 87.1 for carriers of 2 SPINK1 mutations.[31] Multiple studies support comparable ages of disease onset and severity among homozygous and heterozygous N34S carriers.[22–26] However, coinheritance of SPINK1 and additional pathologic variants, in particular CFTR, are implicated in earlier onset and more aggressive pancreatitis.[31] In a study to investigate the role of CFTR and SPINK1 variants in idiopathic CP, results from subjects with sporadic and familial idiopathic CP versus control populations revealed a striking increase in pancreatitis risk with combined CFTR and SPINK1 mutations and was influenced by the type of CFTR alteration (**Table 2**).[31] Lastly, concurrent use of alcohol may precipitate episodes of acute pancreatitis in individuals with SPINK1 mutations. In a case-control study of individuals with acute pancreatitis, the N34S mutation was found in 29 (7.8%) of patients and 12 (2.6%) of controls, and mutation carriers were more frequent in subgroups with severe AP (15/164; 9.1%) and alcohol-induced AP (21/229; 9.2%), although the results were not statistically significant.[32]

Cystic Fibrosis Transmembrane Conductance Regulator

In addition to cystic fibrosis (CF), pancreatitis can be caused by alterations in the CFTR gene and its manifestation and severity is related to the specific variant involved, as well as zygosity. There are nearly 2000 gene variants associated with *CFTR*, and the gene encodes an anionic channel involved in chloride and bicarbonate secretion in the duct cells of the lung, pancreas, digestive system, and other organs, allowing it to control intraluminal pH, thereby affecting the production of sweat, digestive fluids, and mucus. Different mutations cause different defects in the CFTR protein, sometimes causing a milder or more severe phenotype of the disease (see **Tables 1–3**).[33,34]

Mechanism of action

Within the pancreas, bicarbonate secretion is particularly important for the secretion of pancreatic zymogens. A dysfunction in the *CFTR* gene leads to failure of the alkalization of the acinar cells, resulting in retention of zymogens in the duct, where they can become active and begin digesting the surrounding pancreas tissue, thus leading to pancreatitis (see **Fig. 1**). Furthermore, the loss of alkalization can lead to the formation of protein plugs in the pancreatic ducts.

A molecular classification system has been developed to define how the *CFTR* gene defect affects protein expression and total CFTR activity, and subsequently phenotypic expression (see **Table 3**). The CFTR class system groups mutations by the primary molecular defect in the CFTR protein. Total CFTR activity, which is mainly determined by *CFTR* genotype, is one of the few factors that influence the phenotype of an individual and determines if they will develop CF disease and to what degree. The degree of reduction in total CFTR activity, which is regulated mainly by the *CFTR* genotype, relates to the extent of CF manifestations. Mutations that reduce but retain some residual *CFTR* activity can be associated with a variation in symptoms and a spectrum of phenotypes.[33–40]

Epidemiology and prevalence

CF has an incidence of 1/2500 among individuals of Northern European descent and the incidence varies globally. *CFTR* mutations have been identified in approximately 35% of families with pancreatitis who do not have a *PRSS1* mutation.[1] Although all *CFTR* mutations that cause CF are also risk factors for pancreatitis, those less penetrant *CFTR* alleles that do not cause classic CF may still increase the risk for pancreatitis. The most common CF-causing mutation, F508del, is present in 70% of individuals with CF and currently accounts for approximately 40% of identified *CFTR* variants in persons with HP.[1] A single mutation in *CFTR* is not considered disease causing but may increase the risk of pancreatitis 2- to 5-fold.[36,38]

Several case-control studies have evaluated the prevalence of *CFTR* gene mutations among individuals with idiopathic pancreatitis. In a study of 134 individuals with CP, 18 (13.4%) were detected to have at least one *CFTR* mutation; carriers had a younger age at presentation, were predominantly nonalcoholic, and more likely to be nonsmokers.[37] In a German case-control study of 67 individuals with idiopathic CP, 25 abnormal *CFTR* alleles were detected, which were twice the frequency than in control groups.[38] In US-based cohort of 96 individuals with idiopathic pancreatitis, 19 were found to carry a *CFTR* mutation compared with 7/198 in the control group, yielding an odds ratio of 6.7.[39] In a similar study performed in Italy, the CP group was more likely to have a *CFTR* mutation compared with the control group (12.2% vs 3.4%).[40] *CFTR*-related mutations were the most frequent alterations than all other pancreatitis-associated gene mutations in a RAP cohort of patients with less than 35 years of age who had an unexplained first episode of pancreatitis.[41]

Clinical manifestations

The features of *CFTR*-related diseases depend on the functional effects of specific pathogenic variants on the 2 *CFTR* alleles, in addition to the presence of other modifier

Table 3
Classification of *CFTR* gene mutation defect

	Class I	Class II	Class III	Class IV	Class V
Molecular Defect	Defective synthesis of CFTR protein	Defect in CFTR protein processing and trafficking	Defective CFTR channel gating	CFTR channel conductance defect	Reduced synthesis of CFTR protein
Molecular Description	A premature stop codon prevents full translation of mRNA, resulting in truncated CFRTR protein. No mature CFTR protein formed	Defective posttranslational processing and transport reduce quantity of CFTR protein sent to cell surface	Reduction in channel open probability for CFTR at cell surface (does not open as much)	CFTR present at cell surface, but impaired ion movement through channels	Splicing defect reduces quantity of CFTR mRNA transcripts, decreasing amount of CFTR at cell surface
Functional Consequence	CFTR function abolished	CFTR function abolished	CFTR function abolished	Residual expression and function	Residual expression and function

Abbreviation: mRNA, messenger RNA.

genes and environmental exposures. Recent data suggest that *CFTR* pathogenic variants that solely affect bicarbonate conductance (*CFTR-BD*) while maintaining chloride conductance have major effects on the pancreas but minimal effects on the lungs because the pancreas uses *CFTR* as a bicarbonate channel (see **Table 2**).[31] Furthermore, the functional effect of *CFTR* genotypes is determined by the least severe pathogenic variant; a pancreatitis-predominant presentation is seen when the *CFTR* gene variants are either 2 bicarbonate-defective variants or 1 bicarbonate-defective variant and 1 severe variant (see **Tables 2** and **3**).

The following patterns represent the association between *CFTR* alterations and different manifestations of pancreatitis:

Classic cystic fibrosis Individuals who carry 2 *CFTR* mutations (homozygous or compound heterozygous) that are categorized by molecular classification as Class I or II, with near total loss of either messenger RNA or protein expression, present with a CF-severe phenotype and usually develop classic CF. These individuals manifest with advanced CP, malabsorption, and failure to thrive in the first few years of life. Exocrine pancreatic insufficiency occurs in up to 90% of patients with CF.[35] Soon after diagnosis, they often have pancreatic insufficiency with an inability to maintain nutritional needs without the use of pancreatic enzyme supplements.

Atypical cystic fibrosis In individuals who carry homozygous or compound heterozygous mutations in which at least 1 of the 2 *CFTR* mutations is categorized by molecular classification as Class III (altered regulation), Class IV (altered conductance), or Class V (leading to exon skipping), a critical level of CFTR function is retained and the CF phenotype is milder with CP and pancreatic insufficiency developing significantly later than CF-severe patients. However, because pancreatic function is retained, CF-mild patients are at risk for episodes of acute pancreatitis. Affected individuals may also manifest with congenital absence of the vas deferens, bronchiectasis, asthma, and chronic sinusitis. A subset of *CFTR*-related disorders that present with atypical CF features occur when an individual inherits at least 1 altered *CFTR* variant that causes selective deficiency in bicarbonate conductance. The limited CF manifestations include chronic sinusitis, infertility, RAP, and CP but minimal pulmonary disease.

Cystic fibrosis carriers Lastly, carriers who inherit only 1 mutated *CFTR* gene do not have clinical manifestations of CF but are at an increased risk of developing CP, which is about 2- to 5-fold higher than the general population.[36–38] However, studies suggest that there are concomitant risk factors among CF carriers that are associated with the development of CP such as the presence of pancreatic divisum[42,43] or coexisting *SPINK1* mutations,[31,44] and that CF carrier status alone is not a sufficient cause in and of itself.

COMPLEX MULTIGENIC DISORDERS

Most of the kindreds with FP can be attributed to complex, multigenic, or gene–environmental disorders with a variable number of germline pathogenic variants in genes that affect trypsin regulation. At least one-third of recurrent acute and CP results from complex genetic mechanisms,[1] where most of the genotypes are combinations of *SPINK1/CFTR* variants. However, recognition of additional low-risk variants may be significant contributors to pancreatic disease. The combination that leads to the development of pancreatitis involves a gene variant that increases the risk of recurrent trypsin activation (*PRSS1*, *CFTR*) and a gene variant that protects the pancreas from active trypsin or chronic inflammation (*SPINK1*).[1]

ADDITIONAL GERMLINE MUTATIONS ASSOCIATED WITH PANCREATITIS

Additional genes have been implicated in the development of pancreatitis among individuals with RAP, CP, and family history of pancreatitis. Although *PRSS1*, *SPINK1*, and *CFTR* genes are the most commonly associated with pancreatitis, a few less-known genes may be related. These genes include *CTRC*, *CASR*, carboxypeptidase A1 (*CPA1*), and *CLDN2* and are considered disease modifying rather than disease causing (see **Table 1**). For gene variants to be disease modifiers, the variant must also be common within the population, and worsen the severity of recurrent trypsin activation. The coinheritance of pathogenic variants and defective protection is therefore common and increases the likelihood that pancreatitis will progress from recurrent mild injury to end-stage disease.

Chymotrypsin C Gene

The *CTRC* gene encodes chymotrypsin C, which is a digestive enzyme involved in trypsin regulation and sensitive to alterations in calcium concentrations. In the normal state, under low calcium levels, trypsinogen activation sites are disabled while cleavage sites prompt trypsinogen degradation. With high calcium levels, activation sites are exposed and cleavage sites blocked resulting in unobstructed trypsin activity. *CTRC* mutations disrupt trypsin destruction and reduce its protective function in decreasing the risk of CP.[45–47] The most common *CTRC* variant is G60G, which is strongly correlated to progression from RAP to CP, especially in smokers.[48] Of note, loss-of-function pathogenic variants in *CTRC* do not seem to cause CP but rather are seen in combination with other variants including *CFTR* or *SPINK1* variants.[44–46]

In a recent study of 342 children with RAP and CP, early onset pancreatitis was associated with the presence of an associated germline mutation and family history of pancreatitis. Seventy-one percent (72/102) of patients tested were found to have at least 1 gene mutation (*PRSS1*, *CFTR*, *SPINK1*, and *CTRC*)[49]; *CTRC* mutations were more likely to occur with early onset pancreatitis in 8/56 (14%).[49]

Calcium-Sensing Receptor Gene

The *CASR* gene encodes the calcium-sensing receptor, which is a plasma membrane receptor that regulates intracellular calcium activity based on extracellular calcium levels. It has been suggested that loss of function *CASR* variants associated with *SPINK1* or *CFTR* may affect pancreatic duct cell function, whereas gain of function *CASR* mutations affect acinar cell function and are associated with alcoholic pancreatitis (see **Fig. 1**). The sentinel study to associate *CASR* mutations with CP was in a family of 5 individuals heterozygous for N34S *SPINK1* polymorphisms of which only 2 developed CP[50]; these 2 individuals carried mutations in the *CASR* gene. A subsequent study confirmed the association between *CASR* mutations and CP and evaluated whether *SPINK1* N34S and alcohol were necessary factors for the development of CP in carriers. Although there was no association between the various *CASR* genotypes and *SPINK1* N34S in pancreatitis, the *CASR* R990G polymorphism was significantly associated with CP with odds ratio (OR) of 2.0, and a stronger association was noted in subjects who reported moderate or heavy alcohol consumption (OR = 3.12).

Carboxypeptidase A1 Gene

The *CPA1* gene maps to 7q32 and encodes for carboxypeptidase A1, which is an abundant pancreatic enzyme second to trypsinogen. The mechanism by which

CPA1 predisposes to CP does not involve trypsin degradation pathway but rather stems from endoplasmic reticulum (ER) stress; pathogenic mutations diminish secretion through protein misfolding and aggregation, thereby causing ER stress.

The novel relationship between the *CPA1* gene and early onset CP was described in 2013 in a case-control study, which analyzed the presence of *CPA1* alterations in a German cohort of 944 patients with nonalcohol-related CP and 3938 German controls. *CPA1* variants with less than 20% functionality were significantly overrepresented in the CP group (29/944, 3.1%) compared with controls (5/3938, 0.1%; OR = 25). Patients exhibiting a defective *CPA1* variant were younger than those without a gene mutation; individuals carrying a nonfunctional *CPA1* variant had an increased risk of pancreatitis by 38-fold and 84-fold when diagnosed younger than 20 years old and 10 years old, respectively.[51] The association between *CPA1* mutations and nonalcoholic CP has been reported in additional cohorts from Europe, India, and Japan, thereby establishing its global role in CP pathogenesis.[52]

Claudin-2 Gene

The *CLDN2* gene encodes claudin-2, which is expressed in the proximal pancreatic duct and facilitates water and sodium transport to counter chloride and bicarbonate secretion through CFTR.[53] Expression of claudin-2 is upregulated during periods of inflammation. Results from the first genome-wide association study to investigate pancreatitis found a high-risk locus near *CLDN2* on the X chromosome that is associated with atypical localization of claudin-2 in pancreatic acinar cells. This gene has been linked to alcohol-related CP as opposed to RAP. The high-risk gene variant confers an increased risk of pancreatitis secondary to alcohol in men compared with women where nearly half of all men with alcoholic pancreatitis are carriers of this specific variant.[53–55] This association has been confirmed by recent studies in Europe, Japan, and India.

RISK OF PANCREATIC CANCER

The highest risk of pancreatic cancer is reported with HP where the cumulative risk of pancreatic cancer by age 70 years is up to 53-fold greater than the general population.[56,57] Among gene mutation carriers with HP, the incidence of pancreatic cancer increases following a 20 to 40 year history of CP and markedly increases after 50 years old (**Fig. 2**).[56,58,59] A higher incidence with an earlier age of onset is related to a prior smoking history.[17] Based on an expert consensus, pancreatic cancer surveillance has been recommended for individuals with a 5-fold increased relative risk of pancreatic cancer compared with the general population[57,60–62] in order to detect early pancreatic lesions that can be surgically intervened on. However, the challenge with surveillance of patients with HP for pancreatic cancer is the gross distortion of the pancreatic architecture by CP.[59] In turn, a potential consideration for select individuals with HP is total pancreatectomy with or without islet autotransplantation (TP-IAT).[59,63,64]

Genetic Testing and the Diagnosis of Hereditary Pancreatitis

Genetic risk assessment for HP involves a detailed review of the individual's medical history of pancreatitis and related clinical manifestations, radiographic imaging or diagnostic endoscopic procedures for evidence of AP or CP, and a comprehensive family history of pancreatic disease and cancer. Germline testing for the most common etiologic mutations associated with pancreatitis includes evaluation for pathogenic variants in the *PRSS1, CFTR, SPINK1, and CTRC* genes in symptomatic individuals.

Current guidelines related to genetic testing for HP were developed based on expert consensus and are recommended in adults with pancreatitis who meet one or more of the following criteria[60,65]:

- RAP or CP of uncertain cause
- Early age onset of idiopathic CP when younger than 25 years old
- Unexplained pancreatitis as a child
- Family history of idiopathic CP, RAP, or childhood pancreatitis involving FDR or SDR
- At-risk family members of individuals with an identified pathogenic gene mutation associated with HP
- Patients eligible for participation in approved research protocols

It is recommended that genetic testing be performed with pretest evaluation by a certified genetic counselor or an experienced health care provider who can provide appropriate information related to the appropriateness of genetic testing and education related to inheritable risk. Pretest counseling ensures that patients understand the benefits, limitations, and implications of testing. Posttest counseling is of equal importance for the interpretation and disclosure of genetic testing results and implications and recommendations for the tested individual and any at-risk family members. Genetic testing is useful not only to help make a diagnosis but also to anticipate and manage complications of CP. When patients are identified early in the time course of the disease, they are advised to reduce additional risk factors that may accelerate the progression to CP. This includes alcohol and smoking cessation because the genes are modified by these additional environmental risk factors and increase an individual's susceptibility to pancreatitis.

Genetic testing in asymptomatic individuals is currently limited to at-risk family members of individuals with an identified pathogenic gene mutation associated with HP. The decision to test asymptomatic patients younger than 16 years should be individualized and can be considered in a symptomatic child who has met any of the following criteria[65]:

- An unexplained episode of pancreatitis requiring hospitalization
- Two or more unexplained episodes of pancreatitis
- An episode of pancreatitis occurring in a child who has a relative with an HP mutation
- Unexplained CP

There is ample support to extend the assessment of genetic risk for HP beyond the pediatric cases of pancreatitis because adult-onset RAP and CP is often multifactorial in cause and includes gene–environment and gene–gene interactions. In a study to assess the frequency of germline mutations among 197 cases of RAP and idiopathic CP, 58% of individuals with RAP had identifiable genetic variants as did 27% with idiopathic pancreatitis.[41] In addition, 63% of patients with unexplained first episode of acute pancreatitis before age 35 years also had identifiable genetic variants. This evidence may support extending genetic evaluation to individuals with CP diagnosed before 35 years as opposed to 25 years, which is currently recommended.

Lack of family history of pancreatitis should not preclude genetic evaluation and clinical testing because the penetrance of non-*PRSS1* genes is variable within families. In the same study, family history of pancreatitis was not associated with identifiable genetic variants due to possible risk factor exposure of FDRs.[41] However, additional studies have demonstrated that with an extensive family history that includes 2 or more FDRs or 3 or more SDRs over 2 generations, genetic testing may be useful.

Clinical and Surgical Management of Gene Mutation Carriers

Once the diagnosis of HP has been made through predictive genetic testing, treatment should be tailored to each patient's particular needs. Lifestyle modifications, including smoking and alcohol cessation, are recommended for all identified mutation carriers and may improve outcomes in symptomatic individuals. However, no specific treatment exists and can be proposed to individuals with HP. Management of symptoms, in particular chronic pain, can be optimized by a multidisciplinary approach by health care providers, in addition to screening for and treatment of pancreatic exocrine and endocrine insufficiencies. The response to medical, endoscopic, and/or surgical treatment may differ between carriers and noncarriers of pancreatitis-related germline mutations, and clinical management needs to be individualized.

A consideration for select carriers of germline mutations associated with HP is TP-IAT. With the advent of total pancreatectomy for pain management caused by the CP, and auto islet cell transplantation to simultaneously reduce the severity of the pancreatectomy-induced diabetes, this surgical approach may be considered in the management of patients with HP and advanced disease. Performing islet auto transplantation before the pancreas is irreparably fibrosed may offer preserved glycemic control and better quality of life after total pancreatectomy. In addition, total pancreatectomy can potentially eliminate the increased risk of pancreatic cancer development in those with pathogenic gene alterations related to pancreatitis and advanced disease.[59,64,66]

However, strict selection criteria and an interdisciplinary management team are crucial in the consideration of TP-IAT because this surgery carries lifetime health consequences. The long-term outcomes of TP-IAT for CP due to hereditary and gene-associated pancreatitis were reported in a review of a prospectively collected database of 484 TP-IAT subjects from 1977 to 2012 at a single US center.[66] The outcomes of pain relief, narcotic use, and β cell function in patients who received TP-IAT for hereditary/genetic causes (*PRSS1* [n = 38], *SPINK1* [n = 9], *CFTR* [n = 14], and familial [n = 19]) were evaluated and compared with those without a recognized genetic predisposition. The cohort with hereditary/genetic pancreatitis was significantly younger and despite having a shorter duration of years with pancreatitis, had a higher pancreas fibrosis score compared with the nonhereditary cases. All 80 individuals with a genetic predisposition were narcotic dependent and had failed all attempts at endoscopic and direct pancreatic surgery before TP-IAT. Following TP-IAT, 90% of these patients reported no pancreatic pain and had sustained pain relief for the 10-year follow-up, and more than 65% had either partial or complete β cell function. With respect to gene-specific outcomes, the duration of pancreatitis and the severity of pancreas fibrosis resulted in a higher degree of islet function loss in *PRSS1* and *CFTR* carriers but not *SPINK1* carriers. Important considerations in achieving the most favorable outcomes related to TP-IAT were related to the duration of increased pancreatic fibrosis and prior surgical procedures. The increased fibrosis by the time patients receive TP-IAT in the cohort resulted in a lower islet yield and lower percent of patients becoming insulin independent. In addition, previous surgical procedures, in particular the Puestow procedure, resulted in statistically lower islet cell yield and insulin dependence in long-term follow-up.

SUMMARY

Genetic risk assessment for individuals with suspected hereditary and familial pancreatitis provides an opportunity to discover a causative cause for disease. Early identification of HP, through genetic evaluation and testing, and proper management in gene mutation carriers requires a multidisciplinary approach in order to be complete and most effective. Continued advances in genomic technologies with complete genotyping can establish additional associations between complex genetic causes and environment interactions, which may provide personalized management and preventive strategies for pancreatitis in the future.

REFERENCES

1. LaRusch J, Solomon S, Whitcomb DC. Pancreatitis Overview. In: Adam MP, Ardinger HH, Pagon RA, et al, editors. GeneReviews® [Internet]. Seattle (WA): University of Washington, Seattle; 1993–2018.
2. Howes N, Lerch MM, Greenhalf W, et al. Clinical and genetic characteristics of hereditary pancreatitis in Europe. Clin Gastroenterol Hepatol 2004;2(3):252–61.
3. Whitcomb DC. Mechanisms of disease: advances in understanding the mechanisms leading to chronic pancreatitis. Nat Clin Pract Gastroenterol Hepatol 2004;1(1):46–52.
4. Whitcomb DC. Genetic risk factors for pancreatic disorders. Gastroenterology 2013;144(6):1292–302.
5. Shelton CA, Whitcomb DC. Hereditary pancreatitis. pancreapedia: the exocrine pancreas knowledge base. Available at: https://www.pancreapedia.org/reviews/hereditary-pancreatitis. Accessed May 30, 2018.
6. Solomon S, Whitcomb DC. Genetics of pancreatitis: an update for clinicians and genetic counselors. Curr Gastroenterol Rep 2012;14:112–7.
7. Comfort MW, Steinberg AG. Pedigree of a family with hereditary chronic relapsing pancreatitis. Gastroenterology 1952;21(1):54–63.
8. Whitcomb DC, Gorry MC, Preston RA, et al. Hereditary pancreatitis is caused by a mutation in the cationic trypsinogen gene. Nat Genet 1996;14(2):141–5.
9. Gorry MC, Gabbaizedeh D, Furey W, et al. Mutations in the cationic trypsinogen gene are associated with recurrent acute and chronic pancreatitis. Gastroenterology 1997;113:1063–8.
10. Whitcomb DC, Preston RA, Aston CE, et al. A gene for hereditary pancreatitis maps to chromosome 7q35. Gastroenterology 1996;110:1975.
11. Zator Z, Whitcomb DC. Insights into the genetic risk factors for the development of pancreatic disease. Therap Adv Gastroenterol 2017;10(3):323–36.
12. Whitcomb DC. Value of genetic testing in the management of pancreatitis. Gut 2004;53(11):1710–7.
13. Etemad B, Whitcomb DC. Chronic pancreatitis: diagnosis, classification, and new genetic developments. Gastroenterology 2001;120(3):682–707.
14. Nemeth BC, Sahin-Toth M. Human cationic trypsinogen (PRSS1) variants and chronic pancreatitis. Am J Physiol Gastrointest Liver Physiol 2014;306(6):466–73.
15. Hegyi E, Sahin-Tóth M. Genetic risk in chronic pancreatitis: the trypsin-dependent pathway. Dig Dis Sci 2017;62(7):1692–701.
16. Whitcomb DC. Genetic aspects of pancreatitis. Annu Rev Med 2010;61:413–24.
17. Rebours V, Boutron-Ruault MC, Schnee M, et al. The natural history of hereditary pancreatitis: a national series. Gut 2009;58(1):97–103.
18. Joergensen MT, Brusgaard K, Cruger DG, et al. Genetic, epidemiological, and clinical aspects of hereditary pancreatitis: a population-based cohort study in Denmark. Am J Gastroenterol 2010;105(8):1876–83.
19. Teich N, Rosendahl J, Tóth M, et al. Mutations of human cationic trypsinogen (PRSS1) and chronic pancreatitis. Hum Mutat 2006;27(8):721–30.
20. Sossenheimer MJ, Aston CE, Preston RA, et al. Clinical characteristics of hereditary pancreatitis in a large family, based on high-risk haplotype. The midwest

multicenter pancreatic study groups (MMPSG). Am J Gastroenterol 1997;92: 1113.

21. Rebours V, Levy P, Ruszniewski P. An overview of hereditary pancreatitis. Dig Liver Dis 2012;44(1):8–15.

22. Witt H, Luck W, Hennies HC, et al. Mutations in the gene encoding the serine protease inhibitor, Kazal type 1 are associated with chronic pancreatitis. Nat Genet 2000;25(2):213–6.

23. Raphael KL, Willingham FF. Hereditary pancreatitis: current perspectives. Clin Exp Gastroenterol 2016;9:197–207.

24. Whitcomb DC. How to think about SPINK and pancreatitis. Am J Gastroenterol 2002;97(5):1085–8.

25. Fink EN, Kant JA, Whitcomb DC. Genetic counseling for nonsyndromic pancreatitis. Gastroenterol Clin North Am 2007;36:325–33.

26. Pfützer RH, Barmada MM, Brunskill AP, et al. SPINK1/PSTI polymorphisms act as disease modifiers in familial and idiopathic chronic pancreatitis. Gastroenterology 2000;119(3):615–23.

27. Joergensen MT, Brusgaard K, Novovic S, et al. Is the SPINK1 variant p.N34S overrepresented in patients with acute pancreatitis? Eur J Gastroenterol Hepatol 2012;24(3):309–15.

28. Threadgold J, Greenhalf W, Ellis I, et al. The N34S mutation of SPINK1 (PSTI) is associated with a familial pattern of idiopathic chronic pancreatitis but does not cause the disease. Gut 2002;50(5):675–81.

29. Schneider A, Barmada MM, Slivka A, et al. Clinical characterization of patients with idiopathic chronic pancreatitis and SPINK1 mutations. Scand J Gastroenterol 2004;39(9):903–4.

30. Shimosegawa T, Kume K, Masamune ASPINK. ADH2, and ALDH2 gene variants and alcoholic chronic pancreatitis in Japan. J Gastroenterol Hepatol 2008; 23(Suppl 1):S82.

31. Schneider A, Larusch J, Sun X, et al. Combined bicarbonate conductance-impairing variants in CFTR and SPINK1 variants are associated with chronic pancreatitis in patients without cystic fibrosis. Gastroenterology 2011;140(1): 162–71.

32. Tukiainen E, Kylanpaa ML, Kemppainen E, et al. Pancreatic secretory trypsin inhibitor (SPINK1) gene mutations in patients with acute pancreatitis. Pancreas 2005;30(3):239–42.

33. Zielenski J. Genotype and phenotype in cystic fibrosis. Respiration 2000;67(2): 117–33.

34. Rowntree RK, Harris A. The phenotypic consequences of CFTR mutations. Ann Hum Genet 2003;67:471–85.

35. Cohn JA, Friedman KJ, Noone PG, et al. Relation between mutations of the cystic fibrosis gene and idiopathic pancreatitis. N Engl J Med 1998;339:653–8.

36. Cohn JA, Neoptolemos JP, Feng J, et al. Increased risk of idiopathic chronic pancreatitis in cystic fibrosis carriers. Hum Mutat 2005;26:303–7.

37. Sharer N, Schwarz M, Malone G, et al. Mutations of the cystic fibrosis gene in patients with chronic pancreatitis. N Engl J Med 1998;339(10):645–52.

38. Weiss FU, Simon P, Bogdanova N, et al. Complete cystic fibrosis transmembrane conductance regulator gene sequencing in patients with idiopathic chronic pancreatitis and controls. Gut 2005;54(10):1456–60.

39. Choudari CP, Imperiale TF, Sherman S, et al. Risk of pancreatitis with mutation of the cystic fibrosis gene. Am J Gastroenterol 2004;99(7):1358–63.

40. Castellani C, Bonizzato A, Rolfini R, et al. Increased prevalence of mutations of the cystic fibrosis gene in idiopathic chronic and recurrent pancreatitis. Am J Gastroenterol 1999;94(7):1993–5.
41. Jalaly NY, Moran RA, Fargahi F, et al. An evaluation of factors associated with pathogenic PRSS1, SPINK1, CTFR, and/or CTRC genetic variants in patients with idiopathic pancreatitis. Am J Gastroenterol 2017;112(8):1320–9.
42. Gelrud A, Sheth S, Banerjee S, et al. Analysis of cystic fibrosis gene product function in patients with pancreas divisum and recurrent acute pancreatitis. Am J Gastroenterol 2004;99:1557–62.
43. Bertin C, Pelletier AL, Vullierme MP, et al. Pancreas divisum is not a cause of pancreatitis by itself but acts as a partner of genetic mutations. Am J Gastroenterol 2012;107:311–7.
44. Rosendahl J, Landt O, Bernadova J, et al. CFTR, SPINK1, CTRC, and PRSS1 variants in chronic pancreatitis: is the role of mutated CFTR overestimated? Gut 2013;62:582–92.
45. Masson E, Chen JM, Scotet V, et al. Association of rare chymotrypsinogen C (CTRC) gene variations in patients with idiopathic chronic pancreatitis. Hum Genet 2008;123(1):83–91.
46. Rosendahl J, Witt H, Szmola R, et al. Chymotrypsin C (CTRC) variants that diminish activity or secretion are associated with chronic pancreatitis. Nat Genet 2008;40(1):78–82.
47. Beer S, Zhou J, Szabo A, et al. Comprehensive functional analysis of chymotrypsin C (CTRC) variants reveals distinct loss-of-function mechanisms associated with pancreatitis risk. Gut 2013;62(11):1616–24.
48. LaRusch J, Lozano-Leon A, Stello K, et al. The common chymotrypsinogen C (CTRC) variant G60G (C.180T) increases risk of chronic pancreatitis but not recurrent acute pancreatitis in a North American population. Clin Transl Gastroenterol 2015;6:e68.
49. Giefer MJ, Lowe ME, Werlin SL, et al. Early-onset acute recurrent and chronic pancreatitis is associated with PRSS1 or CTRC gene mutations. J Pediatr 2017; 186:95–100.
50. Felderbauer P, Hoffmann P, Einwachter H, et al. A novel mutation of the calcium sensing receptor gene is associated with chronic pancreatitis in a family with heterozygous SPINK1 mutations. BMC Gastroenterol 2003;3:34.
51. Witt H, Beer S, Rosendahl J, et al. Variants in CPA1 are strongly associated with early onset chronic pancreatitis. Nat Genet 2013;45(10):1216–20.
52. Saito N, Suzuki M, Sakurai Y, et al. Genetic analysis of Japanese children with acute recurrent and chronic pancreatitis. J Pediatr Gastroenterol Nutr 2016; 63(4):431–6.
53. Whitcomb DC, LaRusch J, Krasinskas AM, et al. Common genetic variants in the CLDN2 and PRSS1-PRSS2 loci alter risk for alcohol-related and sporadic pancreatitis. Nat Genet 2012;44(12):1349–54.
54. Derikx MH, Kovacs P, Scholz M, et al. Polymorphisms at PRSS1-PRSS2 and CLDN2-MORC4 loci associate with alcoholic and non-alcoholic chronic pancreatitis in a European replication study. Gut 2015;64(9):1426–33.
55. Masamune A, Nakano E, Hamada S, et al. Common variants at PRSS1-PRSS2 and CLDN2-MORC4 loci associate with chronic pancreatitis in Japan. Gut 2015;64(8):1345–6.
56. Lowenfels AB, Maisonneuve P, DiMagno EP, et al. Hereditary pancreatitis and the risk of pancreatic cancer. International hereditary pancreatitis study group. J Natl Cancer Inst 1997;89:442–6.

57. Syngal S, Brand RE, Church JM, et al. ACG clinical guideline: genetic testing and management of hereditary gastrointestinal cancer syndromes. Am J Gastroenterol 2015;110(2):223–63.
58. Rebours V, Boutron-Ruault M, Jooste V, et al. Mortality rate and risk factors in patients with hereditary pancreatitis: uni- and multidimensional analyses. Am J Gastroenterol 2009;104:2312–7.
59. Solomon S, Siddhartha D, Brand R, et al. Inherited pancreatic cancer syndromes. Cancer J 2012;18(6):485–91.
60. Brand RE, Lerch MM, Rubinstein WS, et al. Advances in counselling and surveillance of patients at risk for pancreatic cancer. Gut 2007;56:1460–9.
61. Canto MI, Harinck F, Hruban RH, et al. International cancer of the pancreas screening (CAPS) consortium summit on the management of patients with increased risk for familial pancreatic cancer. Gut 2013;62:339–47.
62. Bartsch DK, Gress TM, Langer P. Familial pancreatic cancer—current knowledge. Nat Rev Gastroenterol Hepatol 2012;9:445–53.
63. Ulrich CD, Consensus Committees of the European Registry of Hereditary Pancreatic Diseases, Midwest Multi-Center Pancreatic Study Group, et al. Pancreatic cancer in hereditary pancreatitis – Consensus guidelines for prevention, screening, and treatment. Pancreatology 2001;1:416–22.
64. Sutton JM, Schmulewitz N, Sussman JJ, et al. Total pancreatectomy and islet cell autotransplantation as a means of treating patients with genetically linked pancreatitis. Surgery 2010;148:676–85.
65. Ellis I, Lerch MM, Whitcomb DC. Genetic testing for hereditary pancreatitis: guidelines for indications, counselling, consent and privacy issues. Pancreatology 2001;1(5):405–15.
66. Chinnakotla S, Radosevich DM, Dunn TB, et al. Long term outcomes of total pancreatectomy and islet auto transplantation for hereditary/genetic pancreatitis. J Am Coll Surg 2014;218(4):530–43.

Total Pancreatectomy with Autologous Islet Cell Transplantation

Beth Schrope, MD, PhD

KEYWORDS

- Chronic pancreatitis • Autologous islet cell transplantation • Type 3c diabetes
- Islet isolation

KEY POINTS

- Total or near-total pancreatectomy is a viable treatment option for patients with end-stage chronic pancreatitis but carries with it the inevitability of insulin-dependent diabetes mellitus.
- The adjunct of autologous islet cell transplantation offers the potential for mitigation or even complete avoidance of insulin use, for a time.
- This highly specialized procedure is performed only in select centers world-wide.
- Both islet isolation and perioperative management require attention to numerous specific details and protocols.
- Further research to optimize islet yield, survival, and function is ongoing, including search for ideal implantation site as well as process tweaks and adjunctive medications.

INTRODUCTION

After decades of research, Najarian and colleagues[1] published the first series of successful autologous human islet cell transplantation for chronic pancreatitis in 1980. Since that time the technique has been sparsely applied due to the complexity of the patient population, surgical techniques, and islet isolation. Yet, despite many nuances and technical considerations, thousands of patients worldwide have successfully undergone this procedure.

Treating severe chronic pancreatitis with total pancreatectomy carries the promise of improved quality of life, with the trade-off of brittle or type 3c diabetes (marked by the paucity or absence of not only insulin but also of the counterregulatory hormone glucagon). Isolation and reimplantation of pancreatic islet cells from the resected specimen offers the hope for relief from diabetes, if not complete then partial, if not

No disclosures.
Department of Surgery, Columbia University College of Physicians and Surgeons, 161 Fort Washington Avenue, 8th Floor, New York, NY 10032, USA
E-mail address: bs170@cumc.columbia.edu

Gastrointest Endoscopy Clin N Am 28 (2018) 605–618
https://doi.org/10.1016/j.giec.2018.05.003
1052-5157/18/© 2018 Elsevier Inc. All rights reserved.

lifelong then for a period of time. In this treatise the author describes the indications for the procedure, including classic and expanded. Particular surgical considerations as well as details of islet isolation are reviewed. Results for both the primary indication of symptom relief as well as the secondary measure of insulin production are summarized. Finally, current considerations and research as well as future directions are identified.

INDICATIONS

Autologous islet cell transplantation was initially conceived as an adjunct to total pancreatectomy for chronic pancreatitis, which can be an unrelenting, progressive disease, one for which the trade-off of brittle diabetes is worth the cost for patients in the end stages. These patients face significant detriment in quality of life, with chronic or recurrent severe pain and nausea, frequent hospitalizations, inability to work or be an otherwise productive member of society, and often opiate dependence.

In certain circumstances, where maximal medical and endoscopic therapies have become ineffective at symptom control, surgical intervention becomes indicated. Choice of surgery depends on several factors, including anatomic features of the pancreas. For example, a fibrotic pancreas with an enlarged duct may benefit from a surgical drainage procedure, or one with a dominant inflammatory mass may benefit from a partial resection, or some combination of both. Yet not infrequently the gland seems "normal", or diffusely fatty, without the above-mentioned characteristics. Patients with these glands may be particularly helped by a total pancreatectomy.

Causes for chronic pancreatitis vary, with the most frequent being alcohol use and cholelithiasis. Less common causes include hereditary pancreatitis (characterized by specific mutations in the PRSS1, CFTR, SPINK, or CTRC genes), autoimmune pancreatitis, hypertriglyceridemia, congenital ductal anomalies, and medication-related, to name a few; all too often (20%–30%) an identifiable cause is never found, and we are left with the ubiquitous "idiopathic" moniker. Although ultimately any given patient regardless of cause may proceed to total pancreatectomy, cause affects expectations for islet yield and procedural "success."

Sporadic publication of expanded indications is noted in the literature. Because chronic pancreatitis is generally a benign disease (although does carry the harbinger of increased risk of malignant transformation over a patient's lifetime), it is comfortable to reimplant islets with concomitant and unavoidable acinar debris back into the patient. Other conditions of the pancreas may merit consideration of islet autotransplantation, including intraductal papillary mucinous neoplasms and even possibly carcinoma, although currently not enough data are available for the widespread recommendation in these circumstances.

PATIENT SELECTION

TPAIT is a radical, "last-resort" treatment for end-stage chronic pancreatitis. As stated earlier, patients should generally have been through the gamut of symptom management strategies, including dietary management, medications (opiates, nonsteroidal antiinflammatory drugs, neuropathic medications, muscle relaxants), chemical neurolysis, endoscopic retrograde cholangiopancreatography, and regional pain relief therapies (spinal cord stimulator or intrathecal drug delivery devices). Once most of these options have failed, surgery can be considered. Possible leniency of this requirement is applied to cases of hereditary pancreatitis (particularly PRSS1 mutation) where a real risk of malignant transformation exists.

Absolute contraindications are prohibitive medical comorbidities, islet cell failure as evidenced by poorly controlled insulin-dependent diabetes (or poor response to stimulated C-peptide testing), steatohepatitis, or portal vein thrombosis. Caution should be exercised in patients on high-dose opiate medications or those in whom weak evidence of pancreatitis is found as the cause of their "visceral hyperalgesia." The former, even if radiographic or other evidence of pancreatitis is definitive, often have extreme difficulty weaning off opiates once the pancreas has been removed. **Box 1** is provided for guidance in patient selection.

Because TPAIT centers are few and far between and attract patients from considerable distances at times, local relationships with a pain management provider and an endocrinologist should be in place before embarking on a surgical journey. Finally, a reasonable social support network is required to assist in the successful recovery and return to productive lives for these patients.

PROCEDURE

In the most basic sense this procedure involves the removal of the entire (or a portion of) host (patient) pancreas, followed by isolation of the islets in solution, and then reintroduction of the islet product into the host tissue. Clearly, however, this is an extraordinarily complex process with many moving parts. Each element will be described in detail henceforth.

Pancreatectomy

Classically a total pancreatectomy, or removal of the entire gland, is preferred, yet there are variations dictated both by surgeon preference and individual patient anatomy. A conventional, en bloc total pancreatectomy entails removal of all pancreatic tissue, the duodenum, the pylorus, and the spleen. Various parenchymal and organ sparing approaches have been proposed and practiced, including duodenum-sparing pancreatectomy, pylorus-sparing pancreatectomy, and spleen-preserving

---

Box 1
Patient selection criteria and contraindications for TPAIT

Patient selection criteria

- Proven diagnosis of chronic pancreatitis or acute relapsing pancreatitis (cross-sectional imaging, Rosemont criteria by EUS, genetics)

- Failure of maximal medical and endoscopic therapy to control symptoms

- Adequate glycemic function on preoperative C-peptide stimulation testing

- Reasonable social and financial support

- Established relationship with pain management provider and endocrinologist

Absolute contraindications

- Active alcoholism

- Beta cell failure (poor or no C-peptide on provocative testing)

- Poorly controlled psychiatric disease

Relative contraindications

- Insulin use

Abbreviation: EUS, endoscopic ultrasound.

pancreatectomy. These ambitions, although admirable, are likely to offer a mostly theoretic advantage.

Literature on pylorus-sparing pancreaticoduodenectomy versus limited distal gastric resection is mixed. Maintaining the pylorus has the theoretic advantage of preventing bile reflux gastritis and complications such as peptic ulcers. Yet, it has been estimated that up to one-third of normal subjects do not have a competent pylorus, and in most cases of peptic ulceration duodenogastric reflux is not present.[2] What has been shown in many series of pancreaticoduodenectomy is that pylorus-sparing procedures have a higher incidence of delayed-gastric emptying, longer average duration of hospitalization, and poorer nutrition at 1 month postoperatively.[3]

Sparing the duodenum for benign disease is of course a valid endeavor, and indeed European surgeons use duodenum-preserving pancreatic head resections with equivalent results in terms of pain relief and pancreatic enzyme use, with decreased intraoperative blood loss and operating times when compared with pancreaticoduodenectomy.[4] However, the advantage of the duodenum-preserving technique cannot necessarily be extrapolated to total pancreatectomy; indeed, the most prolific group in TPAIT (University of Minnesota) had altered their practice to remove at least a portion of the duodenum due to a higher incidence of postoperative complications.[5]

In the case of elective splenectomy where recommended vaccinations can be administered preoperatively, incidence of postsplenectomy infectious complications is uncommon, up to 5% lifetime risk (calculated with any variety of vaccine regimens). This may be decreased further with patient education and proper antibiotic prophylaxis.[6] Indeed, preserving the spleen with sacrifice of the main splenic artery and vein thus relying on the short gastric vascular bundles ("Warshaw" technique) can lead to late complications such as gastric varices, risking hemorrhage and pain from splenomegaly.

Partial pancreatectomy for chronic pancreatitis may also be appropriate, where a discrete anatomic abnormality can be identified, or in the case of near-total pancreatectomy (Child procedure), where a sliver of pancreatic tissue is retained along the duodenum. In the former case one might question the added complexity and risk of islet autotransplantation when in fact in situ islets are retained, although certain scenarios may lend themselves to this proposal. For example, a pancreatic head resection to treat an inflammatory mass in the head of the gland may be proposed, with the uncertainty that chronic inflammation in the remaining gland may lead to ongoing pain. In this case, autologous islet transplantation might be considered a method of "banking" the islets in the best possible state (easily achievable postoperative normoglycemia due to the "native" islets), should symptoms persist after recovery and completion pancreatectomy become necessary. Certainly a patient who had undergone partial pancreatectomy (without islet transplantation) and now requires completion pancreatectomy for ongoing symptoms may be considered for islet transplantation, if only to mitigate (not eliminate) insulin requirements after surgery. Because the mechanism for pain in end-stage chronic pancreatitis is poorly understood, if one assumes all pancreas tissue is affected and potentially responsible for symptoms (on a histologic level, perhaps), one can argue that a total pancreatectomy is required, until data for comparison are available or mechanisms of pain are understood.

Regardless of the extent of resection, unlike a typical pancreatectomy without plans for islet autotransplantation, the surgeon must maintain organ perfusion throughout mobilization of the gland and surrounding organs to minimize warm ischemic time, which can result in islet cell demise. In the case of a total pancreatectomy, this requires preservation of the splenic artery and gastroduodenal artery until the remainder of the organ is completely mobilized. Although it is not practical to preserve individual branches of the superior mesenteric artery to the uncinate process of the pancreas, this dissection is undertaken last to reduce warm ischemia time in this region.

With the final division of the splenic artery, splenic vein, and gastroduodenal artery, the specimen is passed off sterilely to a back table to an ice bath, where the extraneous tissues including the duodenum, bile duct, splenic artery and vein, and any lymphoid or fatty tissues are carefully removed. The pancreatic duct is cannulated and the organ is flushed with cold preservation solution. It is then transported on ice to the islet isolation facility.

While the islets are being isolated, restoration of biliary and enteric continuity is undertaken. Splenectomy or cholecystectomy may be completed at this time, if not done during mobilization of the pancreas (to deliver the organ to the islet isolation laboratory as early as possible, the author prefers to defer removal of these organs to this time of the operation if at all feasible). At this point, because islet isolation takes longer than surgical reconstruction, the patient may remain in the operating room, under anesthesia, to wait for the islet product to be delivered. This is generally no more than an hour or two, and thus is a reasonable option to proceed. Some surgeons prefer, however, to close the patient at this time with the intent for percutaneous access for islet implantation when the product is ready. Indeed, with the possibility of remote isolation this would be the preferred approach. Both scenarios have comparable results[7,8]; the option of remote isolation is described elsewhere in this article.

Islet Isolation

Pancreatic islet isolation for human transplantation should be performed in a laboratory that is in compliance with Food and Drug Administration good manufacturing practice (GMP) regulations, including maintenance of sterility, rigorous process validation, adequate and thorough process documentation, and other steps to maintain quality assurance. When the pancreas in received in the laboratory for processing, the organ is weighed, and the preservation solution is used to inoculate bacterial and fungal culture bottles. The pancreatic duct is perfused with collagenase for tissue digestion. The resulting pancreatic tissue is cut into small pieces and placed into the digestion chamber. This device was specifically created for semiautomated extraction of human pancreatic islets and consists of 2 compartments separated by a fine mesh screen (280 microns).[9] Stainless steel or glass balls are placed into the lower compartment of the chamber with the pancreatic tissue to facilitate mechanical separation of the islets from the acinar tissue. Additional collagenase solution is placed into the lower compartment. Hank's solution is circulated through the chamber, and the system is heated to 37°C (**Fig. 1**). The chamber is then gently agitated (by hand or with an automated agitator). As islets are liberated from the acinar tissue they float to the top compartment. To assess the extent of tissue digestion, a small sample is periodically removed from the top compartment and stained with dithizone, which chelates the zinc of the insulin granules in beta cells of the pancreatic islets, staining separated islets red (**Fig. 2**). As tissue digestion progresses, more intact islet clusters are separated from the surrounding acinar tissue. These islets are collected from the chamber into a separate collecting flask, which is cooled to preserve the islets. Once no more islets are observed in the sample (~30–60 min), the process is terminated. Our criteria for halting digestion are at least 50% of the 40x field is covered with tissue, there are more than 45 islets, more than 50% free islets, and less than 10% fragmented islets.[10] The collected islets are concentrated by centrifugation. Heparin is added to the isolated islets in order to prevent clumping before reinfusion. The islet cell product is issued from the processing laboratory to the operating room for

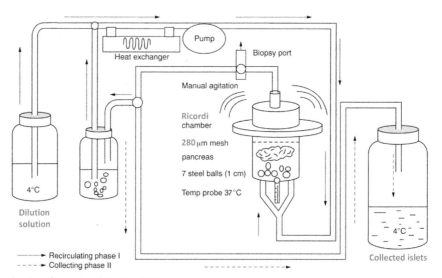

Fig. 1. Schematic of islet isolation apparatus.

reinfusion. Once the product is issued from the processing laboratory, islet yield, purity, and viability are determined. Microbiology testing is also performed on the final product; however final culture results are not available at the time of infusion.

Islet Purity, Quantification, Yield, and Viability

Islet purity is a subjective measure, determined by visual inspection of the dithizone-stained sample and comparing the red-stained (islet) to unstained (acinar) tissue. When large tissue volumes are processed, volume reduction of the product may be desired in order to avoid increased portal pressures during portal vein reinfusion, which may result in loss of islet cells. In this circumstance (ie, if pellet volume is large or >20 mL), islet purification may be performed. The COBE 2991 cell processor (CaridianBCT, Lakewood, CO, USA) is the instrument used for density gradient islet

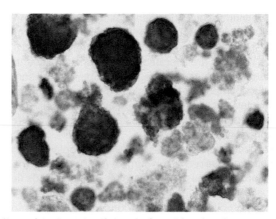

Fig. 2. Hematoxylin and eosin stain of sample from islet chamber. Free islets are dark red; acinar tissue debris is lighter yellow.

purification. The number of individual islets is quantified under the microscope and the diameter of the individual clusters is recorded. The Islet Equivalent (IEQ) is the most commonly used estimate of islet volume.[11] One IEQ represents a typically sized islet (~150 μm in diameter). This scale was introduced to account for variation in islet size and is used by all islet isolation laboratories as a standard convention.[12] The islets cell clusters are enumerated and categorized into groups of 50 μm increments based on their diameters. The numbers of islets in each size group is multiplied by a volume correction factor that allows for the conversion to IEQ. Islet "dose" is expressed as IEQ per kg of recipient weight (IEQ/kg). The viability of the islets is determined by staining with fluorescein diacetate (inclusion dye) and propidium iodide (exclusion dye). An islet score (0–10), which is based on size distribution, fragmentation, density, border, and shape, is assigned to each product.[10]

Islet Implantation

As stated earlier, there are 2 options for islet implantation, in terms of technique: direct access through the open abdomen or percutaneous access in a patient in whom the abdomen has been closed and surgery is complete. The latter is the procedure of choice in cases of remote access where longer delays related to transport are anticipated. Although the search for the perfect implantation site is ongoing, most often the islet product is infused into the portal circulation.

An intravenous bolus of heparin (70 IU/kg up to 5000 IU) is given immediately before infusion to prevent intraportal clotting from tissue thromboplastin present in the islet preparation, and to a lesser extent as prophylaxis for portal venous manipulation. Access to the portal circulation is achieved (direct venotomy, splenic vein cannulation, percutaneous), with means for intermittent pressure measurement in the infusion circuit. Adequate caliber of cannula is necessary to avoid damage to the islets; generally 5 Fr or 16 gauge is sufficient. Too large a cannula may result in islet clumping and the potential for inadequate exposure to passive diffusion for oxygen and nutrients before engraftment. The islet product is gently agitated throughout infusion to avoid clumping in the bag. Baseline and intermittent portal pressure measurements are acquired; in the event of significant portal hypertension (>25 mm Hg) the portal infusion is either suspended and reattempted after a few minutes or ceased. Any remaining islet product is implanted in an alternate site, such as the peritoneal cavity (pelvis) or omentum. Once the islet product is exhausted, the cannula is removed and venous access is closed (primary repair of the venotomy, ligation of splenic vein [when the splenic vein stump was cannulated], or manual pressure [percutaneous access]). If applicable the abdomen is then closed.

Postoperative Considerations

To maximize islet engraftment and function several specific maneuvers are used. First, most surgeons will continue low-dose anticoagulation for 48 to 72 hours postoperatively, for goal-activated partial thromboplastin time 1.5 to 2.0 × normal, both for postportal manipulation thrombotic prophylaxis as well as to mitigate the effects of instant blood-mediated inflammatory reaction (IBMIR). The author screens for large vessel portal venous thrombosis with transabdominal ultrasound on postoperative day #3, and if negative, heparin infusion is discontinued and standard subcutaneous venous thromboembolism prophylaxis is instituted.

Many studies have been undertaken on animal models that reveal the exquisite sensitivity of transplanted islet grafts to hyperglycemia.[13-16] It has been observed that islets exposed to hyperglycemic conditions experience a greater rate of apoptosis, and the remaining islets are resistant to glucose-activated insulin release.

Following the model of the University of Minnesota group (personal communication, David Sutherland, MD, 2008) and others, the author follows protocols to maintain strict glucose control in the 80 to 110 mg/dL, typically with an insulin drip while oral feeding is suboptimal and unpredictable (7 days), with transition to long-acting daily insulin with short-acting coverage as appropriate.

Finally, because many patients with chronic pancreatitis have undergone prior endoscopic manipulations of their pancreatic duct, the organ is frequently colonized with bacteria. Premanipulation and postmanipulation Gram stains are sometimes positive. Because final bacterial culture results may take several days, the author prefers to continue antibiotic prophylaxis for up to 7 days postop, with a drug active against usual gut flora.

RESULTS

It cannot be stated enough that the primary goal of TPAIT is treatment of end-stage chronic pancreatitis, where the major debilitating symptom is pain, and the aspiration for insulin production with autologous islet cell transplantation is secondary. Overall, specific goals for TPAIT include pain relief with reduction in pain medications, beta cell function, and improved quality of life.

With regard to narcotic independence after TPAIT, reported results are highly variable and likely are heavily influenced by patient selection (and reported follow-up). Patients with hereditary pancreatitis are more likely to achieve durable narcotic independence,[17] with 90% of the 80 patients in this series declared pancreas pain free with sustained pain relief. On the contrary, Dunderdale and colleagues[18] reported no improvement in pain scores and no improvement in quality of life postoperatively in patients with alcoholic pancreatitis compared with nonalcoholic pancreatitis. These patients also had much poorer islet cell harvest and function, with none of them achieving meaningful benefit from autologous islet cell transplantation. A recent meta-analysis revealed that for nearly all patients, intensive narcotic use decreases after procedure, with 23% to 82% achieving complete narcotic independence.[19] In the remainder, the inability to fully wean from narcotics has been attributed to opiate-induced hyperalgesia, neurologic central sensitization, gastrointestinal dysmotility, and/or chronic postsurgical pain.

Postoperative glycemic function is correlated well with islet yield, with stratification most commonly presented as less than 2500 IE/kg, 2500 to 5000 IE/kg, and greater than 5000 IE/kg. However, insulin independence is not guaranteed even with maximum IE retrieval. According to the University of Minnesota experience, TPAIT has been successful in preventing brittle diabetes in most patients undergoing this procedure with up to 71% of patients in the recent era (2001–2007, n = 106) demonstrating either full islet function (ie, insulin independence, 33%) or partial islet function (euglycemia on once-daily long-acting insulin, 32%) at 1 year posttransplant. Durability was also demonstrated in those who displayed islet function, with rates of 85%, 68%, and 57% continued function at 2, 5, and 10 years, respectively.[20] A more recent meta-analysis of TPAIT[21] selected 35 single-center studies and reported complete insulin independence ranging from 0% to 83% for total pancreatectomy; no data on C-peptide production (indicating at least partial response) were presented.

SPECIAL CONSIDERATIONS AND FUTURE DIRECTIONS
Expanded Access

With reasonable results in the right patient population, enthusiasm is increasing for TPAIT to expand beyond certain populations and even certain geographic areas.

Remote processing

Islet cell isolation is a complex process, requiring specific expertise, equipment, and facilities, and is thus a limiting factor in delivery of the technique to patients. Recently several centers have published successful islet transplantation (allogeneic and autologous) using remote isolation laboratories, where the pancreatectomy is performed in one location and the islet isolation is performed in another.[7,22–24] The islet transplantation is then done after surgery is complete (in cases of autologous transplantation), via percutaneous technique. These studies have shown comparable results in terms of insulin independence, with perhaps a slight advantage of the local isolation group in terms of C peptide production. Transport cost and time were analyzed and found not to be prohibitive.

Alternative applications

As expertise with TPAIT accumulates, other applications beyond treatment of adult chronic pancreatitis are being considered. These include forays into the pediatric population, and for certain premalignant conditions. Also, very few select cases of autologous islet cell transplantation for malignancy have been described.

Experience in using this technique for children is growing. In a recent review of 75 patients for more than 2 decades, general pain relief is better and islet yield and glycemic function are better than that seen in the adult population.[25] Ninety percent achieved sustained pain relief and 41.3% achieved insulin independence. As with adults total number of islet equivalents per kilogram body weight was the most predictive factor of insulin independence. A meta-analysis of the results of 4 centers worldwide mirrored the generally favorable results, albeit in the short term.[26] These investigators do caution careful selection by a multidisciplinary team and restriction to highly specialized centers with pediatric expertise.

Cases of transplantation of islets from remnant pancreas after known cancer resection have been described. Liu and colleagues reported a case where pancreaticoduodenectomy was performed for pancreatic adenocarcinoma of the head of the pancreas; the procedure was complicated by uncontrolled leak at the pancreaticojejunostomy that was salvaged with completion pancreatectomy and islet autotransplantation. He survived this procedure but ultimately succumbed from local tumor recurrence 2.5 years after transplant without radiographic evidence of tumor metastases in the liver.[27] Another case involved the presence of necrotizing pancreatitis in an ampullary adenoma with high-grade dysplasia, where a pancreatic anastomosis is doomed to fail and thus a total pancreatectomy was advised; final pathology revealed a small focus of invasive carcinoma in the ampulla.[28]

Recently a case of metastatic pancreatic adenocarcinoma in the liver after autologous islet cell transplantation has been reported.[29] This was a 43-year-old man without obvious risk factors for pancreatic ductal adenocarcinoma (PDAC); no cause for pancreatitis was described. Serum tumor markers were negative preoperatively and imaging failed to pronounce a malignant tumor. Biopsies of pancreas and ampulla were negative at the time of TPAIT. Ten months postoperatively on workup for abdominal pain and malaise, several necrotic liver lesions were noted and biopsy proved PDAC. He received several cycles of chemotherapy but ultimately succumbed to his disease. The only notable difference in data from this patient compared with other patients s/p TPAIT is differences in microRNA −10b, −30c, and −106b levels, which were markedly elevated. Importantly, this case demonstrates that malignant cells can survive enzymatic digestion and embolize to the liver during autotransfusion into the portal venous system.

Currently however given the risks of transmission of cancer cells to the liver it is not universally a recommended practice to offer TPAIT in patients with known malignancy. Enhanced screening may provide more comfort in certain circumstances but this will likely not reach widespread adoption, particularly because most pancreatic cancers can be effectively treated with partial resection, and the risk of developing diabetes after partial resection is low. Alternatively in special circumstances perhaps a remnant pancreas could be treated in some way, infused with cytotoxic chemotherapy or irradiated, to eradicate cancer cells yet maintain islets. Certainly more research needs to be completed before recommendation for this indication.

Improvements in Islet Isolation

As it is well established that greater numbers of islets generally produce better islet functional results, clearly the islet isolation laboratory is a key player in optimization of results. In the first few decades of islet isolation there was much discussion about quality and batch difference in the digestive enzymes. More recently it seems that available enzymes are of more uniform quality,[30] although a standardized enzyme formulation has not been realized.[31] Delivery of the enzyme into the pancreatic duct with good distension of the organ seems to be superior to direct injection of the organ with enzyme solution[32]; more complete extracellular matrix digestion, decreased autolysis, and increased islet yield are observed with this technique.

Maximizing Islet Survival

It is clear that greater islet yield generally translates to better glycemic function. By measuring unmethylated insulin DNA in serum after islet cell transplantation it is estimated that 50% or more of the isolated islets die within 24 hours of implantation.[33] Numerous strategies have been proposed to maximize islet survival, including maintenance of normoglycemia, combating IBMIR, and perhaps implantation outside of the portal circulation.

IBMIR is a phenomenon following intraportal infusion of islets occurring 1 to 6 hours after infusion whereby direct contact of islet graft clusters with intraportal blood causes platelet consumption and activation of complement and coagulation cascades and entrapment of islets in clots of platelets and leukocytes.[34] This results in immediate and significant islet cell loss through disruption of islet integrity and islet destruction. Over about the past 2 decades this phenomenon has been well described in both allogeneic and xenographic settings. Recently evidence of its occurrence in autologous islet transplantation was reported[35] with the observation of increased thrombin-antithrombin III complex and C-peptide as well as a decrease in platelets during infusion and up to 3 hours postcompletion. Proinflammatory cytokines interleukin 6 (IL-6) and IL-8 and interferon-inducible protein 10 were also increased.

It has been well recognized that IBMIR is a significant impediment to islet cell engraftment and clinical success.[36] To combat islet loss due to IBMIR, in addition to heparin infusion, an indirect thrombin inhibitor, investigators have experimented with numerous aspects of inhibiting the complement cascade, including direct thrombin inhibition with melagatran with the observation in vitro of diminished leukocyte infiltration and near null platelet adherence.[37] Low-molecular-weight dextran sulfate has also been studied and has been shown in vitro and in vivo with porcine islets to totally abrogate IBMIR[38] as well as in a nonhuman primate model[39] and in an in vitro model of autologous islet transplantation.[35] Further studies proving the safety and efficacy of these additional maneuvers are ongoing.

Recently Dunn and colleagues[40] summarized active clinical trials investigating improving islet function and engraftment. Numerous antiinflammatory drugs are under investigation to combat IBMIR, including alpha1-antitrypsin, etanercept, reparixin, Prolastin, and Arolast. Others acting at various levels of the complement cascade are also under investigation, such as glucagon-like peptide 1 agonist sitagliptin or C5 inhibition with eculizumab. Alternative sites are also being investigated that will specifically reduce this problem.

Alternative Implantation Sites

Many options for anatomic site of islet implantation have been described. In general, the criteria for optimum site for islet transplantation are adequate blood/oxygen perfusion, ease of access, large volume capacity, minimal inflammatory/immune reaction, and access (either direct, via imaging or biochemical assay) for postimplantation assessment.[41] Important factors include availability to nutrient diffuse early to individual islets (avoid clumping) and opportunity for neovascularization as the islets seek to engraft. Most widely used is transplantation of the islet product into the portal circulation, either via direct venotomy, cannulation of the splenic vein stump, or image-guided percutaneous access. Under normal conditions insulin is secreted directly into the portal circulation and is metabolized largely by the liver. Thus insulin secretion directly in liver by in situ islets has the appeal of mimicking most closely unaltered physiology. This site also has the advantages of easy access via percutaneous means and capacity for large volume infusion. Periprocedural period can potentially lead to, however, hemorrhage and portal venous thrombosis, albeit small.

Once implantation has been safely achieved there may exist further negative consequences of portal transplantation. Native islets are well vascularized by arterial supply in the pancreas, but in the liver they are now relatively hypoxic, depend on portal blood, which is lower in oxygen tension, until neovascularization by the hepatic arterial system occurs. The portal circulation also carries toxins absorbed from the intestinal circulation, resulting in a robust hepatic innate immunity; hepatic macrophages (Kupffer cells) play an important role in the initial local inflammatory response after islet transplantation. IBMIR is a well-documented phenomenon that occurs when free islets are directly exposed to the circulation.[35] Avoiding contact with portal blood while maintaining oxygen and nutrient delivery may represent the ideal, but elusive, transplantation site.

A fairly recent review discussed alternative sites for allogeneic islet transplantation.[42] Early investigation into alternative abdominal organ sites including kidney and spleen led to disappointing results in animal studies. Using sites such as intestinal or gastric submucosa or muscle is likely limited in autologous transplantation due to the large tissue volume typically produced. The investigators conclude that a subcutaneous implantation may be the safest approach, but research on host matrix for delivery of oxygen and nutrients is still needed. The omentum provides a favorable microenvironment and has been reported more recently.[43] Clearly a greater understanding of islet engraftment as well as technology advances in tissue engineering will steer us toward an "ideal" site.

SUMMARY

Pancreatic resection is frequently the standard of care for end-stage chronic pancreatitis, in the right anatomic and clinical circumstances. Obviously with resection comes the potential for (in the case of partial resections) or certainty of (for total pancreatectomy) type 3c diabetes. For decades TPAIT has provided hope for cure or near cure for one debilitating disease without exchange for another, namely brittle type 3c diabetes. Many factors are involved during this complex process to affect glycemic results, from patient selection, to preisolation graft handling and preservation, to isolation techniques, infusion site, and postoperative management. Experience and expertise is growing internationally, with promise that new research into many aspects of this complex procedure will provide more patients with better results.

ACKNOWLEDGMENTS

Monika Paroder, MD, Department of Pathology and Cell Biology, Columbia University Medical Center, New York, NY, participated in writing islet isolation section of article.

REFERENCES

1. Najarian JS, Sutherland DE, Baumgartner D, et al. Total or near total pancreatectomy and islet autotransplantation for treatment of chronic pancreatitis. Ann Surg 1980;192(4):526–42.
2. Keet A. The pyloric sphincteric cylinder in health and disease. Berlin: Springer-Verlag; 1993.
3. Huang W, Jiong J, Szatmary P, et al. Meta-analysis of subtotal stomach-preserving pancreaticoduodenectomy vs pylorus preserving pancreaticoduodenectomy. World J Gastroenterol 2015;21(20):6361–73.
4. McClaine R, Lowy A, Matthews J, et al. A comparison of pancreaticoduodenectomy and duodenum-preserving head resection for the treatment of chronic pancreatitis. HPB (Oxford) 2009;11(8):677–83.
5. Farney AC, Najarian JS, Nakhleh RE, et al. Autotransplantation of dispersed pancreatic islet tissue combined with total or near-total pancreatectomy for treatment of chronic pancreatitis. Surgery 1991;110(2):427–37.
6. Okabayashi T, Hanazaki K. Overwhelming postsplenectomy infection syndrome in adults - A clinically preventable disease. World J Gastroenterol 2008;14(2):176–9.
7. Tai DS, Shen N, Szot GL, et al. Autologous islet transplantation with remote islet isolation after pancreas resection for chronic pancreatitis. JAMA Surg 2015; 150(2):118–24.
8. Rabkin JM, Olyaei AJ, Orloff SL, et al. Distant processing of pancreas islets for autotransplantation following total pancreatectomy. Am J Surg 1999;177(5): 423–7.
9. Ricordi C. Quantitative and qualitative standards for islet isolation assessment in humans and large mammals. Pancreas 1991;6(2):242–4.
10. Tanhehco Y, Weisberg S, Schwartz J. Pancreatic islet autotransplantation for nonmalignant and malignant indications. Transfusion 2016;56:761–70.
11. Huang HH, Ramachandran K, Stehno-Bittel L. A replacement for islet equivalents with improved reliability and validity. Acta Diabetol 2013;50(5):687–96.
12. Ricordi C, Lacy P, Finke E, et al. Automated method for isolation of human pancreatic islets. Diabetes 1988;37(4):413–20.
13. Korsgren O, Jansson L, Andersson A. Effects of hyperglycemia on function of isolated mouse pancreatic islets transplanted under kidney capsule. Diabetes 1989; 38:510–5.
14. Ling Z, Pipeleers D. Prolonged exposure of human beta cells to elevated glucose levels results in sustained cellular activation leading to a loss of glucose regulation. J Clin Invest 1996;98(12):2805–12.
15. Biarnes M, Montolio M, Nacher V, et al. Beta-Cell death and mass in syngeneically transplanted islets exposed to short- and long-term hyperglycemia. Diabetes 2002;51:66–72.

16. Juang J, Bonner-Weir S, Wu Y, et al. Beneficial influence of glycemic control upon the growth and function of transplanted islets. Diabetes 1994;43:1334–9.

17. Chinnakotla S, Radosevich DM, Dunn TB, et al. Long-term outcomes of total pancreatectomy and islet auto transplantation for hereditary/genetic pancreatitis. J Am Coll Surg 2014;218(4):530–43.

18. Dunderdale J, McAuliffe JC, McNeal SF, et al. Should pancreatectomy with islet cell autotransplantation in patients with chronic alcoholic pancreatitis be abandoned? J Am Coll Surg 2013;216(4):591–6.

19. Kessell S, Smith K, Gardner T. Total pancreatectomy with islet autologous transplantation: the cure for chronic pancreatitis? Clin Transl Gastroenterol 2015;6(1):e73.

20. Sutherland DE, Gruessner AC, Carlson AM, et al. Islet autotransplant outcomes after total pancreatectomy: a contrast to islet allograft outcomes. Transplantation 2008;86(12):1799–802.

21. Kumar R, Chung WY, Dennison AR, et al. Current principles and practice in autologous intraportal islet transplantation: a meta-analysis of the technical considerations. Clin Transplant 2016;30:344–56.

22. Goss JA, Goodpastor SE, Brunicardi FC, et al. Development of a human pancreatic islet-transplant program through a collaborative relationship with a remote islet-isolation center. Transplantation 2004;77(3):462–6.

23. Khan A, Jindal RM, Shriver C, et al. Remote processing of pancreas can restore normal glucose homeostasis in autologous islet transplantation after traumatic whipple pancreatectomy: technical considerations. Cell Transplant 2012;21(6): 1261–7.

24. Kesseli SJ, Wagar M, Jung MK, et al. Long-term glycemic control in adults patients undergoing remote vs. local total pancreatectomy with islet autotransplantation. Am J Gastroenterol 2017;112(4):643–9.

25. Chinnakotla S, Bellin M, Schwarzenberg S, et al. Total pancreatectomy and islet auto-transplantation in children for chronic pancreatitis. Indication, surgical techniques, post operative management and long-term outcomes. Ann Surg 2014; 260(1):56–64.

26. Azhari H, Rahhal R, Uc A. Is total pancreatectomy with islet autotransplantation a reasonable choice for pediatric pancreatitis? JOP 2015;16(4):335–41.

27. Förster S, Liu X, Adam U, et al. Islet autotransplantation combined with pancreatectomy for treatment of pancreatic adenocarcinoma: a case report. Transplant Proc 2004;36(4):1125–6.

28. Iyegha UP, Asghar JA, Beilman GJ. Total pancreatectomy and islet autotransplantation as treatment for ampullary adenocarcinoma in the setting of pancreatic ductal disruption secondary to acute necrotizing pancreatitis. A case report. JOP 2012;13:239–42.

29. Muratore S, Zeng X, Korc M, et al. Metastatic pancreatic adenocarcinoma after total pancreatectomy islet autotransplantation for chronic pancreatitis. Am J Transplant 2016;16(9):2747–52.

30. Rheinheimer J, Ziegelmann PK, Carlessi R, et al. Different digestion enzymes used for human pancreatic islet isolation: a mixed treatment comparison (MTC) meta-analysis. Islets 2014;6(4):e977118.

31. Brandhorst D, Brandhorst H, Johnson PRV. Enzyme development for human islet isolation: five decades of progress or stagnation? Rev Diabet Stud 2017;14(1): 22–38.

32. Shimoda M, Itoh T, Sugimoto K, et al. Improvement of collagenase distribution with the ductal preservation for human islet isolation. Islets 2012;4(2):130–7.

33. Bellin MD, Clark P, Usman-Brown S, et al. Unmethylated insulin DNA is elevated after total pancreatectomy with islet autotransplantation: assessment of a novel beta cell marker. Am J Transplant 2017;15:1112–8.
34. Bennet W, Groth CG, Larsson R, et al. Isolated human islets trigger an instant blood mediated inflammatory reaction: implications for intraportal islet transplantation as a treatment for patients with type 1 diabetes. Ups J Med Sci 2000; 105(2):125–33.
35. Naziruddin B, Iwahashi S, Kanak M, et al. Evidence for instant blood-mediated inflammatory reaction in clinical autologous islet transplantation. Am J Transplant 2014;14:428–37.
36. Nilssom B, Ekdahl KN, Korsgren O. Control fo instant blood-mediated inflammatory reaction to improve islets of Langerhans engraftment. Curr Opin Organ Transplant 2011;16(6):620–6.
37. Ozmen L, Ekdahl KN, Elgue G, et al. Inhibition of thrombin abrogates the instant blood-mediated inflammatory reaction triggered by isolated human islets: possible application of the thrombin inhibitor melagatran in clinical islet transplantation. Diabetes 2002;51(6):1779–84.
38. Goto M, Johansson H, Maeda A, et al. Low-molecular weight dextran sulfate abrogates the instant blood-mediated inflammatory reaction induced by adult porcine islets noth in vitro and in vivo. Transplant Proc 2004;36(4):1186–7.
39. Johansson H, Goto M, Dufrane D, et al. Low molecular weight dextran sulfate: a strong candidate drug to block IBMIR in clinical islet transplantation. Am J Transplant 2006;6(2):305–12.
40. Dunn T, Wilhem J, Bellin M, et al. Autologous islet transplantation: challenges and lessons. Curr Opin Organ Transplant 2017;22:364–71.
41. Zhu H, Li W, Chen N, et al. Selection of implantation sites for transplantation of encapsulated pancreatic islets. Tissue Eng Part B Rev 2018;24(3):191–214.
42. van der Windt D, Echeverri GJ, Ijzermans JN, et al. The choice of anatomical site for islet transplantation. Cell Transplant 2008;17(9):1005–14.
43. Schmidt C. Pancreatic islets find a new transplant home in the omentum. Nat Biotechnol 2017;35(1):8.

Moving?

Make sure your subscription moves with you!

To notify us of your new address, find your **Clinics Account Number** (located on your mailing label above your name), and contact customer service at:

Email: journalscustomerservice-usa@elsevier.com

800-654-2452 (subscribers in the U.S. & Canada)
314-447-8871 (subscribers outside of the U.S. & Canada)

Fax number: 314-447-8029

Elsevier Health Sciences Division
Subscription Customer Service
3251 Riverport Lane
Maryland Heights, MO 63043